Botany and Healing

Botany and Healing

MEDICINAL PLANTS OF NEW JERSEY AND THE REGION

Cecil C. Still

Rutgers University Press
New Brunswick, New Jersey, and London

Library of Congress Cataloging-in-Publication Data

Still, Cecil C., 1931–
    Botany and healing : medicinal plants of New Jersey and the region
/ Cecil C. Still.
        p.   cm.
    Includes bibliographical references (p. ••) and index.
    ISBN 0–8135–2507–1 (cloth). — ISBN 0–8135–2508–X (pbk.)
    1. Medicinal plants—Northeastern States.   2. Materia medica,
Vegetable—Northeastern States.   I. Title.
RS172.N67S75   1998
615'.32'0974—DC21   97–45725
                                                                     CIP

British Cataloging-in-Publication data for this book is available
from the British Library

Manufactured in the United States of America

For Leonora and the family

Contents

Preface

Plants have always been important in medicine, but with the development of "modern" medicine and the then new chemotherapeutic agents such as the sulfa drugs and penicillin, public perception of the value of medicinal plants diminished. The pharmaceutical industry's renewed interest in medicinal plants can be attributed to the costs associated with the development and marketing of new synthetic drugs and with meeting the regulatory demands of governmental agencies. Current regulations permit the approval of a new drug from a natural source in much less time, saving millions of dollars. The current popular interest in medicinal plants for personal use and in alternative medicine can be viewed as a desire to return to aspects of the medicine of earlier times. This renewed interest has also led to an increasing regard for wild plants as positive contributors to the environment.

My interest in the medicinal plants of northeastern America, especially those of my home state of New Jersey, stems from both my family heritage in herbal medicine and my work as a plant scientist. In the nineteenth century, one of my ancestors, James Still (1812–1885), a self-taught healer, traveled the New Jersey pinelands and practiced what was, in its time, an alternative to the accepted modern medical practice. People from all over southern New Jersey and Philadelphia sought out his herbal preparations and medical advice. Although Still's direct descendants did not carry on his herbal medical practice, I feel that knowing about his achievements stimulated my own early interests in looking for local medicinal plants and growing them myself.

As important as James Still was in his time, I am convinced that the only reason we are aware of his life and medical practice is that he left a *written* record of his activities. I was never quite convinced of his achievements, nor indeed his existence, until the Medford Historical Society published a facsimile edition of his autobiography, originally copyrighted in 1877. That book, and later the original version, convinced me that most, if not all, of the oral history I had heard was reasonably accurate.

I have always wanted to be involved in medicine or plant science. As a child I ordered seeds from catalogues and planted gardens before I had ever heard of James Still. It is entirely possible that older family members were reminded of James Still and began telling stories of this man who was so famous in his time when they noted my interest in plants. I spent my summers as any other child but also tended my garden and, under the direction of my mother, buried many fishheads in the sandy soil of South Jersey under her rose bushes.

Although I began as a Ph.D. plant physiologist, my research interests have broadened to include every aspect of plant biology—from chemistry to taxonomy and ecology. My research on pesticide resistance and naturally occurring insecticides in plants brought me back to the study of plants of New Jersey and the surrounding region. I hoped to identify plants that might produce chemicals with toxic effects on the pests that damage other agriculturally important plants. Rather than taking a random walk through all of the globally estimated 250,000 to 750,000 species of higher plants, it made sense to look at the plants known or suspected to contain active chemicals—those that have been used medicinally.

So I began to generate a list of plants found in New Jersey that, according to the literature, my own knowledge, and folklore, had been used for medicinal purposes. I also made note of plants whose medicinal properties were unknown, but whose close relatives had been used for medicinal purposes. I soon discovered that the plants I had encountered while growing up in southern New Jersey were a small part of the regional flora that had been employed medicinally by native Americans and European settlers in the region.

My fascination with medicinal plants of New Jersey and the Northeast soon expanded beyond its original research purpose of identifying plant species that might have insecticidal uses to include those with potential in the rapidly developing "phytochemical" industry. To that end, I hope, this book will be useful to the future "bioprospectors" in the Northeast.

I originally conceived this book as a textbook to be titled *Medical Botany*. Encouraged by a number of African and Caribbean students, I had begun teaching a one-credit course on medicinal plants, but could not find an appropriate text. I began collecting and refining my lecture notes with the intent of filling this need. The year after the course was initiated, however, an excellent text (Lewis and Elvin-Lewis 1977) appeared, and I abandoned my plan for the medical botany text.

Each year, courses at Rutgers are evaluated by students. I repeatedly received the suggestion to concentrate on local plants, perhaps with field trips, rather than on the more exotic plants of Africa, China, India, or the Yucatan. At first, I dismissed the suggestion, believing that doing so would severely limit the number of plants for consideration, but then decided to explore the local plants that James Still might have used in his medications. A library search led me to Mary Y. Hough's *New Jersey Wild Plants* and other local and regional plant books, but I did not find a title that focused on medicinal plants of New Jersey. I felt that I had discovered a worthwhile pursuit, a project that could build on my expertise and interests and on the current interest in local flora.

Dr. Ralph Good (a now-deceased botanist who was instrumental in the establishment of the New Jersey Pinelands Commission) requested my participation in a symposium on the pinelands to be held at the Rutgers Camden campus on April 25, 1991. We agreed that my presentation should include the story of James Still and the medicinal plants of the pinelands. After all, the pinelands (pine barrens) represent a vast expanse of unique land, rich in plants with medicinal properties, and certainly Still, born and raised in the area, used many of these plants in his practice—several are mentioned in his autobiography. I eventually expanded the pinelands manuscript to include plants statewide, and the result is this book. It is written, not as a textbook, but for a wider audience interested in local plants and their historical uses.

This book focuses on native and naturalized plants that have been found in New Jersey (Hough's book has been an invaluable resource). Almost all of them can be found in other parts of northeastern and east-central North America, including Canada. Many were introduced to our region from Europe, Asia, and other parts of the world. Therefore, the book will be useful well beyond the borders of New Jersey, although other states in the region have medicinal plants not found in New Jersey.

The U.S. Northeast—like every other part of the world—faces the loss of native species. In New Jersey, some of these plants have not been recorded locally by botanists for many years and may no longer exist in the state or perhaps even the region. With the rapid development of residential communities and the consequent destruction of local flora, it is important that we regularly survey native and introduced species to gauge the rate of loss or gain of biodiversity. We must be as concerned with such changes in the ecosystem of our own backyard as we are with the changes in the Amazonian rainforests.

Acknowledgments

I am appreciative of Karen Reeds's initial encouragement and editing of the original manuscript. My present editor, Doreen Valentine, is responsible for maturation and fruition of the manuscript to the present form. I could not have completed the first draft of the manuscript without my wife, Delores, who read and criticized every version from lecture notes to the first submitted draft. Joanne, the best ten-month secretary in all of New Brunswick, has been a partner and, with Amy, my fan club.

Botany and Healing

Introduction

A Historical Sketch of the Use of Medicinal Plants

Any statement about the earliest origins of knowledge of the healing properties of plants has to be speculation. It is, however, reasonable to infer from the behavior of certain wild and domesticated animals today that ancestral forms of *Homo sapiens* as well as other animals could distinguish plants (based on trial-and-error experiences?) that are safe to eat from those that are not. Many cats and dogs seem to know when to become herbivorous and chew on specific grasses. Many of us have observed domestic cats who attempt to protect patches of grass from destruction by humans. Observations of wild chimpanzees seem to indicate that they can identify and seek out plants to alleviate digestive complaints and to remedy other illnesses. The term "zoopharmacognosy" was proposed by Rodriguez and Wrangham (1993) to describe the process by which animals select medicinal plants.

We can imagine that early humans had similar instincts or learned to recognize useful plants by observing other animals and each other. In their constant search for food, these hominids could have sampled plants and remembered them for their singular taste, aroma, or dramatic physiologic responses such as vomiting, diarrhea, or even death. Even deadly plants have found uses as poisons in hunting, fishing, and warfare. From our earliest historical records, we know that the bitter-tasting poison hemlock (*Conium maculatum*, a plant found in New Jersey), for example, was used by the ancient Greeks for executions: Plato's account of the death of Socrates is an accurate description of the action of the alkaloid coniine, found in poison hemlock. It also seems reasonable that some individuals' especially acute sensitivity to taste, smell, and visual detail made them particularly suited to pay attention to plants.

Two very important professions developed very early in civilization: farming and medicinal healing. From archeological evidence, we know that plants were cultivated for food more than 15,000 years ago. The Hearst papyrus, from ancient Egypt (written sometime between the twelfth and eighteenth dynasties—2400–2200 B.C.E.), lists many plant-based remedies and proves that the medicinal uses of plants were systematically studied, recorded, and transmitted from one generation to the next at least 5,000 years ago in the Nile Valley.

Evidence also shows that the Chinese had developed systems of agriculture and medicine very long ago. It is said that the Emperor Shennung (2700 B.C.E.) was the father of Chinese agriculture and medicine. Although the date of the first Chinese herbal is unknown, all of the oldest available herbals mention plants indigenous only to China, suggesting that the knowledge also arose indigenously. Knowledge of the use of medicinal plants, gained empirically by the ancient Chinese, remains useful today. For instance, a small desert plant known as ma huang has been known in China for thousands of years and was used to relieve respiratory complaints such as asthma. Today that plant is known as ephedra and yields the commercially important alkaloid ephedrine, used today for the same purposes worldwide and increasingly used (abused?) today by athletes and exercise enthusiasts.

The ancient medicine of Japan was introduced from China by way of Korea. The oldest surviving medical compendium in Japan was compiled in 984 C.E. by a Japanese physician who was a descendant of a naturalized Chinese. It is the oldest Japanese publication on medicine.

Traditional medicine in India has been passed along from one generation to another in what has been a highly organized written form for 3,000 to 5,000 years. The medical system is still used today in a health care system known as Ayurveda. One of Ayurvedic medicine's great discoveries was the use of the plant *Rauvolfia serpentina*, used for its tranquilizing effect. Rediscovery of this plant and the isolation of the active alkaloid, reserpine, were pivotal events in the modern rebirth of scientific and commercial interest in the medicinal properties of plants. Reserpine continues to be used to control hypertension.

Traditional medicine in sub-Saharan Africa is clearly based on herbal remedies and may ultimately derive from the earliest human observation of medicinal plants. As in many cultures, however, this body of knowledge was usually regarded as secret and privileged information, and as such, subject to all the hazards of oral transmission: the medicine man or woman might die without teaching a successor, or a young apprentice might misunderstand or forget what had been taught about names, smells, tastes, preparation, and administration of the medication. Without a written record, there was always the chance that the inheritors of knowledge would lose or distort it. Also, without a written record, many of these ancient secrets may still be unknown to us—or are now being revealed as we systematically study the medicinal properties of plants in their natural environments.

For the same reasons, we know little about the ancient traditions of herbal healing in the Americas before the European conquest. Dating of ancient campsites suggests that the first Americans arrived in Alaska from Siberia at least 12,000 years ago and moved southward and eastward, eventually populating all parts of the Western Hemisphere. Wherever they went, they encountered new plants and had to adapt their earlier traditions to local flora.

In the case of the Aztecs, written records reveal just how well they succeeded in understanding the plants around them. The Spanish conquistadors and missionaries who first encountered Aztec civilization in the early 1500s marveled at the Aztecs' elaborate botanic gardens—far more sophisticated than any in Europe at that time. The newcomers took pains to prepare illustrated herbals, with commentaries in Nahuatl by native informants, that preserve Aztec names, explanations, and various uses of native plants in medicine and religion, and as food.

When European explorers and settlers came to North America, their survival often depended on native American knowledge—freely shared—of plants unfamiliar to the foreigners. We get glimpses of the uses of these healing plants from the colonists' reports back to Europe. For example, in 1678, a merchant in Virginia wrote to the English scientist Robert Hooke about the practice of burning of dried plant material on the skin as a moxa (cauterizing agent), a practice that appears similar to the ancient Chinese and Japanese tradition of moxibustion.

The Europeans who colonized the Americas also transplanted their own rich herbal traditions. The herbals of sixteenth- and seventeenth-century Europe are largely founded on accounts written down by Greek and Roman physicians and natural historians in the first century of the Christian era (notably Dioscorides, c. 60 C.E.; Pliny, c. 77 C.E.; and Galen, born 129 C.E.). These Renaissance herbals also incorporated folklore, explorers' reports of plants from other lands, and contemporary experience with plants. Beginning in 1530, European herbals included printed illustrations of plants, making it possible to have, for the first time, a visual check on the often ambiguous descriptions of plants named in the manuscript and oral transmissions. The extent and character of European herbal knowledge at the beginning of the seventeenth century are well displayed in the 1,600–plus pages of the best-known English-language herbal of this period, John Gerard's *Herball* (first published in 1597 and enlarged in 1633). The "receipts to cure various disorders" were copied from Gerard's herbal and sent to New England.

The first steps toward an American herbal were taken in Philadelphia by Benjamin Franklin, who saw the need for an herbal that described American as well as European plants. Franklin himself had sold imported and indigenous herbal medicines in a store he owned in the late

1720s. He commissioned John Bartram, who had begun to collect native plants at his farm outside of Philadelphia, to assemble the botanical descriptions of a number of medicinal plants "peculiar to America" for an appendix to the 1751 edition of *Medica Britannica.*

This interest in a distinctly American medical botany was picked up by another Philadelphian, Benjamin Smith Barton, born in 1766. His father, an Episcopal clergyman, was a member of the American Philosophical Society and corresponded with Linnaeus, the father of modern botany. The young Barton, discontented with the fact that his early knowledge of medicine and botany came entirely from European books, took the opportunity at age 19 to travel in western Pennsylvania with his uncle. There he became acquainted with native Americans—then often called "doctors by instinct"—and began his lifelong research into native American medicines, customs, and history that was ultimately published posthumously in 1798–1804 as *Collections for an Essay towards a Materia Medica of the United States.* After taking his medical degree in Germany, the twenty-four-year-old Barton returned to Philadelphia, where the first chair of Natural History and Botany in America was created specifically for him at the Medical College of Philadelphia.

The teaching of materia medica had been standard in European medical schools for two centuries before Barton's appointment in Philadelphia, and it became a normal part of American medical education as well. American medical botany then gradually became an admixture of native American and European practice as European plants were transported across the Atlantic and became naturalized. (One example of a highly successful European introduction is the common plantain, now viewed as an annoying weed of lawns and gardens, but so highly valued in European materia medica that seeds were planted throughout colonial America. Native Americans gave plantain the name "white man's foot" because it appeared wherever Europeans appeared.)

The growth of chemistry in France and Germany in the late eighteenth century and the first half of the nineteenth century, however, had a profound effect on medical botany. Where botany and medicine had long been closely intertwined, now the subjects diverged. Botanists concentrated more on names, classification, and structure of plants, and less and less on their medicinal properties. Determining the medicinal value of plants was chemical and became the field called pharmacognosy. The analysis of the chemical basis of the plants' medicinal properties became the special province of pharmacology (the name "pharmacology" was suggested by Dr. E. R. Squibb in an address before the New York Medical Society in 1866).

Graduates of the new scientifically based medical schools practiced "heroic" medicine. They relied on purgation, bloodletting, and heavy doses of medications containing poisonous chemicals such as arsenic, mercury, and antimony. The aim was to "kill the disease" and hope that the patient would survive the cure. This represented a drastic change in direction: old medical traditions were thrown out for the new scientific approach. Not surprisingly, a movement arose in reaction to such drastic methods, with patients seeking out healers who claimed that in contrast to the new chemicals, their herbal drugs would at least do no harm.

Perhaps the most famous of these herbalists was Samuel Thomson (1769–1843) of Massachusetts, the founder of what came to be known as "Thomsonianism" or the "Botanic System." Despite Thomson's almost complete lack of formal education, he and many others claimed the title of "doctor" and succeeded in propagandizing effectively for the botanic medications and therapies that he espoused and patented. Thomson's theory of health and disease owed much to native American beliefs that heat is life and cold is death. He argued that giving a febrifuge (a fever reducing agent) to someone with a fever was tantamount to taking the side of death in the war between life and death that was being fought within the patient's body. Thomson advocated the use of native American "sweat-herbs," plants that would induce sweat, to treat fevers and thus would enter the "war" on the side of life.

For all the fierce antagonism between the Thomsonians and the orthodox medical profession, most Americans had little choice about their doctor. Outside of big cities, where formally trained physicians tended to settle, the only medical practitioners were likely to be self-taught herbalists who turned to books like Barton's, Jacob Bigelow's three-volume, illustrated *American Medical Botany* (published between 1812 and 1820), or Thomson's *New Guide to Health; or Botanic Family Physician* (first published in the early 1800s). One such practitioner was my kinsman, James Still (1812–1885). Thanks to his published memoirs, we have a detailed personal account of the life and work of a nineteenth-century self-taught doctor.

Still was born near Medford, in the New Jersey pinelands, one of eighteen children born to Charity and Levin Still, ex-slaves from Maryland. Still became interested in medicine at the age of three, when he was vaccinated against smallpox. At the age of eighteen, he became an indentured servant for three years, and as a condition of his indenture, he received three months of education; one month each winter. After finishing his service, he worked at various jobs in Philadelphia and around Medford, hoping to earn enough money to enter medical school. By 1843, he had given up on the dream of a medical education and instead bought a distilling apparatus. He began his business career by distilling and selling extracts of sassafras root and various herbs. Once he learned how to make essence of peppermint, he was able to deal with druggists in Philadelphia, and regular visits to the drugstore revived his interest in becoming a physician.

For one dollar, Still obtained a "medical botany," that is, a botany book devoted to medicinal plants, and two weeks later, for a dollar and a quarter, a second book which contained "formulas for preparing medicines." A third book "of only one hundred and sixty-four pages" gave "instructions for making pills, powders, tinctures, salves, and liniments." I suspect that one of these books was an edition of Thomson's *Guide*.

He then prepared some tinctures for his own family and soon became the neighborhood physician. He obtained yet another book "which contained the history and description of all diseases" and began practicing medicine. (Unfortunately, these books are not described in sufficient detail to positively identify any of them.)

After practicing for some time, Still was told that he could be fined for practicing medicine without a license (the New Jersey Medical Society had supported the passage of this law in 1772). He sought legal advice and learned that he could not be fined but could "not collect for medical services without a licence." He could, however, legally sell medicine and charge for delivering it. By the time he died in 1885, Still had the second or third most successful business in Burlington County and was renowned throughout South Jersey and Philadelphia as the "Black Doctor of the Pines." In the Still family, he is still highly respected and known as the "cancer doctor."

The practice of herbal medicine has not changed significantly over thousands of years. The same plants and uses described by ancient societies are apt to show up in today's field guides to medicinal plants, although typically with less detailed descriptions. One interpretation of this lasting quality is that the remedies have survived because they appear to be effective. An alternative, more skeptical, view is that after herbal medicine became separate from botany, chemistry, and medicine, herbal preparations were accepted because they could "do no harm" but were not considered "serious" medicines. Any discussion at this level predictably leads to inclusion of the "placebo" effect. That situation is changing as we see a resurgence of interest in herbal medicine and a search for remedial chemicals in the developed parts of the world. In developing countries, 70 percent to 80 percent of the medicinal products are herbal, and interests have not changed significantly over the years. In India and Pakistan, the Ayurvedic, Unani, and Tibbi systems of medicine, while not strictly herbal, are probably more widely practiced and accepted than orthodox medicine is. In China, the longstanding use of medicinal herbs and traditional practices such as acupuncture, acupressure, and moxibustion have attracted Western physicians eager to find "new" ways to treat conditions that baffle biomedical science. In the Philippine Islands, a major effort is being made to disseminate knowledge and create awareness of the abundance and importance of locally available medicinal plants: extension agents are trained to identify, prepare, and use the locally available plants for medication and then are sent out to teach others with slide shows and demonstrations that stress the value of traditional medicine to health and the family budget.

In African countries, the practice of traditional herbal medicine has been legalized after years of being prosecuted during colonial times. From my own experience observing practicing herbalists near Nairobi, Kenya, and Dar es Salaam, Tanzania, I can readily understand why traditional medicine is so popular today. The medicines these doctors administer have been harvested from the wild and prepared by hand. The remedies appear to be efficacious, and the cost to the patient much less than commercially available pharmaceuticals. A 500–bed hospital near Nairobi, run by one doctor with nurses and former patients, has won an international reputation.

In Europe and America, herbal medicine continues to be used within the home and by self-taught practitioners, but it has also found new acceptance as the holistic health movement grows. Many physicians are choosing to augment their formal medical training by studying herbal and other forms of alternative medicine. The National Institutes of Health have established a department for alternative medicine, and it seems likely that the modern and traditional in Western medicine will come back together after years of separation. Each will find ways to learn from the other. My hope is that this book will contribute to that reunification and to a renewed appreciation for the plants in our own backyards worldwide.

How to Use This Book

The heart of this book is the list of about 495 species of medicinal plants found in New Jersey and the northeastern U.S. (out of about 2,500 to 3,000 of the total native and introduced plant species in the state). The list is arranged by family and, within each family, by genus and species. Arrangement by family and genus is familiar to every botanist and easy for the amateur naturalist to use in conjunction with standard field guides; at the same time, it highlights relationships that have medicinal significance for the herbalist and the pharmacologist. If one is considering a plant not found in the list but that is a member of one of the families, one might reasonably expect familial medicinal (chemical) potential.

Botanists have grouped plants into families, genera, and species on the basis of similarities of form—especially distinctive shapes and arrangements of leaves, flowers, fruit, stems, and roots. If you see a plant with many flowers arranged like an umbrella and leaves composed of many leaflets, you would be making a good guess that it might be in the same family or genus as another plant displaying different flowers but in a similar umbrellalike arrangement and leaves divided into a slightly different pattern—and that it is not closely related to a plant with a single flower at the top and a stalk with broad, heart-shaped leaves.

The common features that relate groups go deeper than surface appearances, however. Species within a single genus, or genera within a single family, often have biochemical similarities as well. These common features can be revealed in the taste, smell, and physiological effects of the plants. If you know by experience or training that the juice of one species in a plant genus or family can produce itchy blisters on the skin, you will be careful about touching or tasting other plants of the same genus or family. If you know that the bitter-tasting bark of one species can relieve headaches and fevers, you will look for related species that might produce the same result, perhaps with fewer side effects.

The families are arranged in alphabetical order by their most widely used botanical names. All family names end with the suffix "-ae" or "-aceae." Family names are not italicized. For each family, a common name is given, derived from a familiar member of the group, for example, the daisy family (Compositae) or the maple family (Aceraceae). Also mentioned are some well-known plants, genera, and distinctive features of the group as a whole.

Under each family, one or more scientific names of each species are listed. The species are listed alphabetically by scientific name: the first word of each name gives the genus, the second denotes the particular species within that genus. Both genus and species names are italicized.

For most plants, several common names are listed. Some names, like "wormwood," "birthwort," and "liverwort," go back centuries in herbal tradition ("wort" means "root" or "plant" in Old English); others, like "buttercup" and "Queen Anne's lace," are interesting descriptions of flowers; some, like "pipsissewa" and "wahoo bush," reflect native American names. Anyone who deals with plants quickly learns how confusing the multiplicity of common names can be and how critical it is to use scientific names for reliable identification. For some entries, I have given more than one family or generic name, but generally, I have used the names as found in *Gray's Manual of Botany*, vol. 2, as rewritten and expanded by Merritt Fernald, and the second edition of Gleason and Cronquist's *Manual of Vascular Plants of Northeastern United States and Adjacent Canada*.

For each species, the entry provides a brief account of the plant's size, range, habitat, and season of flowering/fruiting in New Jersey. By giving the global range of the family, the entry serves as a reminder of how widespread some of these plant groups are and how the medicinal or food uses of a plant in one culture can suggest uses of its relatives on a different continent. I have also indicated whether the plant is a perennial, biennial, or annual, and whether it is native or imported to New Jersey. Space does not allow more than a brief description of each plant, but the reader is referred to other references cited above and in the sources at the end of the text. (Descriptions in these references often resort to some technical botanic terms, but a glossary of terms and definitions is usually included.) The drawings in this volume indicate important features of the family and genus. They complement but should not be substituted for the much more detailed descriptions and illustrations in standard field guides. For serious botanical and pharmacological research, plants must be checked against herbarium specimens and documentation.

The Glossary serves as a guide to some of the specialized vocabulary that Western physicians and pharmacists have created over the centuries to describe the effects of medicinal drugs.

I report the medicinal uses and preparations listed for each family or species without any guarantee of their safety or efficacy. I urge you, however, to take indications of toxicity seriously. Because it is very difficult to be certain of the role of an individual plant in a preparation made up of several plants (a "compound" preparation), few such preparations are included.

The details of gathering and preparing the plants are usually omitted, in part because such directions were written in such vague terms or not at all, in part because mistakes in preparation can be dangerous, and in part because I want to discourage the indiscriminate harvesting of plants—wild plants deserve all the protection they can get. I have, however, provided a general sketch of the methods used to prepare medicinal plants and for testing their biological activity.

In most cases, only native American uses of plants are given—usually those of the Iroquois and Cherokee. (My debt to *Medicinal Plants of Native America* by Daniel E. Moerman is acknowledged.) There is, unfortunately, no systematic record of plants used by the Lenape, the tribe that lived throughout what now includes the state of New Jersey. When Jacob Bigelow's *American Medical Botany* and other works of materia medica support or add to the native American uses, I have included their comments. Other information on the herbal uses of wild plants comes from a variety of sources: personal experiences, oral tradition passed on to me by family members, friends, students, colleagues, popular articles in general media, technical articles in scientific media, and books and pamphlets purchased from book sales and rare-book dealers.

I report a few food uses of medicinal plants for the reader interested in wild-food plants, again excluding fungi such as wild mushrooms. Many of the plants are the subjects of current research projects (including my own), with new information generated almost at a daily rate. New findings are reported in monthly professional journals, but future books of this type will hopefully disseminate this knowledge.

Currently, in Europe and increasingly in the United States, leaf extracts of the ginkgo tree (*Ginkgo biloba*) are being used, and the ginkgo tree is found throughout the region. I have not included the ginkgo in this list because it is an introduction from China, and although it is grown commercially as a crop in other areas, it is only an urban ornamental at this time in New Jersey.

PART I

Medicinal Plants and Their Preparation

❧

Centuries of human experience with plants have demonstrated that some plants have strong physiological effects that can relieve or cure disease. The task of the herbalist and the researcher in pharmacognosy is to separate from the quarter-million-plus species of higher plants (although their medicinal properties have been clearly established, the fungi, lichens, algae, and microorganisms will not be considered in this book) the comparatively small number, perhaps 1 or 2 percent, that are likely to have medicinal properties and to report on how to use them safely and efficaciously.

What Makes a Plant Medicinal?

Folk medicine practitioners sometimes claim that every kind of plant has medicinal value. For our purposes though, the term "medicinal" must be more clearly defined. For example, when therapeutic effects are attributed to the mere presence of certain plants, the healing is more likely to be the result of an improved environment than to medicinal properties of those plants. Plants used for food are not strictly medicinal, although it is clear that they may contain factors that prevent disease. Vitamins and minerals are the best-known examples, but scientists are uncovering other naturally occurring components of food plants that induce resistance to disease or that interfere directly or indirectly with carcinogens and other environmental poisons. In the past, plants have been employed as remedies simply because the plant part resembled the sick part of the body—a plant with a liver-shaped leaf was used to treat liver problems, a plant with milky sap was used for difficulties in breast feeding, and so on. The logic here has rarely led to a successful remedy.

Most students of pharmacognosy would agree that many plants re-garded as medicinal are set apart by their unique chemistry. All plants, and indeed all living organisms, are characterized by a common set of biochemical reactions. If we consider various groups of living organ-isms, we can biochemically define, within those groups, those products that are essential to normal growth, reproduction, and survival of indi-vidual plants and species, and those that are of secondary importance to the plant that contains them. Natural product plants (which include those regarded as medicinal) are those whose composition includes a significant accumulation of products of secondary importance. All plants are potentially food plants, but not all plants have a buildup of distinc-tive secondary products. Many scientists feel that there must be a reason for the existence of secondary products in plants; the usual explanation is that the products somehow help the plant to defend itself against the environment and other organisms.

For our purposes, we will limit the definition of medicinal plants to two groups: (1) those producing biologically active secondary products whether or not they account for the claimed therapeutic effects and (2) those in which we assume the presence of biological activity because of traditional claims of remedial effects, even when the active agent is un-known.

Of the 310 or so families of seed plants, medicinal plants occur in perhaps 200 to 250. The daisy family (Compositae), the mint family (Labiatae), the bean family (Leguminosae), the lily family (Liliaceae), the buttercup family (Ranunculaceae), the rose family (Rosaceae), and the carrot family (Umbelliferae) are especially rich in medicinally use-ful species.

Effects of Context on Plant Efficacy

Part of my interest in concentrating on local plants was the probability of success in isolating active chemicals in the laboratory, which is greatly increased when plants are harvested directly from their natural environ-ment, in the proper season and developmental stage. Plants can be thought of as beginning life as an embryo, in a seed form, then either developing into an adult that produces the next generation of seed and dies (an annual plant), or winters over and begins new growth in the spring (a perennial). It also made sense because locally available plants could be cultivated in the necessary quantity for a variety of applications.

Appearance and chemical composition of a plant may be strongly in-fluenced by the local environment in which it grows naturally. Such fac-tors as moisture, light intensity, day length, and neighboring plants are four of the major local environmental factors affecting the appearance or chemical composition of a plant. If such a plant is moved, say from one continent, country, state, or county to another where it has not been found naturally, it may grow and appear normal but differ drastically in chemical composition. It is also true that the chemical composition of a plant usually varies from season to season and from organ to organ within the same plant. It may well be that the compound of interest occurs in signficant concentration in the flower or seed, and also at a certain season only.

It is very important to know where the plant was harvested. Plants growing near heavily traveled roads, incinerators, or landfills should be avoided: they may have absorbed heavy metals or other environmental toxins. Plants grown in a garden should be maintained in as near a natural state as possible. In no case should one attempt to "help" the plants along with high-nitrogen fertilizers. Nitrogen may be toxic to wild plants and may also accumulate to levels within the plant that are toxic to humans.

Being fully aware of potential effects of a foreign environment on chemical composition, I grew in my garden some of these plants (purchased as seeds or plantlets from commercial suppliers). Some I harvested and used, with questionable efficacy, as cures and preventives: boneset, joe-pye weed, and echinacea, for example. Others, such as plantain, dandelion, fox grape, sassafras, elderberry, mulberry, strawberry, and groundnut, were harvested from the wild as curatives and interesting foods. Conscious of the potential toxic effects of other medicinal perennials—ginseng, blue cohosh, black snakeroot, New Jersey tea, redbud, pawpaw, wild ginger, bloodroot, rue, goldenseal, celandine poppy, and doll's eyes, to name just a few—I cultivate these for their interesting forms and as photographic subjects rather than for medicinal use.

Preparation of Plants for Medicinal Uses

The medicinal effects of a plant depend not only on its particular metabolic products and on the circumstances in which the plant grew, but also on the way it is prepared for use. Whole plants collected from the garden or field are used fresh, or washed, blotted dry, and then, as quickly as possible, dried to a brittle state at as low a temperature as possible to protect heat-sensitive components and to stop the plant from decomposing or becoming moldy. The best way to dry plants for medicinal use is in a 50°C to 80°C (120°F to 175°F) oven, with circulating air, and for not more than twenty-four hours. (Most workers have noted that drying changes the natural state of chemicals within the plant.)

Just as some parts of a plant are more suitable for food than others, the concentration of biologically active product often varies markedly from one part of the plant to another. The concentration may also change over the lifetime of the plant. So it is important to know what part of the plant to harvest and when and how to handle it once it has been harvested. Leaves are usually collected at the time of flowering, the leaf stalk removed, and the blades quickly dried. Flowers are usually picked and dried soon after they open. Bulbs and roots are generally dug up in autumn. Bulbs need to be cleaned and, for long term storage, sliced and dried. The bark and inner parts of roots are often separated before they are dried. The bark of stems and twigs is usually peeled from the wood before drying.

In general, one should assume that for each step of preparation the product loses some of its efficacy—or may gain in toxicity. But there are many exceptions: when the biologically active components are stable and nonvolatile, the activity may be greatly concentrated by drying. Consider the differences between fresh kitchen herbs and the dried herbs sold in stores—many of the nuances of flavor and aroma vanish with drying, but the key flavors become stronger, so recipes specify much smaller amounts of the dried product. It is convenient to buy dried medicinal plants and products from a supplier or health food store, but then you have to trust in someone else's identification of the plant and method of harvest and preparation. For centuries, herbalists, pharmacists, and physicians have warned consumers to be wary of unscrupulous purveyors of dried herbs that have been adulterated with cheaper, inactive plant material. Today's high-demand market has the same problems.

Once the medicinal plant or plant part has been dried, the material can be ground to a powder and then swallowed in a gelatin capsule. More likely though, the active components have to be extracted before they can be used or stored.

There are four widely used basic techniques for extraction: infusion, decoction, maceration, and juicing. (With technological advances, newer methods of extraction using electric fields, membranes, and so on will not be described here.) Infusion usually requires nothing more than pouring hot water over the plant materials (fresh or dry). Decoction means boiling the plant material in water for period of time; evaporation concentrates the active products in the remaining liquid. The most concentrated decoctions are sometimes referred as "plasters" (see red clover cancer remedy). In maceration (also called cold-water infusion), as the plants steep in cold water, the less heat-stable and highly water-soluble components are extracted into the liquid. All three kinds of water extracts are often simply called "teas," although infusion is the most familiar technique. Juicing may extract the active components in near-natural state and concentration: the fresh plant material is ground in a cold glass mortar and pestle or in a blender, and the juices are then collected crude or by filtration through clean cheesecloth or a paper filter. The juice is highly subject to decomposition by bacteria or fungi during storage.

A less common method, solvent extraction, is accomplished with alcohol (ethanol) or another volatile organic solvent. The solvent is then evaporated to produce a concentrate that is usually very viscous and quite stable. In research laboratories and commercial production, a maximally concentrated, solvent-free extract can also be obtained using high pressure and gases such as carbon dioxide in relatively sophisticated techniques. Volatile compounds are collected by various techniques of distillation. Oils and other products for external use are best prepared from dried materials in mineral oil, cooking/salad oil, white petrolatum, or other solvents such as lanolin.

With the exception of high-pressure gas extraction, the processes described have long traditions behind them. For centuries, herbalists, pharmacists, doctors, and housewives have prepared infusions, decoctions, teas, distillates, and extracts of small quantities of medicinal substances.

The United Nations and the World Health Organization, which have longstanding interests in medicinal plants and traditional medicine, estimate that 80 percent of the world's population uses crude extracts of plants as therapeutic agents. The pharmaceutical industry, however, has had to approach the identification, extraction, and testing of plant-derived medicines in a much more systematic way and on a larger scale. The United Nations Industrial Development Organization proposed a nine-step procedure for establishing the medicinal value of plants:

1. Collect biologically active plant material.
2. Authenticate the plant's botanical identity.
3. Extract the biologically active chemicals.
4. Separate the chemical constituents.
5. Identify the active chemicals.
6. Synthesize active chemicals and analogues.
7. Select compounds for evaluation in animals.
8. Select compounds for evaluation in humans.
9. Carry out Phase I clinical trials.

Isolating the pure compound makes it possible to prepare standard doses of the drugs. By synthesizing analogues—chemicals with similar structures but not identical to the natural compound—it may be possible to minimize side effects or increase efficacy.

It is also true that the organic chemist's choices of compounds for synthesis and production of analogues may depend more on the compounds' chemical suitability for all these processes than strictly on their actual biological activity. The biological activity of the crude extract may, in fact, have been the result of the interaction and synergy of several components—once the material is purified, it may be inactive or even toxic in tests. We still have much to learn from traditional methods of preparation, unsophisticated though they may seem by comparison with the high technology of the modern laboratory.

Cautionary Note

Many herbalists encourage the prophylactic use of herbal medicines, arguing that you should not wait until you are thirsty before digging a well. But from my personal experiences of the effects of herbs and my knowledge of the biochemistry of plant products, I urge great caution in the use of these plants. I have found, for example, that two plants with long histories of medicinal use in Asian civilizations—the neem tree (*Azadirachta indica*) and ginseng (*Panax ginseng*)—have a strong effect on my blood pressure. The neem tree has been used for centuries in India and Africa. There is good evidence that it is effective against pathogenic fungi, bacteria, viruses, and insects. Neem twigs used as toothbrushes prevent dental diseases, and oral preparations have been used to treat malaria. For myself, chewing a small amount of the fresh leaf appears to lower my blood pressure immediately. Consuming fresh or dried ginseng root for a prolonged period, a cure-all which has an equally valued place in Chinese herbal medicine, raises my blood pressure.

This book is not intended to be used for self-medication, nor are the preparations described intended to replace or supplement medications prescribed by a physician. It is not intended to be used as a field guide for the harvest of plants for personal use or sale. Many plants can be poisonous or confused with poisonous plants. Do not taste, handle, or use a plant unless you are absolutely certain of its botanical identity— and then only with great caution. Amateur botanists and herbalists should never ingest medicinal plants without first consulting a professional. Much of the chemistry of these plants is still unknown. Many plants used for food or medicine may eventually be shown to be unsafe. People vary in their sensitivity to chemical components of plants, and responses—especially allergic responses—can be fatal.

Although one can find a reasonable number of edible and medicinal wild plants in the region, it should be kept in mind that in urban areas and along highways, these plants (e.g. ginkgo) are most likely to have been contaminated by environmental pollutants and should not be consumed. In addition, some plants, such as the green violet, the angelica tree, and the Norway pine, are rare and considered endangered. It is probably best to regard wild plants generally as representing emergency medicines or foods.

PART II

Medicinal Plants of New Jersey and the Region

∾

001 Aceraceae

The maple family of flowering trees and shrubs. Aceraceae occur as native and as escaped plants. The leaves are opposite and may be either simple or pinnate. There are no stipules. The fruit is winged (a double or triple samara), splitting into sections at maturity. The family consists of two genera, both of which are found in the Northern Hemisphere. The most common genus is *Acer*, which includes the box elders. Species of *Acer* occur in all of the moist regions of North America, but the sugar maple (*Acer saccharum*) is limited to the eastern portion of the continent. The sugar maple produces not only sap for the production of maple syrup, but also very valuable hardwood. The most recognizable morphological characteristics of the genus are the winged fruit and the leaf shape.

Roots and leaves of several members of the family contain inhibitory compounds that have allelopathic effects on other plants; that is, the roots and leaves contain chemicals that enter the soil and inhibit or otherwise control the growth of other plants.

When injured, all maples exude watery sap that can be used as food. It varies in quality depending on the species. The best quality comes from the sugar maple and is best collected on sunny days following freezing nights. A trough pounded into the tree about 4 feet from the ground and below a vertical slash in the trunk allows for the collection of sap. Maple sap can be consumed fresh or allowed to ferment, producing maple wine or vinegar. Prolonged boiling produces maple syrup and, on drying, maple sugar. Cracked corn (grits) can be boiled in two volumes of water to produce a firm mass that is then mixed with maple

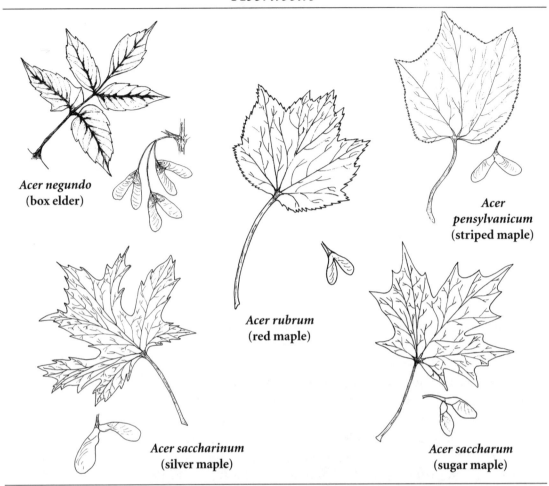

Acer negundo
(box elder)

**Acer
pensylvanicum**
(striped maple)

Acer rubrum
(red maple)

Acer saccharinum
(silver maple)

Acer saccharum
(sugar maple)

syrup or sugar to produce a nutritious food. Maple vinegar can be mixed with maple syrup or sugar to produce a flavorful sauce for cooking meats.

The inner bark of maple trees may be dried, powdered, sifted to remove woody elements, and baked to produce a flat bread. Seeds can be removed from the samara, boiled, and eaten hot. Newly sprouted maple seedlings can be eaten fresh, or dried and stored for consumption later.

Acer negundo (ashleaf, box elder, water ash) is a 40- to 70-foot native and escaped tree found in both northern and southern New Jersey along river banks and in fertile woods. Twigs are green and glossy, and leaves are pinnate, with three to seven leaflets, (with three leaflets it has been mistaken for poison ivy), the end leaflet larger than the lateral leaflets. Leaflets may be toothless or coarsely toothed. The fruit is a double samara.

Native Americans prepared a decoction or infusion of the inner bark as an emetic to treat stomach disorders that might be relieved by vomiting.

Acer pensylvanicum (moosewood, striped maple, whistlewood) is a 15-foot, relatively slender, native maple found in wooded areas of northern New Jersey. The bark is greenish with longitudinal white stripes. Leaves are 5 to 8 inches wide and finely toothed. The fruit is a double samara.

Native Americans used moosewood as they used box elder. In addition, they used the inner bark for pulmonary complaints (colds, coughs, bronchitis, and the like) and the wood to treat gonorrhea and kidney disorders. A bark poultice was used externally as a wash and for paralyzed or swollen limbs. A strong decoction prepared from the leaves and twigs was used as an emetic, and a weaker preparation was taken to relieve nausea.

Acer rubrum (red maple, scarlet maple, swamp maple) is a 20- to 80-foot native tree found in low-lying woods and swamps, and along streams in northern and southern New Jersey, including the pinelands. The bark is smooth and light gray on young trees, but rough and dark gray-brown on older trees. Twigs and buds are reddish, and leaves have three to five toothed lobes. The fruit is a double samara.

Native Americans prepared an astringent infusion from the inner bark and leaves for menstrual cramps, dysentery, and for application to sore eyes, measles, hives, and gunshot wounds. The inner bark can also be boiled to a syrup and used as a wash for sore eyes.

Acer saccharinum (silver maple, soft maple, white maple) is a 120-foot native and escaped tree found in dry and clay soils but usually in floodplain and alluvial soils of northern New Jersey. The leaves of the silver maple are 4 to 6 inches long, with five deep lobes, and serrate. The upper side of the leaf is green while the lower is white, turning clear yellow in fall. The flowers are greenish yellow and pubescent when young. The fruit is a double samara.

Native Americans used preparations of the inner bark and roots as medicines. The bark was used primarily as an astringent infusion or decoction for diarrhea and other disorders as described for *A. rubrum*. A root bark infusion was taken for gonorrhea.

Acer saccharum (hard maple, rock maple, sugar maple) is a 60- to 130-foot native tree found in the rich-soiled, hilly woods and fields of northern New Jersey. The twigs are glossy, and the leaves are green on both sides. The leaves are five-lobed, and the fruit is a double samara.

Native Americans used the inner bark for pulmonary complaints and to control diarrhea. The preparation is diuretic and expectorant. Native Americans referred to it as a "blood purifier." Maple syrup was taken as a "spring tonic" and used in cough syrups.

002 *Adiantaceae*

A fern family previously considered a branch of the Polypodiaceae, see the description of that family.

Adiantum pedatum (maidenhair fern) is an easily identified native fern found in moist, rich soils in deep woods of northern and southern New Jersey, including the pinelands. The fronds, which are about 1 foot high, are flat, with shiny, black stalks. The leaflets are alternate and lobed on the upper edge.

The leaves are aromatic and bitter. Native Americans prepared a whole-plant decoction to be taken internally for relief of symptoms associated with head and chest colds, influenza, pleurisy, and asthma. A whole-plant decoction or infusion was also used as an emetic. A root decoction was used externally or taken internally for rheumatism. The powdered plant was inhaled or smoked for asthma and heart trouble. A leaf infusion, when prepared as a hair tonic, is described as making the hair shiny.

Adiantaceae

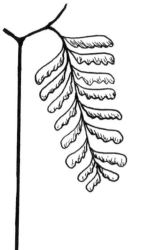

Adiantum pedatum
(maidenhair fern)

003 *Alismataceae*

The monocotyledonous water-plantain or arrowhead family of aquatic or marshland herbs. These plants are usually identified by their leaves, which are basal, simple, linear, and ovate or arrow-shaped. The main veins are parallel, a characteristic of monocots, with smaller veins pinnate or crosswise. The family distribution is worldwide but concentrated in the Northern Hemisphere.

Alisma plantago-aquatica (A. triviale) (common water-plantain, large water-plantain) is a native, erect perennial found in shallow water or mud and was reported to exist in Sussex County. The leaves are characteristic of the species, but they are more oval than sharply arrow-shaped, as is typical of the family.

Native Americans used a root decoction for pulmonary and kidney complaints and for tuberculosis. A plant infusion was used as a gynecological aid in "womb troubles."

Alisma subcordatum (devil's spoon, small water-plantain) is a native, erect perennial found in shallow-water and muddy areas in northern and southern New Jersey. Although the leaves are oval, they are more heart-shaped than those of the large water-plantain and thus more characteristic of the family.

Leaves and roots were used by native Americans to prepare a diuretic for kidney stones and urinary tract disorders. A poultice prepared from the root was used for bruises and wounds. The leaves are rubefacient.

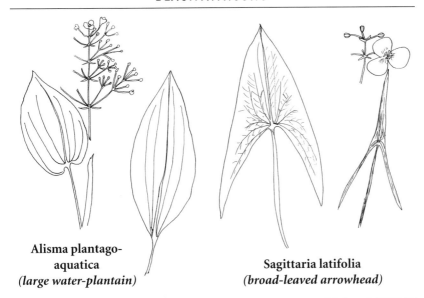

**Alisma plantago-
aquatica**
(large water-plantain)

Sagittaria latifolia
(broad-leaved arrowhead)

Sagittaria latifolia (arrowhead, broad-leaved arrowhead) is one of several native species of erect, deep-water perennials with distinctly arrow-shaped leaves found throughout the state in marsh areas and peaty bogs, and along the edges of streams, ponds, and lakes. The tubers are edible.

Native Americans used the leaves and tubers to prepare an infusion for fevers, rheumatism, and indigestion. As with the water-plantain, a poultice was applied for bruises and wounds. A leaf poultice was used to control lactation. The leaf infusion was used as a wash for feverish babies.

004 *Amaranthaceae*

The amaranth family of herbs and, rarely, shrubs, trees, or vines. Leaves are simple, entire, and alternate or opposite. It is a family of weeds and is most abundant and used medicinally in Africa and tropical America. *Amaranthus caudatus* is used in East Africa as a vermifuge and in tropical America for pulmonary complaints. The root is diuretic. More than 20 Amaranthaceae are used for medicinal purposes in the Americas, the Caribbean, the Philippines, and Indonesia.

Amaranthus retroflexus (green amaranth, pigweed, wild beet) is a 6-inch to 2-foot native, gray, downy, annual weed found throughout the state. Leaves are alternate, and the stems are covered with fine hairs. The flower spikes are up to $2^{1}/_{2}$ inches long and appear between August and October.

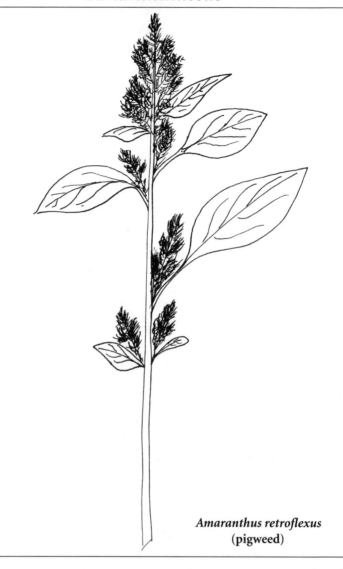

Amaranthus retroflexus
(**pigweed**)

Native Americans prepared an astringent infusion from the flowers and leaves to control diarrhea, excessive menstrual flow, and bowel hemorrhage.

005 *Anacardiaceae*

The cashew family of flowering trees and shrubs. The bark is usually resinous. Leaves are simple to pinnate and alternate. The family is primarily tropical in distribution, but extends into the temperate regions of the Northern Hemisphere. The family includes mango, pistachio, and

Anacardiaceae

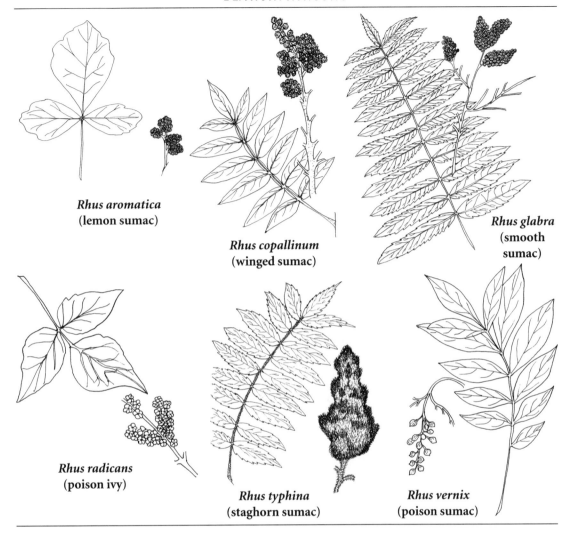

Rhus aromatica
(lemon sumac)

Rhus copallinum
(winged sumac)

Rhus glabra
(smooth
sumac)

Rhus radicans
(poison ivy)

Rhus typhina
(staghorn sumac)

Rhus vernix
(poison sumac)

the sumacs. They have dioecious or perfect flowers and drupaceous fruits. Astringent preparations from the leaves and bark of this family probably owe their activity to the presence of tannins and gallic acid, and they have been used for tanning leather. In tropical areas, many Anacardiaceae, including the cashew-nut tree, are used for many medicinal purposes.

Rhus aromatica (fragrant sumac, lemon sumac, polecat bush) is a 2- to 7-foot native and partially naturalized bush or shrub found in dry woods and dry, open areas of northern New Jersey. Leaves are composed of three leaflets. Yellow flowers appear on short spikes in May as the leaves develop. Red, hairy, oily fruits appear in August.

Native Americans used all parts of the plant in medicine. The root bark tea is astringent and was used to treat diarrhea, genitourinary tract problems, and bedwetting in children. Leaves are diuretic and were chewed for colds and stomachache. The bark was also chewed for colds, and the fruit was chewed for toothache and stomachache. Dried, powdered fruit was used on smallpox sores.

Rhus copallinum (*R. copallina*)(dwarf sumac, shining sumac, winged sumac) is a 2- to 10-foot native shrub or tree, found in dry woods and clearings of northern and southern New Jersey. Leaves are composed of 9 to 31 shiny, toothless leaflets. There is a prominent wing along the midrib. The branches are covered with fine hairs, and the fruit is covered with red hairs.

The root infusion is astringent and was used for diarrhea. The fruit was chewed to control bedwetting and for the treatment of mouth sores. An infusion prepared from the bark was used to stimulate milk flow.

Rhus glabra (scarlet sumac, smooth sumac) is a 3- to 10-foot native shrub found in fields and open areas of northern and southern New Jersey. Leaves are composed of 11 to 31 toothed leaflets. The branches are very smooth, without hairs, while the fruit is red with short hairs. It is especially important to recognize the distinguishing morphological characteristics of *R. glabra* and *R. vernix*, the poison sumac.

Native Americans used the entire plant as medicine. The fruit was used to control bedwetting. The leaves were smoked for asthma and prepared as an infusion for diarrhea and mouth diseases. The root decoction was used as an emetic and diuretic, while the bark infusion or decoction was used for diarrhea and fevers.

Bigelow described the berries of *R. glabra* and other species as refrigerant for fevers and a gargle for sore throats.

Rhus radicans (*Toxicodendron radicans*) (cow itch, poison ivy) is a common, native trailing or climbing vine or erect shrub found in all areas of New Jersey, although rare in the pinelands. Leaves are alternate and glossy, and composed of three leaflets. The flowers and fruit are white, with fruit appearing in August through November, providing food for birds through the winter.

Poison ivy is so troublesome and widespread that it is known to the majority of local residents; however, even professional botanists new to the area have been attracted to its waxy and colorful fall foliage. In one case, a professor of pharmacognosy discovered the poisonous nature of this plant by performing a classic test for alkaloids: when plant tissue is chewed, released alkaloids impart a characteristic bitter taste. Needless to say, one should not perform this taste test on unfamiliar plants or on seemingly familiar plants in an unfamiliar environment.

Poison ivy contains an oil that, on simple contact with the plant by sensitive individuals, will cause small, watery pimples or eruptions to appear on the skin, accompanied by severe itching and burning. These plants also may cause a severe reaction in the oral cavity, the gastrointestinal tract, or the respiratory tract when the oil is inhaled as a volatile. The oil may be volatilized when plants are burned or shredded. The active principle in the oil is known as urushiol and is composed of derivatives of catechol and other phenolic resins that on skin contact act as a powerful hapten. Urushiol is present in the rash and spreads to other parts of the skin by scratching.

Leaf preparations were once rubbed on the skin in attempts to induce immunity and used medicinally for the treatment of paralytic and liver disorders. A poultice prepared from the leaves was used for the treatment of chronic running sores and swollen glands.

Rhus typhina (staghorn sumac, velvet sumac) is a 5- to 20-foot native shrub or tree found in dry, rocky soils of northern and southern New Jersey. Leaflets are numerous, with sharp teeth. Branches and fruit are covered with hairs. Flowers appear in June, with fruit in September. As the names "smooth sumac" and "velvet sumac" suggest, the major difference between *R. glabra*, discussed previously, and this plant is the lack of hairs, causing smoothness of the one and the velvety hairiness of the other.

Uses by native Americans are similar to those for *R. glabra*. In addition, the berries are used to prepare a cough syrup, and berries and leaves are used to prepare an infusion for sore throat and tonsillitis. An astringent decoction is prepared from the root or bark for control of diarrhea and bleeding.

Rhus vernix (*Toxicodendron vernix*) (poison dogwood, poison sumac, swamp sumac) is a tall, native shrub or small tree found almost exclusively in swamps and very moist habitats throughout New Jersey, including the pinelands. Leaves are divided into 7 to 13 smooth, light green, entire leaflets. The smooth leaf margin is the distinguishing characteristic when compared with the smooth sumac described above. The bark is gray-brown and smooth or rough, depending on the age of the plant. Small, green flowers appear from May through July, with dull white fruit developing in August and through October. The entire plant is poisonous in all seasons. For toxicity see *R. radicans*.

Native Americans used the bark as an emetic, and the plant was also used in some form to prepare a wash for sores ("foul ulcers") and to treat asthma, fevers, and gonorrhea.

Bigelow describes the poisonous character of poison sumac and its introduction into medicine in England and France for the treatment of paralysis and cutaneous eruptions, and the use in America for "consumptive complaints."

Annonaceae

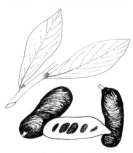

Asimina triloba
(pawpaw)

The pawpaw or cherimoya family of aromatic trees, shrubs, and vines. Leaves are simple, entire, and alternate. The fruit is a berry with large seeds. This is primarily a tropical family, represented in eastern North America by the pawpaw (papaw). In tropical areas, many of the Annonaceae are used for both food and medicinal purposes. They are also used to prepare fragrant, pleasant-tasting beverages. As a family, the Annonaceae contain a large number of alkaloids, including the aporphine and morphine groups. The presence of the former may account for the diuretic activity, while the latter, when present, could account for the reported narcotic effects experienced when the seeds are consumed. Pawpaws seem to be immune to diseases and pest insects.

Asimina triloba (custard apple, pawpaw) is a 10- to 20-foot native, small tree or shrub. It is rare but may be found in rich-soiled, moist, wooded areas of northern and southern New Jersey. The leaves are oblong to lancet-shaped and up to 1 foot long. Appearing in May, the flowers are purple with petals curved backward. The fruit is oblong and green or yellow, with large seeds.

Native Americans apparently did not use pawpaw for medicinal purposes. The fruit is edible and somewhat banana-flavored. Most people find the fruit laxative. Leaves and seeds are insecticidal and were used, as they are in tropical areas, to control head lice. Seeds are emetic and should be regarded as toxic. The leaf infusion is diuretic. It seems to the writer and probably to the reader that this is a promising commercial crop; such research is under way at universities in several of the northeastern states.

007 *Apocynaceae*

The dogbane family of herbs, shrubs, and trees including oleander and periwinkle. Members of this family are mostly tropical, with milky sap and simple, entire leaves. They often have showy flowers and fruit consisting of two follicles or drupes. Many of the Apocynaceae contain poisons that affect the heart. *Nerium oleander* (laurier rose) is native to the Mediterranean and tropical Asia. It is cultivated elsewhere, including California. In colder climates it makes a very attractive plant that is easy to grow and ornamental, with showy flowers produced indoors and out throughout the year; however, all parts of the plant (roots, stems, leaves, and flowers) are poisonous, whether fresh or dry. Even the flower nectar is toxic. It is said that a single leaf can be fatal for a human. Deaths in humans are usually due to chewing leaves, sucking nectar, or eating

Apocynaceae

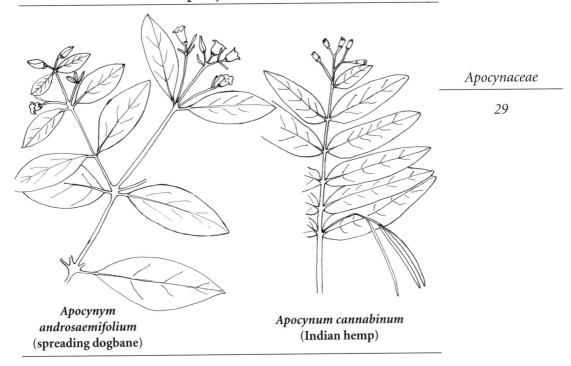

**Apocynym
androsaemifolium
(spreading dogbane)**

**Apocynum cannabinum
(Indian hemp)**

meat cooked on skewers prepared from the stems. The milky latex or clear exudate from cut leaves or the stem may cause contact dermatitis, and the roots are said to be abortifacient. *Nerium indicum* leaves are used in Chinese medicine to treat heart disease, traumatic bruises, and resistant fungus infection, and as an insecticide for killing flies and maggots. Other genera in the family include *Adenium, Acokanthera, Strophanthus, Thevetia,* and *Tanghinia,* which are similar to *Nerium* in their toxicity. Many are used to prepare arrow poisons, and all are used medicinally, it is not unusual for death to result from attempts at medicinal use. *Adenium obesum* (desert rose) seeds or seedlings can be purchased locally; this plant is a popular ornamental because of its unusual shape and showy red-pink flowers. It is native to Africa, used both medicinally and to produce an arrow poison. *Catharanthus major,* listed among the poisonous Apocynaceae, is the source of some of the most effective cancer chemotherapeutic agents available today (vinblastine and vincristine). The antibiotic oleandomycin is produced by the fungus *Streptomyces antibioticus* and not, as the name might suggest, synthesized by the higher plant *Nerium oleander.* There are about 60 species of *Apocynum* in North America, at least 3 of which are native to New Jersey.

Apocynum androsaemifolium (spreading dogbane) is a 1- to 4-foot native, spreading, perennial shrub found in fields and along roadsides throughout the state, although it is rare in the pinelands. Leaves are oblong or egg-shaped, opposite, and smooth. The small (1/8 to 1/4 inch) flowers are pink and bell-shaped, and appear in June and July. The plant contains a milky juice and the cardioactive glycoside cymarin, which has caused toxic symptoms in livestock. Experiments conducted in Arizona show that 15 to 20 grams of green leaves were sufficient to kill a horse or cow, and that 1 to 5 grams would kill a sheep.

Native Americans used dogbane root as a laxative and for other digestive complaints. It was used as an herbal steam, snuff, or poultice for headache. A root preparation was also taken for intestinal worms in humans and mixed with feed for worms in horses. Green berries were taken for heart and kidney problems.

Bigelow described dogbane (frequently called ipecac) as an emetic in large doses, and tonic and stomachic in smaller doses.

Apocynum cannabinum (dogbane, Indian hemp) is native and more shrublike than spreading dogbane. Its distribution is statewide, differing only from spreading dogbane in the pinelands, where the variety pubescens is not rare. Flowers are greenish white, bell-shaped, and terminal, present from June through August. Fruit is present from September through October.

Both spreading dogbane and Indian hemp are described as less toxic in the dried state; poisoning symptoms are similar, and medicinal uses are the same.

Apocynum medium (intermediate dogbane, small-flowered dogbane) is native and considered by some botanists to be a hybrid. Its distribution differs from that of the other dogbanes in that it has not been identified in the northern portions of the state. Pink flowers are present from June through August, with fruit from September through October.

Symptoms of poisoning and medicinal uses are similar to those of the other dogbanes. The large, bitter, milky root, prepared according to an established recipe, was an important food for Native Americans and a celebrated "infallible" remedy for the treatment of venereal diseases. It was also used in the treatment of Bright's disease (kidney diseases), rheumatic gout, and dropsy. The leaves were used as a ceremonial emetic.

Aquifoliaceae

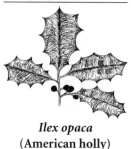

Ilex opaca
(American holly)

008 *Aquifoliaceae*

The holly family of evergreen shrubs and trees. The leaves are alternate, simple, spiny, and lobed. Flowers are small and white. The fruit is fleshy and red or black, with four internal segments. The family consists of three genera, the largest being *Ilex*, which is widely distributed and especially abundant in eastern North America. *I. vomitoria* leaves contain caffeine and were used by Native Americans of the southeastern United States as an emetic, ceremonial tea. *I. aquifolium* is native to Europe.

Ilex opaca (American holly) is a 25- to 50-foot native and escaped evergreen tree found statewide, including the pinelands. The bark is thin and grayish. The leaves have spines along the margins and at the tip. Trees are male or female, with white flowers and bright red berries forming on the female plants, making them a Christmastime favorite for holiday decoration.

Native Americans used the leaves, bark, and berries medicinally. The bark was used to prepare an eyewash, and the leaves were used to prepare eye drops. Leaves were also used to scratch sore muscles and to prepare a wash for measles and sores. The berries, regarded today as poisonous, were chewed for colic and dyspepsia.

009 *Araceae*

The arum family of terrestrial or aquatic monocotyledonous herbs; stems are rhizomes or tubers. Leaves are simple or compound, and flower stems may be leafless or leafy. Juice may be milky and pungent. *Caladium*, *Philodendron*, and species of *Dieffenbachia*, all used as houseplants, contain irritating juices or sharp crystals of calcium oxalate that can produce burning and swelling in the throat severe enough so as to approach asphyxiation. Recovery may require several days. Few of the Araceae are edible, but sweet flag rootstock and stalk interior are sweet-tasting and are used to produce a candy. The base of the stalk and root are sliced and boiled to produce a thick syrup. It is also among those plants known to contain carcinogens.

Acorus calamus (calamus, sweet flag) is a 1- to 4-foot native aquatic, perennial herb growing in colonies found in swamps and along streams throughout New Jersey, including the pinelands. Small, green to yellow flowers appear in the spring or early summer on a dense spadix (characteristic) protruding from the side of a long, swordlike bract.

Native Americans used sweet flag as a panacea. This was among the most widely used medicinal plants, a cure-all root that was chewed, smoked, or rubbed on the skin for any illness. The root was chewed for colds, headache, sore throat, diarrhea, worms, dropsy, yellow urine, gravel, toothache, fever, earache, tuberculosis, lung ailments, rheumatism, and irregular menses. It was used to induce sweat, urination, and hallucinations.

In Chinese medicine, the roots and stems are used to treat epilepsy, strokes, and rheumatoid arthritis; to kill worms; and to relieve toxic dysentery.

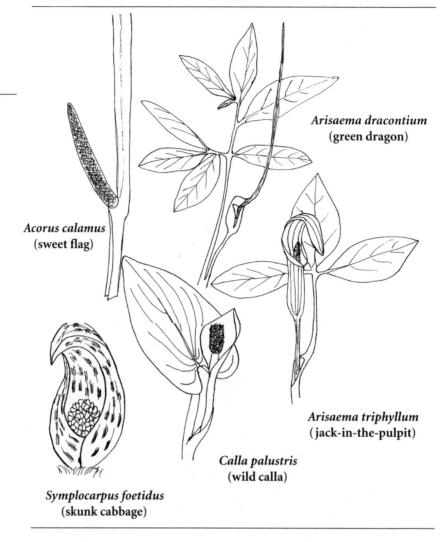

Arisaema dracontium
(green dragon)

Acorus calamus
(sweet flag)

Arisaema triphyllum
(jack-in-the-pulpit)

Calla palustris
(wild calla)

Symplocarpus foetidus
(skunk cabbage)

Bigelow described sweet flag root as a stimulant, a heating agent, and a tonic; it was given in cases of flatulent colic, stomach cramps, and so on.

Today it is described as antispasmodic and anticonvulsant, and it has been found to lower serum cholesterol levels in experimental animals. Hallucinations are probably induced by beta-asarone, present also in oil of calamus. Oil of calamus has been shown to be carcinogenic.

Arisaema dracontium (dragonroot, green dragon) is a 1- to 4-foot native perennial herb found in low woods and along streams of northern and southern New Jersey, flowering in late spring. The characteristic green spadix develops within a hood and protrudes several inches beyond. The single leaf is divided into 5 to 15 leaflets.

Native Americans used dried dragonroot for the treatment of "female disorders" and, when properly prepared, for food. The root contains calcium oxalate crystals that must be removed before consumption.

Bigelow described dragonroot as "too violently acrid to be a safe medicine in its recent [fresh] state," but that the dried root may be grated in milk and given as a carminative and diaphoretic.

Arisaema triphyllum (Indian turnip, jack-in-the-pulpit, wake robin) is a 1- to 2-foot native perennial herb found in moist, wooded areas of northern and southern New Jersey. As with dragonroot, the inflorescence is solitary and composed of a hooded spadix. The hood is nearly black on the undersurface. Flowers appear in spring, with the spadix becoming a cluster of bright scarlet-red berries in the summer. The single leaf is divided characteristically into three leaflets, hence the species name.

Native Americans used a root poultice or decoction for headaches, various skin diseases, colds, dry coughs, diarrhea, and cramps. The root was also stimulant, expectorant, and diaphoretic. Steam was used for sore eyes and to induce sneezing. The root was used after drying and contains calcium oxalate crystals. See the caution above for the family.

Calla palustris (water arum, water dragon, wild calla) is a 2- to 6-inch native perennial herb found usually in bog areas of northern New Jersey. Flowers begin to appear in late spring. The "hood" is white and does not fold over the spadix, which is green, giving the inflorescence the characteristic appearance of the calla lily used by florists. The leaves are stalked and heart-shaped.

Native Americans used the root decoction for hemorrhage, influenza, shortness of breath, and cleaning the eyes of the blind. A decoction prepared from the stem and roots was used as a poultice for snakebites, and a poultice of the crushed root was applied to reduce swelling.

The fresh plant contains calcium oxalate crystals and must be used with caution (see caution for *Arisaema dracontium*).

Symplocarpus foetidus (devil's tobacco, skunk cabbage) is a 1- to 2-foot native perennial herb found in swamps and other wet areas throughout New Jersey, including the pinelands. Flowers appear in very early spring (they produce sufficient heat to melt ice and snow) before significant leaf development. The flowers are clustered in a spadix within a purplish-brown-and-green mottled hood to form the characteristic 2- to 5-inch-long inflorescence, especially striking when seen against a background of snow. The large leaves unfold and develop later, producing an offensive odor when crushed.

Native Americans used the dried root to prepare an infusion for coughs, colds, and convulsions in children and adults. A leaf poultice was used for pain and swelling. Raw leaves were chewed by epileptics.

The plant was also used for worms, rheumatism, weak heart, hemorrhage, headache, cramps, and "falling of the womb."

The roots are mildly narcotic and contain calcium oxalate crystals (see caution for *Arisaema dracontium*).

010 *Araliaceae*

The ginseng family of herbs, shrubs, vines, and trees with pithy stems. Leaves are simple, palmate, or pinnate, but always alternate. Stipules are often present. Fruits are usually berries and rarely a drupe. A large family, primarily tropical, with only four genera found in the United States and Canada. The family is sometimes called the Hederaceae, and the common English ivy, *Hedera helix*, is probably the best-known member. *Oplopanax* occurs from Alaska to northern California and across northern Michigan. *Panax* occurs in eastern North America, and the largest genus, *Aralia*, occurs throughout the United States and Canada. There are at least six Asian medicinal Araliaceae, including the well-known *Panax ginseng.*

Aralia hispida (bristly sarsaparilla, dwarf elder) is a 1- to 3-foot shrubby, native perennial herb with a short, woody, bristly stem, found in sandy, well-drained soils of clearings and open-wooded areas of northern New Jersey. Leaves are bipinnate, 1 to 3 inches long, with five ovate leaflets that are sharply and irregularly serrate. Globe-shaped greenish white umbels of flowers on long stalks extending above the leaves appear in May and June, with malodorous, dark purple fruit forming in August.

Native Americans used the root as an alterative and as a tonic. For dropsy, it was used as a diuretic and to reduce back pain associated with kidney irritation.

Aralia nudicaulis (small spikenard, wild sarsaparilla) is a 1- to 2-foot native, "stemless," perennial herb found in moist, wooded areas throughout New Jersey, possibly including the pinelands. The single leaf is divided into three sets of ovate, quinately pinnate leaflets positioned umbrellalike above the flowers. The greenish flowers, in one to three umbels, appear in May and June on a separate, naked stalk. The berries are purplish black. The root (stem) is horizontal and running.

Native Americans used a root decoction for stomach pain and "stoppage of periods" (abortifacient). An infusion of the root was taken as a "blood tonic," and a root poultice was applied for burns and sores. Chewed fresh root, or dried and powdered root, was used for nose bleeds. Wild sarsaparilla was also made into a pleasant-tasting beverage and used to flavor patent medicines in the nineteenth century.

Araliaceae

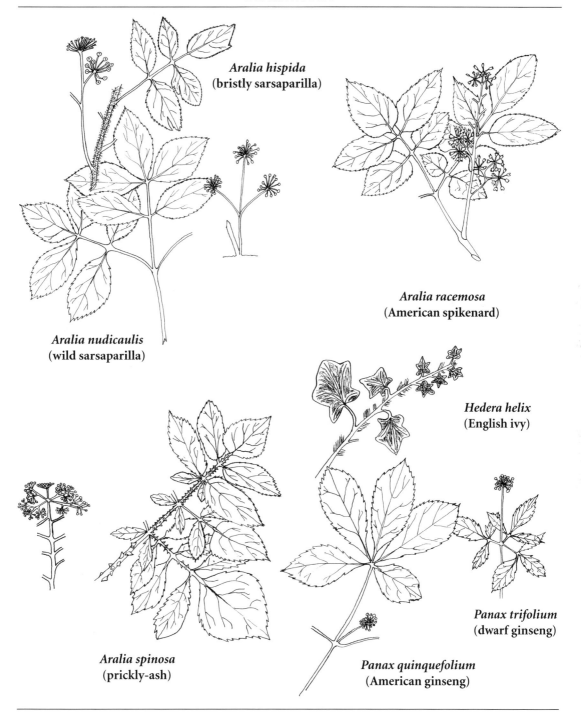

Aralia hispida
(bristly sarsaparilla)

Aralia racemosa
(American spikenard)

Aralia nudicaulis
(wild sarsaparilla)

Hedera helix
(English ivy)

Aralia spinosa
(prickly-ash)

Panax trifolium
(dwarf ginseng)

Panax quinquefolium
(American ginseng)

Bigelow described wild sarsaparilla as a mild diaphoretic and stimulant, with the tea a remedy for catarrh, rheumatism, and some skin disorders. He described *A. hispida* and *A. racemosa* as having similar properties.

Aralia racemosa (American spikenard, life-of-man, petty morrel) is a 3- to 5-foot native perennial shrub found in rich-soiled, wooded areas of northern New Jersey. The widely branched, dark-green or reddish stem is usually described as smooth, but may be somewhat hairy. The leaves are compound, with 6 to 21 large, toothed leaflets, heart-shaped at the base. Flowers are whitish in long, branching clusters of small umbels, beginning to appear in June. The berries are dark purple.

Native Americans used the juice of beaten roots as a wash for burns, to draw and heal boils, and to control diarrhea. The infusion of roots and berries is tonic, diaphoretic, expectorant, and antiseptic. A decoction of the bark was used for uterine prolapse.

Aralia spinosa (angelica tree, devil's walking stick, Hercules club, prickly-ash) is a large, 6- to 30-foot native, spiny-trunked shrub found in rich-soiled woods and clearings of northern and southern New Jersey. Doubly compound leaves are up to 3 feet long, with egg-shaped leaflets on sharply spiny stalks. The flowers are small and white in large, branching clusters of umbels. Flowers appear in July and give rise to black fruit in the fall.

Native Americans used the root to prepare a wash for paralysis and a salve for old sores. Green roots are poisonous, and the roasted and powdered roots are very strongly emetic and purgative. A poultice of pounded roots was applied to swollen leg veins, and a cold root infusion was used as drops for sore eyes.

Bigelow described the fresh-root-bark tea as both emetic and cathartic. The bark was described as "pungent and heating" and was used for rheumatism and skin disorders.

Hedera helix (English ivy) is an evergreen prostrate or climbing, woody vine of indeterminate length, naturalized throughout the state. The leaves are simple and entire, the flowers are small and yellow, the fruit is a black berry.

Native Americans used ivy in scrofula, dropsy, and pulmonary complaints. The leaves contain high concentrations of triterpene saponins and should be regarded as poisonous. A syrup prepared from the bark and twigs shows anticaries activity and is tonic, astringent, and expectorant.

Panax quinquefolium (American ginseng, ginseng, sang) is a 1- to 2-foot native perennial herb with a large, fleshy root, once found in rich-soiled and well-drained hardwood forest areas of northern and southern

New Jersey. Three leaves and one flower stalk arise at the same time from a single stalk, produced annually in April from an underground bud. The leaves are palmate and composed of five leaflets. The flowers are whitish in a single umbel. The fruit is a scarlet-red berry.

Ginseng is another of the widely used panacea or cure-all medicinal plants. Roots are chewed fresh, and leaves and roots are dried for the preparation of infusions and decoctions. Extracts of Asian ginseng may alter the microbial ecology of the intestine, and some researchers suggest that this leads to reduced toxicity, carcinogenesis, aging, and other phenomena in which intestinal bacteria participate. Medicinal benefits are too numerous to list but a caution is necessary: prolonged use may promote hypertension in some individuals.

In Chinese medicine, American ginseng is used to increase energy, calm the nerves, produce saliva, and increase appetite.

Panax trifolium (dwarf ginseng, groundnut) is a 3- to 8-inch rare native perennial herb with a nutlike root found in moist woods of northern and southern New Jersey. Three leaves and a single flower stalk arise at the same time from a single stalk, produced annually from an underground bud. Leaves are divided into three stalkless leaflets. The flowers appear in a single umbel. The fruit is a yellow berry.

Native Americans used the plant for headache, breast pain, rheumatism, dropsy, gout, tuberculosis, venereal disease, and diseases induced by mercury. A poultice of the chewed root was applied to cuts as a coagulant.

011 *Aristolochiaceae*

The birthroot or birthwort family of creeping herbs and woody vines occurring primarily throughout the tropics. Leaves are simple, entire, and alternate.

Aristolochia serpentaria (Virginia snakeroot) is a 2-foot or less rare native, herbaceous, pubescent perennial found in wooded areas of northern and southern New Jersey. It is extremely rare—in more than 10 years of searching in New Jersey, I have not found it, but I have cultivated other closely related species to observe and photograph their unique flower shape. Leaves are simple, entire, elongated, and heart- or arrow-shaped. Flowers are large, spotted, brownish purple, and curved upward in an S shape.

Native Americans used the root in medicine. The root is aromatic and was used fresh or dried. The fresh root was chewed for colds or bruised to produce a poultice for toothache and snakebite. The dried root was

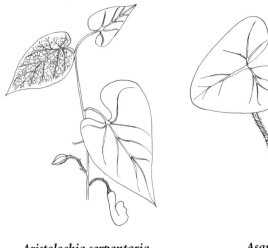
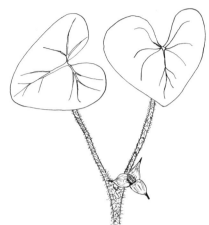

Aristolochia serpentaria
(**Virginia snakeroot**)

Asarum canadensis
(**wild ginger**)

used to produce a diaphoretic, diuretic, weak infusion taken for rheumatism, pains, headache, coughs, sore throat, pleurisy, fevers, snakebite, and intestinal worms. The decoction is antiseptic, probably attributable to the presence of aristolochic acid, an aromatic bitter isolated from many Aristolochiaceae. The acid also shows antitumor activity in experimental systems.

Bigelow described Virginia snakeroot as tonic and diaphoretic, antispasmodic, and anodyne. It was used as a febrifuge but was also regarded as being too stimulating for many diseases. A less-often-used name for the plant, birthwort or birthroot, suggests uses in childbirth as an abortifacient.

Asarum canadensis (asarabacca, Canada snakeroot, wild ginger) is a creeping, native perennial herb found in rich-soiled, wooded areas of northern and southern New Jersey. The leaves, two per plant, are heart-shaped or kidney-shaped and form a Y in which the flower develops. The flower is hidden by the leaves and is described by some as chocolate brown and others as brown-purple. The three "petals" of the flower are actually sepals.

Native Americans usually used the root medicinally, but fresh leaves were applied to wounds and dried leaves were powdered to produce a snuff for head and eyes. The root was highly valued as a flavoring agent for cooked foods and for the preparation of a sweat-producing decoction for indigestion, coughs and colds, worms and "to start periods" or for "scant or painful menstruation" (abortifacient). The cooked root was placed in the ear for earache. Native Americans believed the plant to have "general medicinal properties" and to be a powerful stimulant. It was also used to treat cases of typhus, typhoid, and scarlet fevers. Wild ginger also contains aristolochic acid, described under *A. serpentaria*.

Bigelow described Canada snakeroot as a "warm diaphoretic and stimulant" similar to *A. serpentaria*.

012 *Asclepidiaceae*

The milkweed family of perennial herbs, vines, and, rarely shrubs or small trees with umbellate flowers and a milky sap in most species. Leaves are simple, opposite, whorled, or alternate. The seeds and seed pods are characteristic. The family occurs throughout the tropics, with the genus *Asclepias* being the most numerous in North America. Some milkweeds are dangerous to both humans and other animals. Sheep, goats, cattle, horses, and domestic fowl have been poisoned by the cardiac glycosides they contain. The phenomenon of "puking blue jays" is attributed to the ingestion of larvae that have fed on leaves or butterflies that have fed on the flower nectar of milkweeds. Milkweeds are present throughout the state, including the pinelands, producing flowers from June through July and fruit from June through August.

Asclepias incarnata (swamp milkweed, flesh-colored asclepias) is a 2- to 6-foot native perennial found in wet lowlands and swamps statewide, with the exception of the central pinelands. Leaves are opposite, lance-shaped and entire. Flowers are red (pink to rose purple) with hoods

Asclepidiaceae

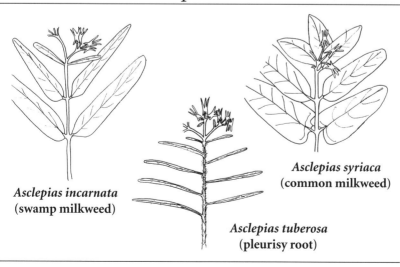

Asclepias incarnata
(swamp milkweed)

Asclepias tuberosa
(pleurisy root)

Asclepias syriaca
(common milkweed)

about 1/8 inch long with longer horns projecting. Flowers appear in July.

Native Americans used the root infusion in a bath for children and adults. It was taken as an anthelmintic for tapeworms and as a diuretic, antidiuretic, carminative, cathartic, and emetic. The root tea was also used to heal the newborn's navel, and cord made from the stems was used for tooth extraction.

Bigelow described flesh-colored asclepias as expectorant, diaphoretic, diuretic, and laxative, to be given in catarrh, asthma, rheumatism, secondary syphilis, and worms.

Asclepias syriaca (common milkweed, silkweed) a 2- to 4-foot native, downy perennial found in fields and along roadsides of northern and southern New Jersey. The leaves are large, oblong or oval, opposite, and attached to the stem with a short petiole. The underside of the leaf is grayish downy. The flowers are dark pink and fragrant, arising from leaf axils and first appearing in June.

Native Americans used the root infusion as a diuretic and laxative. It was taken for gravel and dropsy and has been used for the treatment of asthma, rheumatism, mastitis, and venereal diseases. The milk was used to treat warts and ringworm and was rolled until firm enough to make chewing gum. The roots and young plants were prepared as food.

Bigelow described common silkweed as antispasmodic, expectorant, and useful in catarrh and asthma.

Asclepias tuberosa (butterfly weed, pleurisy root) is a 1- to 2-foot native, herbaceous perennial found along dry roadsides and in well-drained open fields throughout New Jersey, including the pinelands. The leaves are lance-shaped and narrow. This is the only milkweed with alternate leaf arrangement and without a milky juice. The stem is hairy, but the most distinguishing feature is the showy, bright orange flowering head, present from late June through early August.

Native Americans boiled the seeds in milk for the treatment of diarrhea. The seed or root infusion was used as a gentle laxative. The raw root was eaten for bronchial and pulmonary troubles. The root infusion was also used for pleurisy, heart trouble, influenza, and rheumatism.

Bigelow described butterfly weed as a mild diaphoretic, expectorant, and subtonic, used in catarrh, bronchitis, the secondary stages of pneumonia, and in phthisis as a palliative.

013 *Aspidiaceae*

The shield fern family, considered generally as part of the family Polypodiaceae. For a description, see Polypodiaceae.

Athyrium filix-femina (lady fern) is a 3-foot native fern found in moist, shady areas throughout New Jersey, including on occasion the pinelands. The stems are smooth, and the plant grows in circular clumps of leaves (fronds). The fronds are doubly divided, and the leaflets are toothed.

The root decoction is diuretic and induces breast milk flow. A decoction prepared from pounded stems was taken for body pains and to ease labor pain in childbirth. The dried, powdered root was used to promote healing of sores.

Dryopteris cristata (crested shield fern, crested wood fern) is native and found in moist, shady areas throughout New Jersey, perhaps including the pinelands. The fronds are 30 inches long and 5 inches wide at the middle. They are blue-green, doubly divided, and ladderlike.

The root infusion was used to treat stomach trouble.

Polystichum acrostichoides (Christmas fern) is a 1- to 3-foot, shiny, evergreen, native fern found on rich-soiled, wooded slopes throughout the state, including on occasion the pinelands. The fronds are leathery, tapering, and singly divided, with coarsely toothed leaflets showing an upward-pointed, basal auricle.

The root decoction was used externally as a rub for rheumatism. The root infusion was taken internally for pneumonia and stomach or bowel complaints, and to induce emesis. A decoction prepared from the "vine" and small leaves was taken for fevers in small children. A poultice of wet, crushed roots was applied to the back of the head for convulsions in children and to the back and feet for spinal trouble and babies' sore backs.

014 *Aspleniaceae*

A fern family considered generally as part of the family Polypodiaceae. For a description, see Polypodiaceae.

Asplenium trichomanes (maiden fern) is a 2- to 8-inch evergreen fern found in acidic, dry, rocky areas of northern New Jersey. Fronds are all alike and pinnate, with the pinnae nearly opposite and slightly lobed.

Native Americans used maiden fern for irregular menses (abortifacient), breast diseases, liver complaints, "acrid humors," and coughs.

015 *Balsaminaceae*

The balsam or touch-me-not family of herbs with leaves simple, alternate, opposite, or in threes. The fruit is usually an exploding capsule but

Balsaminaceae

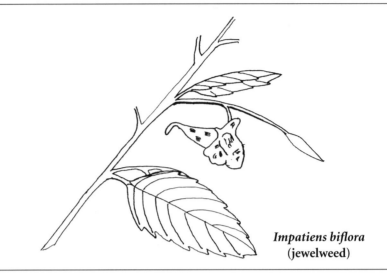

***Impatiens biflora*
(jewelweed)**

sometimes a berry. The family consists of only two genera in tropical and subtropical areas, one being *Impatiens*. Only two species of *Impatiens* are native to the United States and Canada.

Impatiens biflora (*I. capensis*) (jewelweed, spotted touch-me-not) is a 3- to 5-foot smooth, annual native herb found in moist areas throughout the state, including the pinelands. The leaves are oval, toothed, and alternate and opposite on the same plant. The flowers are orange, spotted with red-brown, and present throughout the summer and early fall.

A poultice of freshly crushed stems and stem juice is used for poison ivy rashes, nettle stings, sores, and babies' hives. The poultice is also applied to sore or raw eyelids. The stem tea is taken internally to ease childbirth and as a cleansing bath in childbirth. Crushed flowers are applied to cuts, burns, and bruises. A tea prepared from the roots or whole plant is taken for stricture or difficulty in urination, stomach cramps, chest colds, jaundice, kidney problems, and dropsy.

Impatiens pallida (pale jewelweed, pale touch-me-not, yellow jewelweed) is a 3- to 5-foot native annual herb found in moist, shaded limestone areas of northern New Jersey. The flowers are yellow and less spotted than those of *I. biflora*.

Medicinal uses are similar to those described for *I. biflora*.

016 *Berberidaceae*

The barberry family of shrubs and perennial herbs. The leaves may be simple, pinnate or ternately compound, and alternate. They may be deciduous or evergreen. The family occurs primarily in the temperate regions of the Northern Hemisphere.

Berberis vulgaris (common barberry) is a 3- to 10-foot naturalized branching shrub found in well-drained soils of northern New Jersey. The branches are grayish with three-part spines. The leaves are mostly alternate and spatula-shaped, with spiny teeth. The flowers are yellow, growing from the axils in drooping, multiflowered racemes.

The bark or crushed root is used to treat ulcerated gums and sore throat. The leaf decoction is taken for jaundice and the berry is used to treat sore throat and fever. The roots and bark contain berberine, a yellow antibacterial alkaloid with a broad spectrum of biological activities.

Caulophyllum thalictroides (blue cohosh, papoose root) is a 1- to 2-foot native perennial herb found in moist, rich-soiled, wooded areas of northern New Jersey. Bluish leaves are divided into three to five three- lobed leaflets. Flowers are purplish or yellow-green in branching

Berberidaceae

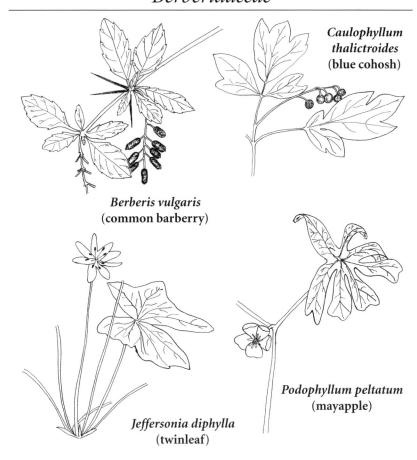

Caulophyllum thalictroides (blue cohosh)

Berberis vulgaris (common barberry)

Jeffersonia diphylla (twinleaf)

Podophyllum peltatum (mayapple)

terminal clusters. Flowers form in early spring and give rise to blue, ber-rylike seeds.

Native Americans used a decoction or syrup prepared from the root to treat epilepsy, fever, and pulmonary complaints; to promote child-birth and remediate excessive menstruation; and also to treat urogenital problems in men. The root decoction was also used as a foot and leg bath for rheumatism.

Blue cohosh produces dark blue seeds containing poisonous compounds (alkaloids such as methylcytisine) that accelerate respiration and raise the blood pressure. These alkaloids also stimulate intestinal and uterine contractions. Poisoning usually occurs in children, who are attracted to the blue seeds.

Jeffersonia diphylla (rheumatism root, twinleaf) is a rare, 8- to 16-inch native perennial herb found in rich-soiled, wooded areas of northern New Jersey. Leaves are divided lengthwise into two leaflets. White flowers appear in April, one to each 6- to 8-inch stalk. The fruit is about 1 inch long, pear-shaped, and opening with a hinged lid.

The whole-plant poultice is used for sores, ulcers, and inflammation. A plant infusion or decoction is used for urinary tract problems, gravel, dropsy, and diarrhea in adults and children.

Podophyllum peltatum (American mandrake, mayapple, wild jalap) is a 12- to 18-inch native perennial herb found throughout the state, including the pinelands. Leaves are in pairs and umbrellalike. The flower is white and solitary, and grows beneath the leaves. The fruit is 2 inches long, yellow, and lemon-shaped. The leaves are characteristic of the species.

Native Americans used the root as a purgative, emetic, and anthelmintic, and to treat rheumatism. The expressed juice of the fresh root was dropped into the ear for deafness and used as a crow and insect repellent in which corn was treated before planting. A decoction prepared from the whole plant was sprinkled on potato plants to kill potato bugs and was used as a laxative for horses. The powdered root was applied to ulcers and sores. The fruit is edible when ripe.

Bigelow described mayapple as "one of the most certain and efficacious of the cathartic vegetables, which have been examined in this country," particularly recommended in dropsy.

All parts of the mayapple except the ripe fruit contain podophyllotoxin, a lignanlike compound that causes gastrointestinal upset. Mayapple is now cultivated for the isolation of chemicals to be used as cancer chemotherapeutic agents.

The birch family of trees and shrubs. The leaves are simple and some-times deeply lobed or divided. Flowers are either staminate or pistillate and appear in conelike structures referred to as catkins. The fruit is a small samara or nut. The family occurs primarily in northern temperate regions, but species extend southward to Argentina and Bengal. Species of *Alnus* are able to obtain nitrogen from the atmosphere through an association between their roots and soil microorganisms known as *Frankia*.

Alnus glutinosa (black alder, European alder) is a naturalized 70-foot tree found in wet, low areas of northern New Jersey. Leaves are dull, dark green, 2 to 5 inches long, rounded, and serrate, with five to seven pairs of veins, nearly smooth on the underside. Leaves and stems are sticky. The male flowers are in pendulous yellow catkins, and the brown, conelike female flowers appear before the leaves.

Native Americans used the bark tea as a panacea for the treatment of any disease.

Alnus serrulata (common alder, smooth alder) is a 6- to 15-foot native

Betulaceae

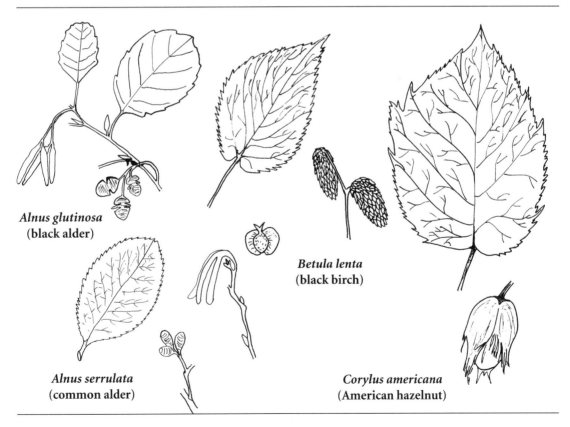

Alnus glutinosa
(black alder)

Betula lenta
(black birch)

Alnus serrulata
(common alder)

Corylus americana
(American hazelnut)

shrub, forming thickets along waterways throughout the state, including the pinelands. Leaves are finely toothed, ovate, and broadest above the middle. The male flowers form long catkins. The fruit is woody and conelike, and persists through the winter.

Native Americans used a bark infusion as a diuretic, emetic, and purgative, as well as for coughs, heart trouble, high blood pressure, and pains associated with childbirth and menstruation. A mouth soreness in babies, "thrash" (thrush?), was also treated with the bark tea. A hot infusion prepared from berries was taken for fever.

Bigelow lists black alder as *Prinos verticillatus*, a native shrub. The bark is described as a moderate tonic used in intermittent fevers, dropsy, and cutaneous diseases.

Betula lenta (black birch, cherry birch, mountain mahogany, sweet birch) is a 50- to 70-foot native and escaped tree found in rich-soiled woods of northern and southern New Jersey. The bark is smooth, black, and nonpeeling, with a strong wintergreen fragrance. The leaves are toothed, oval, and 6 inches in length. The flowers are inconspicuous.

Native Americans chewed the leaves for dysentery and used a leaf infusion for colds. The bark decoction was used for stomach and pulmonary troubles and also for "milky urine."

Corylus americana (American hazelnut) is a 3- to 8-foot native shrub found in shaded edges and well-drained, rich-soiled, wooded areas of northern and southern New Jersey. Leaves are 3 to 6 inches long, heart-shaped or rounded at the base, broadly oval or ovate, serrate, and pubescent. Young branches (branchlets) are pubescent and glandular. Hazelnut flowers in early March to April, with edible fruit ripening in September.

Native Americans used an infusion prepared from scraped bark for hives and a decoction prepared from the inner bark to induce emesis. A poultice of boiled bark was applied to cuts to promote healing. Raw nuts were used for hay fever, prenatal strength, and childbirth hemorrhage.

018 *Bignoniaceae*

The trumpet-vine family of trees, woody vines, shrubs, and herbs, mainly tropical. They have opposite leaves and irregular flowers with two or four stamens.

Catalpa bignonioides (catalpa, Indian bean) is a naturalized, large ornamental tree of up to 45 feet tall found in moist, well-drained areas statewide, including the pinelands. Leaves are large, 10 inches long and 7 inches wide, oval to heart-shaped, and opposite or in whorls of three

Bignoniaceae

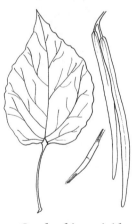

Catalpa bignonioides
(Indian bean)

from each node. They are malodorous when injured. Flowers are white, with two orange stripes and purple spots. They appear in showy clusters from June to July, with long, cigar-shaped fruit from July to August.

Native Americans apparently did not use catalpa for medicinal purposes. An infusion prepared from the seeds has been used for asthma, while the seed pod is mildly narcotic. The bark infusion has been used to reduce fever. Flowers are reported to have caused contact dermatitis.

019 *Boraginaceae*

The borage family of herbs, small trees, shrubs, and vines. Leaves are simple, entire, and alternate. The family is distributed globally, including the deserts.

Boraginaceae

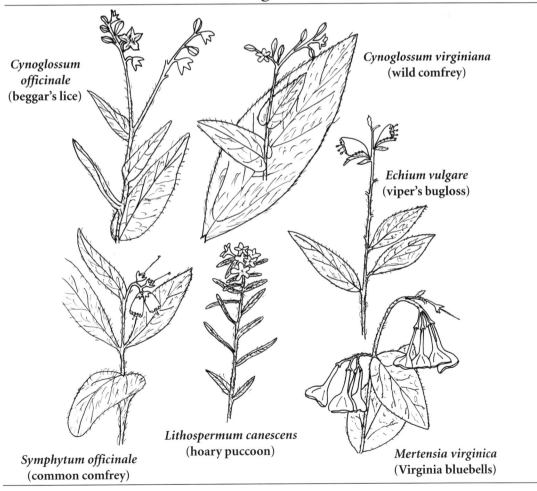

Cynoglossum officinale (beggar's lice)

Cynoglossum virginiana (wild comfrey)

Echium vulgare (viper's bugloss)

Symphytum officinale (common comfrey)

Lithospermum canescens (hoary puccoon)

Mertensia virginica (Virginia bluebells)

Cynoglossum officinale (beggar's lice, gypsy flower, hound's tongue) is a 1- to 3-foot downy, leafy-stemmed, naturalized biennial weed found in open pastures and waste places of northern and southern New Jersey. The basal leaves are in a rosette, and the stalkless stem leaves are oblong and lance-shaped. It is a hairy plant, with reddish-purple flowers enclosed by a soft-hairy calyx.

Native Americans used a whole-plant decoction as a wash and as a poultice for leg cancer. The root decoction was used as a wash and douche for venereal disease.

Cynoglossum virginiana (wild comfrey) is a 1- to 2-foot hairy, native perennial herb found in well-drained open woods of northern and southern New Jersey. The basal leaves are in a rosette, while the few upper-stem leaves have a heart-shaped, clasping base. Flowers, appearing in spring, are blue to pale lilac, in spreading racemes.

Native Americans used the root decoction internally and as a bath for "itching genitals." A syrup prepared from the root was taken for milky urine.

Echium vulgare (blue devil, blue weed, viper's bugloss) is a 1- to 3-foot rough, bristly, naturalized perennial herb found in open limestone fields and waste places of northern and southern New Jersey. Leaves are alternate and lance-shaped. Flowers, appearing in summer, are bright blue, opening one at a time in a series of spikes on curled branches.

Native Americans used a root or leaf infusion for kidney disorders.

Lithospermum canescens (hoary puccoon) is a 6- to 18-inch native perennial herb with very fine, soft white hairs, reportedly found in dry, open areas of northern New Jersey. The lance-shaped leaves and stems are fine-hairy and grayish. Yellow-orange tubular flowers with five lobes appear in April.

Native Americans used hoary puccoon leaf infusion as a wash for fever and in a compound infusion taken internally and rubbed on the body to prevent convulsions.

Mertensia virginica (Virginia bluebells, Virginia cowslip) is a 1- to 2-foot native perennial found in well-drained, moist, rich-soiled, wooded areas of northern New Jersey. Leaves are alternate, egg-shaped, and entire. Flowers are blue or pink in bell-shaped nodding clusters, appearing in April and May.

Native Americans used bluebells as a pulmonary aid in whooping cough and consumption. A root decoction was taken for venereal disease.

Symphytum officinale (common comfrey) is a 2- to 3-foot, large-rooted, escaped perennial found in open, moist fields and waste places primarily in northern New Jersey but also on the inner-coastal plain of southern New Jersey. The leaves are large—3 to 8 inches long—broadly oval to lance-shaped, and rough-hairy. The bell-shaped, tubular summer flowers may be purple, blue, pink, yellowish, or white, in furled clusters.

Native Americans used a comfrey infusion for dysentery, sprains, and bruises, as well as for heartburn and constipation during pregnancy. A root infusion was taken for gonorrhea. Raw leaves are fed to livestock for internal bleeding. Comfrey root contains hepatotoxic pyrrolizidine alkaloids, known to cause liver damage.

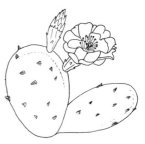

Opuntia compressa
(**prickly pear**)

020 *Cactaceae*

The cactus family of plants, characterized by large, succulent, usually leafless stems with clusters of spines. In North America, major concentrations are in Mexico and throughout the Southwest.

Opuntia compressa (*O. humifusa*) (Indian fig, prickly pear) is a 6-inch to 1-foot native perennial cactus found in dry soils throughout the state, including the pinelands. Jointed pads have tufts of sharply pointed, barbed spines. Large, showy, yellow flowers appear in May and give rise to red fruit in August.

Native Americans used a poultice of peeled stems for wounds, and the fruit juice was rubbed on warts.

021 *Campanulaceae*

The bellflower family of herbs and sometimes shrubs and trees; named for the bell-shaped (hence the name "campana") flowers and also known by the nondescriptive name Lobeliaceae (after Matthias de l'Obel [1538–1616], a Flemish botanist). The leaves are usually alternate, but sometimes opposite or whorled. The family is widely distributed, especially in temperate and subtropical regions. Members of this family contain potentially toxic alkaloids such as lobeline. Although *Lobelia cardinalis* is regarded as less toxic than *L. inflata*, both plants should be regarded as poisonous.

Lobelia cardinalis (red cardinal flower) is a 2- to 3-foot native perennial found statewide, especially along streams and in moist meadows. Leaves are alternate, lance-shaped, and toothed. The striking, showy, scarlet flower spikes appear in late June.

Native Americans applied a poultice of crushed leaves for headache. A leaf infusion was taken for colds, fever, and rheumatism, and a cold infusion was snuffed for nosebleed. A root infusion was taken for stomach trouble and worms and was considered a "strong medicine" for the

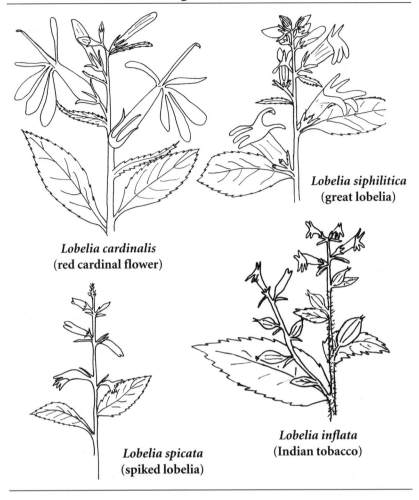

Lobelia siphilitica
(great lobelia)

Lobelia cardinalis
(red cardinal flower)

Lobelia spicata
(spiked lobelia)

Lobelia inflata
(Indian tobacco)

treatment of typhoid; it was also applied externally as a wash and poultice for sores. As a pulmonary aid, it was used for croup, and as a venereal aid, for syphilis.

Lobelia inflata (Indian tobacco) is a hairy native annual, 6 to 18 inches tall, found in waste places, open woods, and fields throughout the state, but rarely in the pinelands. The leaves are oval to lanceolate, toothed, and hairy on the underside. The flowers, appearing in summer, are white or pale blue and inconspicuous. The calyx becomes inflated. Of the New Jersey plants in this family, this is the most used and poisonous.

Native Americans used the leaves as a rub for aches and stiff neck, and in a leaf infusion, it was used as a wash or poultice for abscesses and sores. The root poultice was used for body aches, bites and stings, and venereal disease sores. The plant was chewed for sore throat and smoked "to break tobacco habit." The whole plant infusion is a strong emetic and laxative. The whole plant was also used for the treatment of asthma, croup, and alcoholism.

Bigelow described Indian tobacco as a "prompt emetic, attended with narcotic effects during its operation. If a leaf or capsule be held in the mouth for a short time, it brings on giddiness, headache, a trembling agitation of the whole body, sickness, and finally vomiting." Bigelow acknowledged the usefulness of lobelia for asthma and other pulmonary complaints, but predicted that "on account of the violence of its operation, it is probable that this plant will never come into use for the common purposes of an emetic."

Lobelia siphilitica (great lobelia) is a 1- to 5-foot native perennial found statewide in moist areas and along streambanks. Leaves are alternate, 2 to 4 inches long, and pointed. The flowers are blue (blue-lavender) and appear in late summer. As a member of this family, it should be regarded as dangerous, but less than *cardinalis*.

Native Americans snuffed a cold infusion for nosebleed and also used an infusion internally for rheumatism, colds, fever, croup, and syphilis. The root infusion was taken for stomach trouble and worms.

Lobelia spicata (spiked lobelia) is a 2- to 4-foot native perennial found statewide in fields and meadows. Leaves are oval to somewhat lance-shaped and essentially toothless. Whitish to pale blue flowers appear in June on a slender, leafless, spikelike raceme. As a member of the family, it should be regarded as toxic.

Native Americans used a cold infusion of the roots in scratches for "trembling and shaking" and as an emetic. A decoction of stalks was used as a wash for sores of the neck and jaw and was taken for "bad blood."

022 *Cannabaceae*

The hemp family of herbs, composed of two genera, *Cannabis* and *Humulus*, both occurring in the Northern Hemisphere.

Cannabis sativa (hemp, marijuana) is a 5- to 14-foot naturalized annual weed found throughout the state in areas where it has escaped from illegal cultivation. Leaves are palmate, with five to seven lobes. Leaflets are lance-shaped and toothed. Flowers are greenish and sticky, appearing in August.

Native Americans used marijuana as a psychological aid and stimulant. Today it is also used to prevent nausea and relieve pain. In China, a seed decoction is taken for constipation.

Humulus lupulus (common hops) is a twining perennial vine, without tendrils, found in waste areas and rich thickets throughout the state, including on occasion the pinelands. Leaves are mulberrylike, with three

Cannabaceae

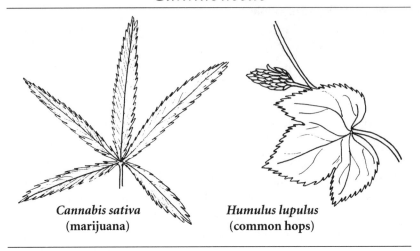

Cannabis sativa
(marijuana)

Humulus lupulus
(common hops)

to five deep lobes. Staminate and pistillate flowers are on separate plants and present from May through August. Flowers are greenish, in loose axillary clusters. The fruit is a 1- to 2^1/$_2$-inch drooping cluster of overlapping bracts.

Native Americans used tea prepared from the flowers for nervous tension and pain. Dried blossoms were applied for toothache and earache. A fruit tea was taken for intestinal pain and fever. The vine was used for kidney and bladder problems, rheumatism, coughs, and influenza; to produce sleep; and to treat breast and womb problems. A poultice of the chewed root was applied to wounds. A poultice of the heated plant in a bag was applied for earache, and a poultice of the soaked plant was applied for pneumonia and to swellings and bruises. Today, dried flowers are used to flavor beer.

Bigelow described hops as preservative, tonic, and salubrious. He also described it as a narcotic acting as an anodyne and soporific, less active than opium but useful in nervous weakness and hysteria.

023 *Caprifoliaceae*

The honeysuckle family of shrubs, woody vines, trees, and herbs. Leaves are simple or pinnate; fruit is a berry or drupe. The family is concentrated in cool or temperate regions.

Lonicera canadensis (American fly honeysuckle) is a 3- to 6-foot rare native shrub found in moist or dry, wooded areas of northern New Jersey. Leaves are egg-shaped, with fine hairs along the edges. Flowers are greenish yellow, appear in spring, and give rise to red berries.

Native Americans used a decoction prepared from stems as a diuretic and for the treatment of syphilitic sores. The bark was used for the treatment of urinary disease and to prepare an infusion for "children who cry all night."

Lonicera japonica (Japanese honeysuckle) is an evergreen, woody, trailing or twining naturalized vine found in thickets and along roadsides throughout the state as noxious weeds. The leaves are oval and toothless, but may be lobed on the lower end. White flowers form in the spring and become yellow. The fruit is a black berry.

Native Americans apparently did not use Japanese honeysuckle for medicinal purposes. The flower nectar is sweet, and the leaves and flowers are used in Asia to prepare a pleasant infusion that is antibacterial, antiviral, and very useful in the treatment of influenza. It is used as a wash for rheumatism, bacterial infection (sores), and cancerous tumors.

In Chinese medicine, decoctions of flowers or the vine are used to treat colds, laryngitis, bacterial dysentery, interitis, skin sores and boils, and rheumatism.

Sambucus canadensis (common elder, elderberry) is a 3- to 12-foot native shrub found in moist, rich soils throughout the state, including the pinelands. Leaves are opposite and compound, with elliptical, sharply toothed leaflets. Flat clusters of fragrant white flowers appear in late spring, giving rise to purplish black fruit.

Native Americans used a berry infusion for rheumatism and a fermented berry infusion for neuritis. Wine prepared from the berries was taken as a tonic. The flower infusion was used to induce sweating in a treatment for fevers, infant colic, and infant constipation. Leaves were used to prepare a wash to prevent infection. A decoction prepared from seeds and roots was taken for liver troubles, and a poultice prepared from branches was applied for severe headache. A bark infusion was used in difficult childbirth, as a wash for pain and swelling, and as a spring emetic. The inner bark of young shoots was used as a repellent for flies and insects and as a diuretic and purgative. A decoction prepared from the pith was taken for gonorrhea. A bark poultice was applied for headache and cuts. Fresh bark was placed in cavities for toothache. Root bark was used to free the lungs of phlegm. A root poultice was applied for swollen breasts. Parts of the plant were also used to prepare a salve for burns and as a treatment for dropsy.

Bigelow described elderberries as moderately laxative and expectorant and described the flower tea as a popular diaphoretic.

Elderberry wood and unripe fruit contain cyanogenic glycosides and other poisonous alkaloids.

Triosteum perfoliatum (fever root, feverwort, scarlet-fruited horse gentian, tinker's weed, wild coffee) is a 2- to 4-foot native perennial found in well-drained, open areas statewide. Leaves are opposite, entire, and

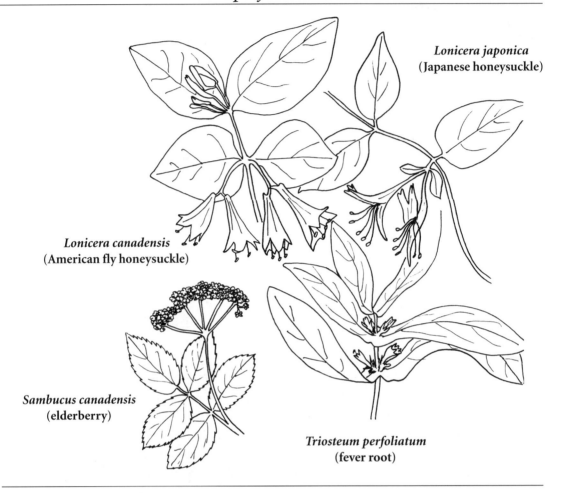

Lonicera japonica
(Japanese honeysuckle)

Lonicera canadensis
(American fly honeysuckle)

Sambucus canadensis
(elderberry)

Triosteum perfoliatum
(fever root)

pierced by the stem. Flowers are purplish brown or greenish, appearing in May and giving rise to orange-yellow berries in August.

Native Americans used feverwort as an emetic and febrifuge. The plant "ooze" was used as a wash for leg swelling, and a plant infusion was used as a foot bath. A root infusion was taken for irregular menses, as a dietary aid for babies and adults for weight gain, and for colds and sore throat. The root poultice was applied to old sores and snakebites.

Bigelow described fever root as a cathartic and emetic.

Viburnum lentago (nannyberry, sweet viburnum, wild raisin) is a 5- to 15-foot native shrub found in rich, moist soils of northern New Jersey. Leaves are 2 to 4 inches long, pointed, ovoid, serrate, and often rust-colored, with winged petioles. Clusters of white flowers are 2 to 5 inches wide, appearing in May. The fruit is oval, bluish black, and edible.

Native Americans took a leaf infusion or applied a leaf poultice in

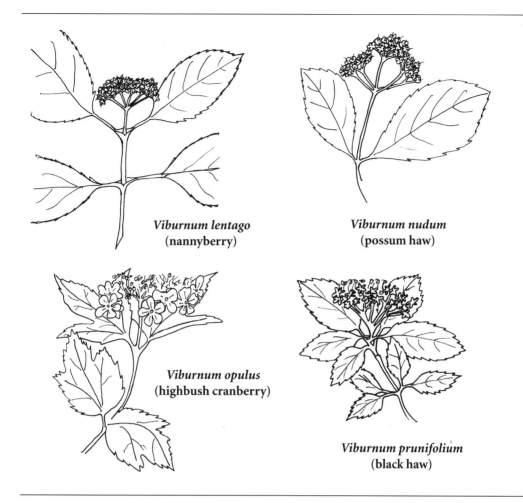

Viburnum lentago
(nannyberry)

Viburnum nudum
(possum haw)

Viburnum opulus
(highbush cranberry)

Viburnum prunifolium
(black haw)

dysuria as a diuretic. An inner-bark infusion was used as a diuretic. A root decoction was taken for consumption and to treat irregular menses.

Viburnum nudum (larger withe rod, naked withe rod, possum haw) is a 12-foot native deciduous shrub found in bogs and wooded swamps throughout the state, including the pinelands. The glossy, leathery leaves are oval and slightly toothed, with a wavy border. Broad, branching, flat clusters of small, white flowers appear in spring, giving rise to small, bluish black fruit.

Native Americans used the bark decoction as a diuretic and antispasmodic.

Viburnum opulus (*V. trilobum*) (highbush cranberry) is a large, erect native shrub up to 12 feet tall found in cool, moist woods and on rocky slopes of northern New Jersey. The leaves, hairy on the underside, are coarsely toothed and have three to five deep lobes, similar to those of maples. Four-inch rounded clusters of white flowers appear in April, giving rise to acidic, red berries.

Native Americans used a bark decoction as an emetic for "bad blood" and fever. The bark decoction was also taken as a laxative, for stomach cramps, and to treat swollen glands and mumps. A berry infusion was used as well for swollen glands and mumps, and a branch decoction was used for uterine prolapse. A root decoction was taken for general body ache and was given to babies for fever.

Viburnum prunifolium (black haw, stagbush) is a 6- to 15-foot native shrub or small tree with stout, spreading branches, found in well-drained soils of thin woods, roadsides, and watersides of northern and southern New Jersey. Most of the leaves are 1 to 2 inches long, ovate, and finely toothed. Flat clusters of white flowers appear in March, giving rise to sweet, edible, blue-black berries.

Native Americans used a bark infusion for a sore tongue and to prevent recurring spasms. The bark infusion was also taken as a tonic and diaphoretic.

024 *Caryophyllaceae*

The pink family of small herbs, widely distributed in temperate areas of the Northern Hemisphere. The family includes carnations, dianthus, and babies'-breath and is distinguished by flowers with five long-clawed petals enclosed in a tubular calyx.

Agrostemma githago (corn cockle; purple cockle) is an upright naturalized annual to 3 feet tall, native to Europe and naturalized in New Jersey. It occurs statewide as a grainfield weed and along roadsides. Four-inch, narrow leaves are opposite, with stems and leaves hairy. Solitary flowers, 1 inch in diameter, appear in early June, producing seed in September. The fruit is a capsule, with many black poisonous seeds. The sapogenin githagenin occurs throughout the plant but especially in the seed. Severe gastrointestinal upset results from ingestion, which may occur when eating ground corn, oats, or wheat contaminated with corn cockle seed. Interestingly, when corn cockle grows as a weed in wheat fields, it stimulates the growth of wheat and increases the yield of the grain.

Native Americans apparently did not use corn cockle for medicinal purposes. In Europe, the seeds have been used to treat cancers, warts, dropsy, and jaundice. The seeds have also been used to produce a diuretic and vermifuge.

Saponaria officinalis (bouncing Bet, soapwort) is a 1- to 2-foot, smooth-stemmed, thick-jointed, naturalized perennial herb found in

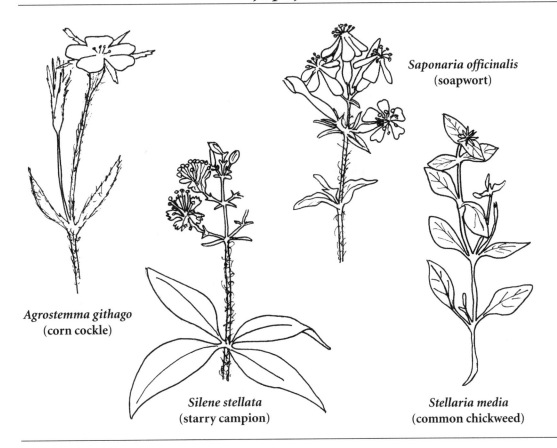

Saponaria officinalis
(soapwort)

Agrostemma githago
(corn cockle)

Silene stellata
(starry campion)

Stellaria media
(common chickweed)

waste places and along roadsides throughout the state, perhaps including on occasion the pinelands. Leaves are opposite, oval, and entire, with three to five prominent ribs. The flowers are 1 inch, pink or white, often double, and clustered; they appear in summer.

Native Americans applied a leaf poultice for boils and for pain in the spleen. The root juice was used as a hair tonic.

Silene stellata (federal twist, starry campion, widow's frill) is a 2- to 3-foot native perennial herb found in dry, open areas statewide. The leaves are opposite in whorls of four, slender, and entire. The flowers are white and nodding in branching racemes, appearing in July.

Native Americans applied a root poultice to dry up running sores.

Stellaria media (common chickweed) is a prostrate naturalized annual weed found in open areas and gardens statewide. The leaves are opposite, oval, and entire. The lower leaves are long-stalked. Flowers with inconspicuous petals form throughout the growing season.

Native Americans used a leaf decoction as an eyewash. Plants are edible and used as salad greens.

The bittersweet or staff-tree family of evergreen trees, shrubs, and woody vines; it is widely distributed. Leaves are simple, and either alternate or opposite. They have small, regular flowers and usually brightly colored fruit with arillate seeds.

Celastrus orbiculatus (Asiatic bittersweet, round-leaved bittersweet) is a high-climbing, 20- to 30-foot naturalized shrub, sometimes described as a vine, found in moist, rich-soiled thickets of northern and southern New Jersey. Leaves are alternate, ovate, fine-toothed, and pointed. Flowers are small and greenish, in small axillary, branched clusters, appearing in late spring, and producing bright orange fruit. This Asian species is naturalized and a more vigorous grower than *C. scandens*. The fruit is hidden by foliage, remaining inconspicuous until the leaves have fallen.

Medicinal uses in Asia are similar to those described for *C. scandens*.

Celastrus scandens (climbing bittersweet) is native and similar to the Asian species in all respects except that the leaves are slightly larger and

Celastraceae

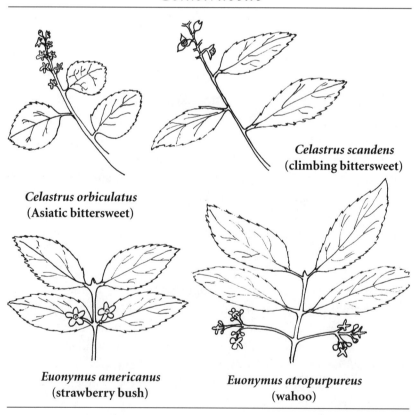

Celastrus scandens
(climbing bittersweet)

Celastrus orbiculatus
(Asiatic bittersweet)

Euonymus americanus
(strawberry bush)

Euonymus atropurpureus
(wahoo)

flowers are formed in terminal, many-flowered panicles or racemes, above the foliage. These plants are commonly brought into the home for dry flower arrangements. The colorful fruit is poisonous and particularly attractive to young children. Climbing bittersweet should not be confused with bittersweet, the common name for *Solanum dulcamara*, which is also a poisonous plant described with the Solanaceae.

Native Americans used the astringent leaf decoction for diarrhea and as a wash for sores. A stem-and-leaf decoction was used to regulate menses, and a root decoction taken for suppressed menses. A root decoction was also used as a diuretic and as a laxative for babies. The boiled root was applied for cancer and to old sores. The root was also chewed for cough.

Euonymus americanus (bursting heart, strawberry bush) is a 3- to 6-foot native shrub found in rich-soiled woods of northern and southern New Jersey. Leaves are nearly evergreen, shiny, finely toothed, sharply pointed, opposite, growing in pairs, and essentially stalkless. Flowers are greenish to purple and single or in small clusters with stalked petals. They appear in late spring and produce a rough, warty pod that splits to expose three to four scarlet seeds becoming purplish black.

Native Americans used a plant decoction for suppressed or excessive menstrual flow. A bark infusion was used as a tonic, an antiseptic, and for urinary troubles. The infusion was sniffed for sinus and taken for stomachache. A root infusion was taken for uterine prolapse.

Euonymus atropurpureus (burning bush, wahoo) is a large, 6- to 25-foot native shrub or tree found in rich-soiled woods of northern and southern New Jersey. Leaves are opposite, oblong to oval, pointed, finely toothed, and hairy on the undersurface. Flowers are small and purple, in axillary clusters, appearing in late spring. The fruit is a smooth, four-lobed capsule with scarlet seeds.

Native Americans used a plant or leaf infusion as a laxative. Bark infusion was used for an eyewash, and an inner-bark decoction was taken for uterine problems. A poultice prepared from pounded fresh bark was applied to old sores.

026 *Chenopodiaceae*

The goosefoot family of herbs, shrubs, and, rarely, small trees. Leaves are simple, somewhat succulent, and alternate or, rarely opposite. Most are weeds, including lamb's-quarters (pigweed). Cultivated plants in the family are the beet (*Beta*) and spinach (*Spinacia*).

Chenopodium album (lamb's-quarters, pigweed) is 6-inch to 6-foot native annual weed found in all environments throughout the state,

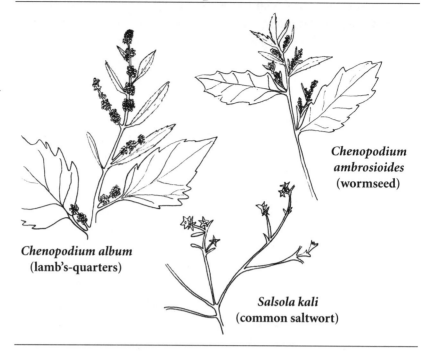

Chenopodium
ambrosioides
(wormseed)

Chenopodium album
(lamb's-quarters)

Salsola kali
(common saltwort)

including the pinelands. The leaves are alternate, egg- or arrow-shaped, and irregularly toothed. Flowers are small and greenish, and in many small clusters.

Native Americans ate the cooked greens as a preventive medicine for scurvy. A cold infusion prepared from the whole plant was taken for diarrhea, and a root infusion was used for urethral itching. A plant poultice was applied to burns.

Chenopodium ambrosioides (Mexican tea, wormseed) is a 2- to 5-foot somewhat woody, aromatic, naturalized annual herb found in all environments statewide, including the pinelands. Flowers are on leafy spikes.

Native Americans used a seed decoction or "stew" for intestinal worms. A poultice of crushed leaves was applied for headache, and the root was used to treat delayed menses (abortifacient).

In Chinese medicine, the whole plant is crushed and mixed with boiling water for tea, and stems and leaves are boiled in water for external uses. The tea is described as bitter, fragrant, anthelmintic (recommended for ancyclostomiasis), stomachic, carminative, and analgesic. The decoction is used as a soak or bath and to treat insect bites.

Bigelow described wormseed as a good vermifuge for lumbrici of children. One "table spoonful" of the expressed juice of the whole plant is the recommended dose for a child 2 or 3 years of age.

Oil of wormwood is 60 to 80 percent ascaridole, an organic peroxide that produces a toxic effect on the central nervous system.

Salsola kali (barilla plant, common saltwort, Russian thistle) is a native and naturalized bushy annual weed found along the coastal areas and railroad right-of-ways of northern and southern New Jersey. The leaves are alternate, entire, prickly, and thornlike. Flowers are loosely branched and green.

Native Americans used an infusion prepared from ashes internally and externally for smallpox and influenza. A poultice of chewed plants was applied to ant, bee, and wasp stings.

027 *Cistaceae*

The rockrose family of herbs and shrubs. The leaves are simple, entire, and alternate or opposite. The family is primarily tropical and subtropical.

Helianthemum canadense (Canada frostweed, long-branched frostweed) is a 6-inch to 2-foot native perennial found in dry, sandy soils throughout the state, including the pinelands. Leaves are alternate, lance-shaped and entire, $1/2$ to $1^1/2$ inches long. Spring flowers are large ($3/4$ to $1^1/2$ inches), solitary, yellow, and five-petaled, lasting one day. Later flowers are apetalous.

A leaf infusion was taken by native Americans for kidney problems and sore throat. A root poultice was applied for sore throat. The plant was generally regarded as a "strengthening" medicine.

028 *Commelinaceae*

The spiderwort family of monocotyledonous herbs in the order Liliales.

Commelina communis (Asiatic dayflower) is a weak-stemmed, 6-inch to 2-foot naturalized perennial that roots at the joints to produce a sprawling plant found in moist, shady areas, especially around buildings, in northern and southern New Jersey. Leaves are alternate and entire. Flowers are $1/4$ to $1/2$ inch, with two relatively large, blue petals above and one small, white petal below. Flowering begins in summer.

In China, a leaf tea is used as a gargle for sore throat and tonsillitis. It is also taken for dysentery and urinary tract infection.

Tradescantia virginiana (Virginia spiderwort) is a 1- to 3-foot native, irislike perennial found in moist soils of northern and southern New Jersey. Leaves are alternate and entire. Flowers are blue to purple, $3/4$ to $1^1/2$ inches, in a terminal cluster, appearing in April. Sepals and flower stalks are hairy.

Cistaceae

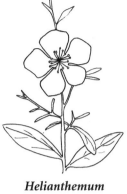

Helianthemum canadense (Canada frostweed)

Commelinaceae

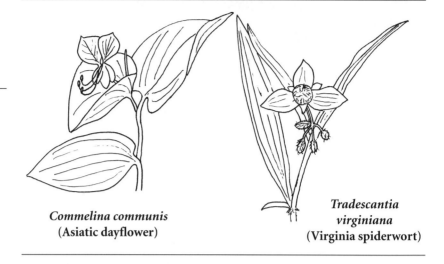

Commelina communis
(Asiatic dayflower)

*Tradescantia
virginiana*
(Virginia spiderwort)

Native Americans used an infusion as a laxative and crushed the plant for application to insect bites. A root poultice was applied for cancer.

029 *Compositae*

The daisy family, a difficult family to describe, even though most of its members are readily recognizable. The name Compositae describes the flower head, which is "composed of flowers." The more recognizable composites are the sunflowers and daisies.

Achillea millefolium (thousand leaf, yarrow) is a 1- to 3-foot delicate, fragrant native perennial found in fields and roadsides throughout the state, including the pinelands. Leaves are lanceolate, alternate, and finely dissected (lacy). Flowers are usually white in flat clusters and appear from late spring through fall. Each flower has four to six toothed rays.

The leaf infusion or decoction is astringent and taken by native Americans for bloody diarrhea and bloody urine, for fever as a sedative, for colds, as an aid during and after childbirth, for liver and kidney complaints, as a wash for sore eyes, as an aromatic bath for sick infants, for worms in children, for poison ivy rash, for earache, and as a hair wash. It is sprinkled on hot stones to produce herbal steam for headache and rheumatism. Crushed leaves were stuffed into the nose to stop bleeding and into tooth cavities or chewed for toothache. The leaf-and-flower tea is taken for chest pains, colds, coughs, and nausea; to produce sweating; as a rub for respiratory disease, an anticonvulsant wash for babies, a wash for affected parts in gonorrhea, an inhalant for headache,

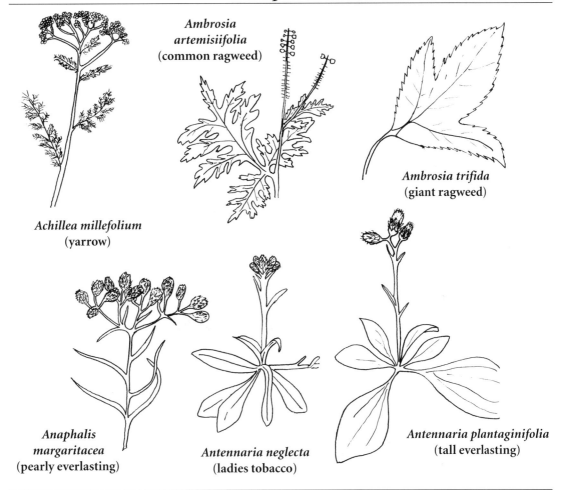

Ambrosia
artemisiifolia
(common ragweed)

Ambrosia trifida
(giant ragweed)

Achillea millefolium
(yarrow)

Anaphalis
margaritacea
(pearly everlasting)

Antennaria neglecta
(ladies tobacco)

Antennaria plantaginifolia
(tall everlasting)

and a wash for insect and snakebites. The root decoction was used as an eyewash, for stomach trouble and tuberculosis, and boiled until dark in color and taken warm for colds. A stem-and-leaf decoction was used to induce abortion. Leaf poultices were applied to burns, swellings, and bruises and rheumatism.

Ambrosia artemisiifolia (bitterweed, common ragweed, Roman wormwood) is a 1- to 6-foot noxious, native annual weed, found in open areas and along roadsides throughout the state, including the pinelands. As the scientific name suggests, the leaves are artemisialike, that is, highly dissected; they may be alternate or opposite. Flowers are green and inconspicuous in erect spikes that are conspicuous. Ragweed flowers in mid-July through October, and although the seeds are valuable wildlife food, the pollen is a notorious allergen. This genus is probable responsible for 90 percent of the pollen-induced allergies in the United States.

Native Americans used crushed leaves for insect stings, hives, and toe infections. The leaf infusion was taken for pneumonia and fever. A root decoction was taken for "menstrual troubles" and stroke.

Ambrosia trifida (buffalo weed, giant ragweed, horse-cane) is native and found in moist areas statewide. It is similar in appearance to common ragweed, but its leaves are much less dissected and the plant is much taller, ranging from 6 to 15 feet. The leaves are opposite and may or may not be lobed. It is an annual, and a prolific pollen producer and potent allergen.

Native Americans used giant ragweed for the same health complaints listed for *A. artemisiifolia*.

Anaphalis margaritacea (pearly everlasting) is a 1- to 3-foot native perennial found in dry soils and open areas throughout the state, including the pinelands. Leaves are alternate, linear, and entire. The stems and leaf undersides are white and woolly. Flower heads are composed of several, pearly white, petallike bracts, with male flowers showing a tuft of yellow in the center. Flowers appear in mid-July.

Native Americans inhaled a steaming infusion for headache and sun blindness. The warm infusion was taken and leaves were smoked or chewed for colds. The flower infusion was used as an herbal steam for rheumatism and paralysis. A poultice of flowers was applied to sores and swellings. Roots and stalks were used for diarrhea and dysentery, and dried leaves were used as a substitute for chewing tobacco.

Antennaria neglecta (field pussy toes, ladies tobacco, mouse-ears everlasting, pussy toes) is a 3- to 18-inch native perennial found in dry, open fields and woods throughout New Jersey, including the pinelands. Leaves are alternate and entire, with the upper surfaces dull green and woolly. The largest leaves are 1 to 2 inches long and $1/4$ to $1/2$ inch wide. Basal stems are slender and prostrate. Flowers are white, in several heads appearing in April.

Native Americans used a leaf decoction for body pains.

Antennaria plantaginifolia (mouse-ears everlasting, tall everlasting, white plantain) is native and often not separated from *A. neglecta*. If it is a separate species, the difference may be that the largest leaves are broader, $1^1/2$ to 3 inches long, and $3/4$ to $1^1/2$ inches wide.

Native Americans used a whole-plant infusion to treat "bowel problems" in children and a decoction as a mouthwash for toothache. A leaf infusion was used for excessive menses and to prevent sickness after childbirth. A root infusion was taken for leucorrhea.

Anthemis cotula (dog fennel, mayweed, stinking chamomile) is an 8-inch to 2-foot naturalized annual weed found in waste places and along roadsides of northern and southern New Jersey. Leaves are finely divided

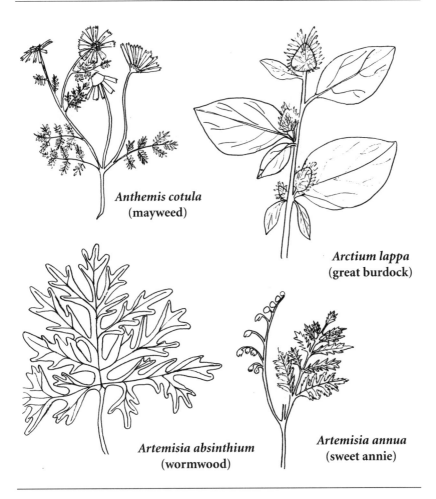

Anthemis cotula
(mayweed)

Arctium lappa
(great burdock)

Artemisia absinthium
(wormwood)

Artemisia annua
(sweet annie)

and malodorous. Flowers, appearing from late May and throughout the summer, are 3/4 to 1 inch, white, and daisylike.

Native Americans used dog fennel as an emetic and a tonic, as a sudorific and pain reliever for colds, and for hysterics, epilepsy, dropsy, asthma, rheumatism, and fevers. A decoction or cold infusion prepared from the whole plant, bark, or root was used as an antiemetic. A cold stalk infusion was taken for ptomaine poisoning, and a cold infusion of roots and stems was taken as a sedative. The root was chewed for toothache. The plant was also regarded as poisonous.

Bigelow described mayweed as tonic, stimulating, and diaphoretic, but in large doses, sudorific and emetic.

Mayweed plants are acrid, causing irritation of the mucous membranes, and may cause the skin to blister.

Arctium lappa (beggars' buttons, great burdock) is 2- to 9-foot naturalized biennial found in waste places of northern and southern New Jersey. Leaves are large, entire or slightly toothed, and largest at the bottom of a solid, deeply grooved stem. Flowers are 1 to $1^{1}/_{2}$ inches wide, pink or purple, and thistlelike, appearing in July on long stalks.

Native Americans used great burdock for rheumatism, gravel, and scurvy. A root or seed infusion was used to treat venereal disease by "cleansing the blood." A boiled-leaf poultice was applied to scrofulous sores on the neck. Buds and roots were used to treat sores and chancres.

In Chinese medicine, seeds, roots, and leaves are used. The seeds are boiled to prepare a decoction. The roots and leaves are crushed for external application. The seed decoction is taken for influenza, tonsillitis, and pertussis. Externally, the roots and leaves are applied for boils and abscesses.

Arctium minus (common burdock) is a 2- to 5-foot naturalized smaller copy of the great burdock and is found in northern New Jersey. The flowers are $^{1}/_{2}$ to 1 inch, the stem is hollow and not grooved, as it is in the great burdock. Flowers appear in late July.

Native Americans used a leaf infusion after coughing spells and a root decoction for whooping cough, pleurisy, and rheumatism. A poultice of leaves was applied for rheumatic pains. Roots were used to treat boils and abscesses, and whole plants were boiled to make "ooze" for the treatment of swollen legs and ulcers.

Artemisia absinthium (wormwood) is a 1- to 4-foot naturalized perennial found in fields and waste places of northern and southern New Jersey. The leaves are strongly aromatic, soft-hairy, white or silver-green, and divided. Small, drooping flowers appear in July.

Native Americans used a warm, boiled plant poultice for muscle pain. A leaf infusion was used for intestinal worms.

Artemisia annua (annual wormwood, fragrant wormwood, sweet annie) is a 1- to 10-foot bushy, naturalized annual found in waste areas and along roadsides of northern and southern New Jersey. Leaves are divided, fernlike, and sharp-toothed. Clusters of small, green-yellow flowers appear in mid-August.

In India and China, sweet annie was considered a good stomachic and diuretic and was used for jaundice and skin diseases. Today, it is used for treatment of colds, influenza, fevers, diarrhea, and dysentery. It is also the source of a very efficacious antimalarial drug.

Artemisia campestris (*A. caudata*) (mugwort, tall wormwood, wild wormwood) is a 2- to 6-foot native biennial found on dry, sandy beaches and in open areas of northern and southern New Jersey. Leaves are divided, and leaf divisions are narrow, but not white-woolly. Flower stalks

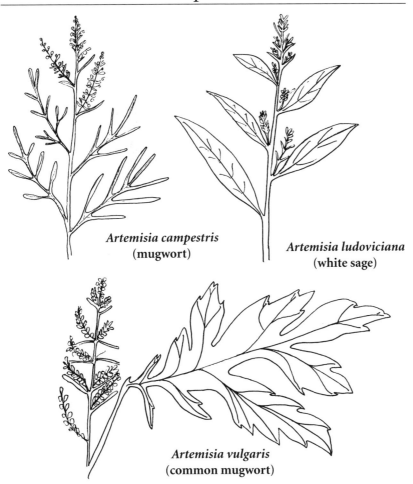

Artemisia campestris
(mugwort)

Artemisia ludoviciana
(white sage)

Artemisia vulgaris
(common mugwort)

are leafy, with the greenish flowers in long clusters appearing in late July.

Native Americans used a plant decoction for coughs, colds, tuberculosis, and "everything." A poultice of steamed branches was applied to bruises and sores.

Artemisia ludoviciana (western mugwort, white sage) is a 1- to 3-foot native perennial found in dry, open waste areas and weedy meadows of northern and southern New Jersey. Leaves are lance-shaped and entire, with soft, white undersurfaces. Flowers are in leaf axils and appear in July.

Native Americans used crushed leaves as a snuff for sinus troubles, nosebleeds, and headaches. For rheumatism and other aches, crushed or steamed plants were used. Branches were used as a bed in the sweatbath for infections and influenza. A leaf infusion was used to regulate menses, and a plant decoction was used to control diarrhea, as a laxative, and a treatment for venereal disease and severe infection. Leaves were smudged to repel mosquitos.

Artemisia vulgaris (common mugwort) is a 2- to 4-foot naturalized perennial found along roadsides and streams and in waste areas of northern and southern New Jersey. Leaves are white-woolly beneath, deeply lobed, and pointed. Flowers appear in early July in erect heads.

Native Americans used a plant infusion for afterbirth pains and to stop excessive menses. A plant decoction was used as a wash for gonorrheal sores. The plant was used to prepare a worm medicine and was placed in the steam bath for pleurisy. A plant poultice was applied to the chest for colds and to the navel of the newborn. Leaves were placed in the nostrils for cold and headache, and pulverized leaves were used to hasten healing of sores.

In Chinese medicine, a leaf decoction is used to control excessive fetal activity, bleeding, and postpartum abdominal cramps. Mugwort is also the plant most often used as fuel in moxibustion.

Aster novae-angliae (New England aster) is a 2- to 8-foot stout, hairy-stemmed native perennial found in moist meadows and swamps of northern New Jersey. The leaves are entire, lance-shaped, and clasping. Flower are 1 to 2 inches, with 40 to 50 violet-purple ray flowers. This is the most showy of asters, with flowers appearing in late August.

Native Americans used a plant infusion for fever and a root decoction for diarrhea. Roots were poulticed for pain, and the ooze of roots was sniffed for catarrh. The plant was smudged to revive an unconscious person.

Bidens bipinnata (soapbush needles, Spanish needles) is a 1- to 3-foot square-stemmed native annual found in moist, sandy or rocky soils throughout the state, including the pinelands. Leaves are opposite and divided, with toothed leaflets. Flowers are yellow, without rays, appearing in late July and producing needlelike, barbed seeds.

Native Americans chewed the leaves for sore throat and used an infusion for intestinal worms.

Cacalia atriplicifolia (pale Indian-plantain, tassel flower) is a 3- to 9-foot native perennial found in dry, open areas of northern and inner-coastal southern New Jersey. Leaves are alternate, broad, lobed, palmately veined, and pale beneath. The stem is round, smooth, and whitish. Tubular, rayless flowers are in flat clusters of five, appearing in late June.

Native Americans used a poultice for cuts, bruises, cancer, and to "draw out blood or poisonous matter."

Chrysanthemum leucanthemum (marguerite, ox-eye daisy, whiteweed) is a 1- to 3-foot naturalized perennial weed found in fields, pastures, and waste areas throughout the state, with the possible exception of the pinelands. Leaves are alternate, elongate, and toothed. Flowers are white,

Compositae

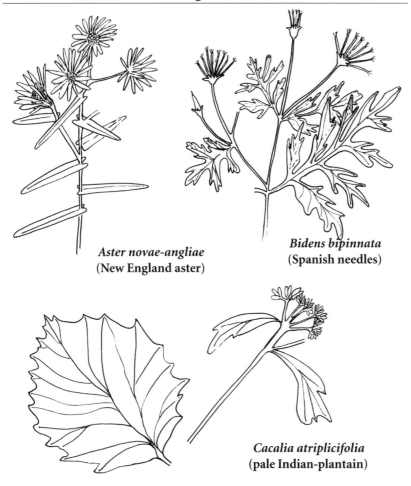

Aster novae-angliae
(New England aster)

Bidens bipinnata
(Spanish needles)

Cacalia atriplicifolia
(pale Indian-plantain)

daisylike, and borne on long stalks. Flowers are present from mid-May through fall.

Native Americans used the flowers to prepare tonic decoctions or infusions and wine. The whole plant was used to treat fevers. Stems and dried flowers were used to prepare a wash for chapped hands.

Chrysanthemum parthenium (feverfew, fever-few) is a 1- to 3-foot bushy, naturalized perennial weed found along roadsides and in waste areas throughout the state, with the possible exception of the pinelands. Leaves are alternate and pinnately divided into toothed, egg-shaped segments. Flowers are white in clusters appearing in May.

The plant was used by native Americans for rheumatism and to prepare a bath for swollen feet.

Cichorium intybus (blue sailors, chicory) is a 1- to 4-foot naturalized perennial weed found along roads and in fields and waste areas state-

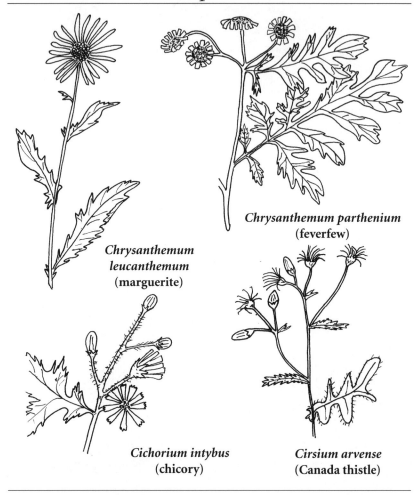

Chrysanthemum parthenium
(feverfew)

**Chrysanthemum
leucanthemum**
(marguerite)

Cichorium intybus
(chicory)

Cirsium arvense
(Canada thistle)

wide, including the pinelands. Basal leaves are lobed and toothed (dandelionlike). Flowers are blue, with petals square-ended and toothed, appearing in late June.

Native Americans used the root infusion as a tonic for nerves and in decoction as a wash and poultice for chancres and fever sores. The roasted root is used as a substitute for or amendment to coffee.

Cirsium arvense (Canada thistle) is a 1- to 5-foot naturalized perennial thistle, a noxious weed of cultivated fields and waste areas throughout the state, including the pinelands. Leaves are alternate, lobed, and spiny. Flowers are thistlelike and pink, and appear in mid-June. This plant is a serious agricultural problem because of a vigorous taproot and a creeping underground stem that produces colonies of plants.

Native Americans used the plant as a "bowel tonic" and to treat consumption. A leaf infusion was used as a mouthwash for infants.

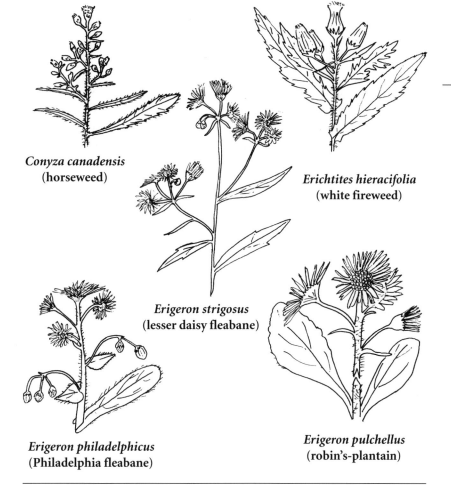

Conyza canadensis
(horseweed)

Erichtites hieracifolia
(white fireweed)

Erigeron strigosus
(lesser daisy fleabane)

Erigeron philadelphicus
(Philadelphia fleabane)

Erigeron pulchellus
(robin's-plantain)

Conyza canadensis (*Erigeron canadensis*) (butterweed, Canada fleabane, hogweed, horseweed) is a 3-inch to 7-foot native annual weed
found statewide, including the pinelands. Leaves are alternate, lance-
shaped, and toothed. Stems are hairy, and greenish white flowers appear in late July.

Native Americans used the plant as a medicine for horses, a steaming agent in sweat baths, a lotion for pimples, and a treatment for diarrhea. A plant poultice was applied for headache and earache, and a root
decoction was taken for stomachache.

Bigelow described Canada fleabane as most useful in acute and
chronic diarrhea and as a diuretic for dropsy.

Erechtites hieracifolia (pilewort, white fireweed) is a 1- to 9-foot native annual found throughout the state, including the pinelands, in moist
areas and along watersides, and in open areas after fires. The leaves are

alternate, 2 to 8 inches long, and toothed. This is a coarse, weedy plant that may be hairy, with a grooved stem. The tubular flowers, appearing in late July, are white and rayless.

Native Americans used the plant and root as astringent tonics that were also emetic and cathartic.

Erigeron philadelphicus (Philadelphia fleabane, skervish) is a 1- to 3-foot native perennial found in well-drained, moist, rich soils of northwestern New Jersey. The leaves are alternate, toothed, and clasping a hairy stem. Flowers are pinkish white, appearing in early May.

Native Americans used skervish as a diuretic and sudorific, as well as for "suppressed menstruation," "dimness of sight," hemorrhages, "spitting of blood," epilepsy, kidney problems, and gout. The root was chewed and a cold root infusion taken for colds. A whole-plant decoction was taken "to open the lungs." The flower infusion was used for fever, and powdered flowers were snuffed for headache and "loosening a head cold." A plant poultice was applied to running sores, and smoke from dried flowers was inhaled for head cold.

Bigelow described Philadelphia fleabane as diuretic, and citing the confusion with a plant known as scabish or skevish (skervish?) wrote, "So great is the uncertainty which belongs to vulgar nomenclature."

Erigeron pulchellus (frost root, robin's-plantain, skervish) is a 6-inch to 2-foot soft-hairy, native perennial found in well drained, rich-soiled, open areas of northern and inner-coastal New Jersey. New rosettes are formed from underground stems. Stem leaves are alternate and fewer than lower leaves, which are larger and toothed. Flowers are clear blue, appearing in early May.

Native Americans used frost root essentially as they did *E. philadelphicus.*

Erigeron strigosus (lesser daisy fleabane, white-top) is a 1- to 3-foot hairy native perennial found in dry, open areas statewide. Leaves are alternate, lance-shaped, and entire or with two teeth. Flowers are white, tinged with pink, and appear in late May.

Native Americans used the plant for headache and a root infusion for heart troubles.

Eupatorium maculatum (joe–pye weed, spotted joe-pye weed) is a 2- to 6-foot native perennial found in wet, open areas statewide, with the exception of the pinelands. Leaves are opposite, lance-shaped, and in whorls of four to five. The stem is deep purple or purple-spotted. Purple flowers in flat-topped heads appear in early August.

Native Americans used the root infusion or decoction as a diuretic and for gout, dropsy, kidney trouble, and rheumatism as well as for chills, fevers, colds, "female problems" after birth, and gonorrhea. The decoction was also used as a wash for inflamed joints and in a quieting bath for children.

Compositae

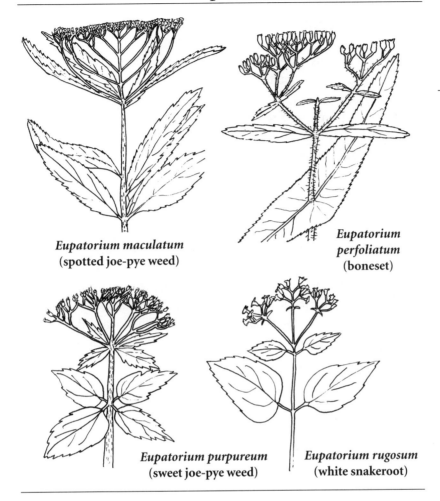

Eupatorium maculatum
(spotted joe-pye weed)

**Eupatorium
perfoliatum
(boneset)**

Eupatorium purpureum
(sweet joe-pye weed)

Eupatorium rugosum
(white snakeroot)

Eupatorium perfoliatum (boneset, thoroughwort) is a 1- to 6-foot native perennial found in wet areas and thickets, with the exception of the pinelands. Leaves are long, tapering, opposite, and continuous across the stem, giving the appearance of perforation. Flowers are white in flat clusters, appearing in late July.

Native Americans regarded boneset as a panacea. It was used as a tonic, sudorific, stimulant, emetic, purgative, antiseptic, and diuretic. Infusions or decoctions were taken for colds, sore throat, influenza, fevers, "ague," "biliary system," kidney trouble, and gonorrhea and were used externally for piles. The root was used to correct irregular menses and urinary problems, as well as for pneumonia and pleurisy. The crushed-root decoction was used to "cure the liquor habit," and a decoction prepared from the crushed whole plant was taken for typhoid, fevers, and headache. A poultice of the boiled plant tops was applied for rheumatism and headaches, and a root decoction poultice was applied to syphilitic chancres.

Bigelow described thoroughwort as a tonic stimulant, useful as a digestive aid but in large doses causing emesis and catharsis, and proved sudorific. It was also useful in intermittent fevers and, when used externally, against some cutaneous diseases.

Eupatorium purpureum (gravel root, green-stemmed joe-pye weed, joe-pye weed, purple boneset, queen of the meadow, sweet joe-pye weed) is a 6- to 12-foot native perennial found in wet roadside ditches, rich open ground, and shaded edges of woods in northern and southern New Jersey. Leaves are in whorls of four or five. The stem is solid and green, but purple at the leaf nodes. Flowers are pink-purple in a slightly rounded cluster, appearing in late July. Dried leaves have a vanillalike sweet aroma.

Native Americans used the root as a diuretic and also for gout, dropsy, rheumatism, and "female problems" after birth as well as an antidote for poison. The root was used as a tonic during pregnancy and as a laxative. Vapors from a plant top decoction were inhaled for colds, and a poultice of fresh leaves was applied for burns. The plant infusion was taken for diseases of the urinary tract and for arrow wounds. A strong solution of roots was used as a wash for babies, and sections of stem were used to blow or spray medicine.

Bigelow described gravel root as bitter, astringent, and aromatic, operating as a diuretic and useful in dysuria and calculous diseases.

Eupatorium rugosum (*E. urticaefolium*) (white snakeroot) is a 1- to 5-foot native perennial found in thickets and well-drained, rich soils of northern and southern New Jersey. Leaves are opposite, somewhat heart-shaped, and toothed. Flowers are white in branched clusters, appearing in early August.

Native Americans used white snakeroot as a diuretic; for diarrhea, gravel, urinary disease, "ague," and fever; a panacea; and as a steaming agent in the sweat bath. The root smudge was used to revive unconscious people, and a root decoction was taken for inflamed or prolapsed uterus and venereal disease. The whole-plant decoction was taken as a laxative.

White snakeroot is said to have caused the death of Abraham Lincoln's mother. In epidemics of the nineteenth century, it was reportedly responsible for the death of 25 percent of the population of certain areas. The disease is known as milk sickness, caused by the ingestion of milk from cows that have eaten enough of the plants to contaminate the milk but not enough to cause death or severe symptoms in the cow.

Gnaphalium obtusifolium (*G. polycephalum*) (cat foot, rabbit tobacco, sweet everlasting, white everlasting) is a 1- to 2-foot native biennial found in dry, open areas throughout the state, including the pinelands.

Leaves are alternate, lance-shaped, and stalkless; gray-green above, whitish underneath, and aromatic when bruised. The stem is soft-woolly, accounting for the generic name (na-FA-li-um). Dirty white flower heads are in branching clusters, appearing in mid-August.

Native Americans used a plant decoction as a face wash for nerves and insomnia. The tea was also taken for coughs and consumption. The plant was chewed for sore mouth or throat and used to prepare a cough syrup. It was also used in the sweat bath. A blossom and leaf decoction was taken for colds and lung pain. The leaf decoction was taken as an antiemetic and as a gargle for mumps or to prepare a poultice for mumps. The dried stems or leaves were smoked for asthma and steamed for headache.

Helenium autumnale (American sneezeweed, false sunflower, swamp sunflower) is a 2- to 6-foot native perennial found in rich thickets and wet areas throughout the state, including the pinelands. Leaves are alternate, lance-shaped, and toothed. Flowers, appearing in mid-August, are yellow with a globular disk. The petals are wedge-shaped, broadest at the tip, three-toothed, and drooping.

Native Americans powdered dried leaves or flowers as a snuff to induce sneezing to clear the head in colds. The stem infusion was used as a wash for fevers and to stop bleeding after childbirth. The plant was known to be poisonous to cattle.

Helianthus annuus (sunflower) is a 3- to 10-foot native annual found in rich-soiled, dry, open areas throughout the state. Leaves are alternate, long-stalked, broadly heart-shaped, and toothed. The yellow flower head is large, 3 to 6 inches wide, with the disk brown, flat, and 1 to 2 inches wide; flowers appear in late July.

A flower infusion is taken for chest pains, and a flower decoction for pulmonary troubles. The seeds were eaten to improve appetite. The leaf decoction was taken for high fevers and was used as a wash for screwworm sores on horses. A root decoction was used as a warm wash for rheumatism. A poultice of warm ashes was applied to the stomach for worms, and a moxa of pith was used on scratched warts for removal.

Helianthus tuberosus (girasole, Jerusalem artichoke) is a 5- to 10-foot native and escaped perennial found in well-drained, moist, rich-soiled areas of northern and southern New Jersey. Leaves are opposite, oval, pointed, and toothed, with a rough upper surface. The stem is hairy. Flowers, appearing in early August, are 2 to 3^1/$_2$ inches wide, and yellow, with long-pointed bracts. Edible tubers are formed underground.

Native Americans used the plant and flower preparations for rheumatism. Flowers were also eaten for rheumatism. Edible tubers contain inulin as the storage carbohydrate, but it is probably not related to medicinal properties.

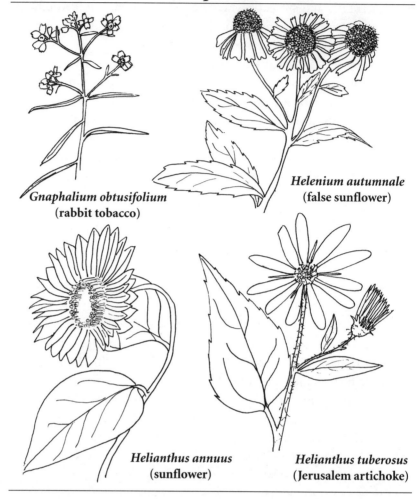

Gnaphalium obtusifolium
(rabbit tobacco)

Helenium autumnale
(false sunflower)

Helianthus annuus
(sunflower)

Helianthus tuberosus
(Jerusalem artichoke)

Hieracium pilosella (mouse-ear hawkweed) is a 1- to 2-foot weedy, naturalized perennial found in open fields of northern and southern New Jersey. Leaves are entire, white-woolly underneath, in a basal rosette. The flower head, appearing in mid-May, is usually solitary, on a slender leafless stem.

Native Americans used a plant infusion for diarrhea.

Hieracium venosum (poor robin's plantain, rattlesnake weed, vein-leaved hawkweed) is a 1- to 2-foot native perennial found in dry, open areas statewide, including the pinelands. Leaves are entire, purple-veined, in a basal rosette. Flower heads are numerous, appearing in late May, on a smooth stem, sometimes bearing a few leaves.

Native Americans used the root in the preparation of a compound infusion taken for bowel complaints.

Inula helenium (elecampane) is a 2- to 8-foot naturalized perennial

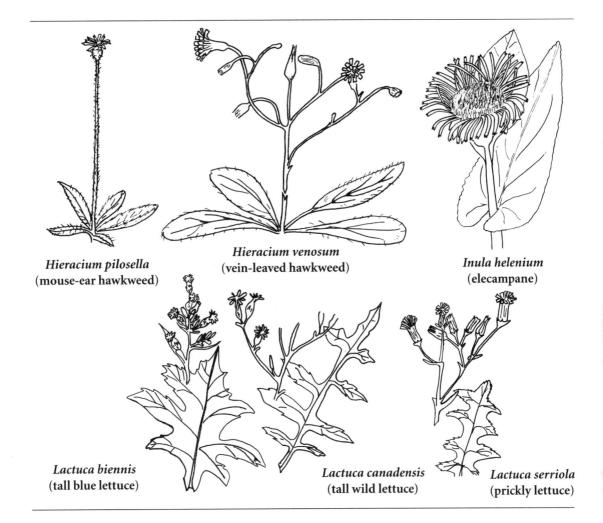

Hieracium pilosella
(mouse-ear hawkweed)

Hieracium venosum
(vein-leaved hawkweed)

Inula helenium
(elecampane)

Lactuca biennis
(tall blue lettuce)

Lactuca canadensis
(tall wild lettuce)

Lactuca serriola
(prickly lettuce)

found in rich-soiled, open, well-drained areas of northern and southern New Jersey. The leaves are alternate, finely toothed, and woolly on the underside. Upper leaves are smaller. Flowers are yellow and large, with rays numerous and stringlike, giving the head a disheveled appearance. Flowers appear in late June.

Native Americans used elecampane root for lung disorders, coughs, asthma, and consumption as well as a tonic to strengthen digestive and reproductive organs. A decoction or cold infusion prepared from the powdered root was taken for fevers, stomach gas, tuberculosis, asthma, heart trouble, stroke, colds, and headache. Dried leaves were given to children for asthma. A poultice of crushed plants, leaves, or roots was applied for arthritis, rheumatism, sores and cuts.

Bigelow described elecampane as tonic and expectorant but inferior to many other similar medicines.

Lactuca biennis (*L. spicata*) (tall blue lettuce, wild lettuce) is a 2- to 15-foot native biennial found in moist, well-drained, open areas of northern and southern New Jersey. Leaves are deeply lobed and coarsely toothed. Flower heads are blue and numerous, in branched clusters, appearing in late June.

Native Americans used a root decoction for body pain, vomiting, diarrhea, heart trouble, and hemorrhage. A plant infusion was used to relieve caked breasts and ease lactation.

Lactuca canadensis (lettuce, tall wild lettuce) is a 3- to 10-foot native biennial found in well-drained, open areas statewide. Leaves are alternate, toothed, clasping, and variable, ranging from deep lobed to lance-shaped. The stem is smooth. Flowers are pale or reddish yellow and dandelionlike; they appear in late June.

Native Americans used an infusion to relieve pain, calm nerves, and produce sleep, and as a stimulant and for "milksick." The milky sap was rubbed on warts and poison ivy rash. A poultice of crushed roots was applied to control severe bleeding from a cut.

Bigelow used the name *L. elongata* for the native wild lettuce [*L. canadensis*], which he recommended as a substitute for *L. virosa* of Europe. He described the properties as of "inferior strength" as an anodyne and in promotion of "excretions of the skin and kidneys."

Lactuca serriola (*L. scariola*) (prickly lettuce) is a 2- to 7-foot naturalized biennial weed found in waste areas throughout the state. Leaves are alternate and highly variable, but always spiny. Flowers are yellow, appearing in late June.

Native Americans used a leaf infusion after childbirth to stimulate lactation.

Matricaria chamomilla (German chamomile, ground apple, pinheads, wild chamomile) is a 6-inch to 2-foot naturalized annual found in waste areas and along roadsides statewide. Leaves are alternate, finely divided, and described as either apple- or pineapple-scented, depending on the individual observer. The stem is smooth; flowers are white, $3/4$ to 1 inch wide, and daisylike, and appear in May.

Native Americans used the infusion or decoction of chamomile as a stomachic, antispasmodic, tonic, carminative, diaphoretic, nervine, emmenagogue, and sedative. The tea was used for childhood complaints such as colds, convulsions, stomach pains, colic, earache, restlessness, and measles. The warm tea was sudorific, and the cold tea was taken for fevers and as a stomach tonic. A syrup of fresh or dried flower juice with white wine was used for jaundice, dropsy, nervousness, and uterine problems.

Matricaria matricarioides (false chamomile, pineapple weed, rayless chamomile) is a 4- to 16-inch naturalized annual found in open areas

Compositae

Matricaria chamomilla (German chamomile)

Matricaria matricarioides (pineapple weed)

Prenanthes alba (white lettuce)

Rudbeckia hirta (black-eyed Susan)

Rudbeckia laciniata (green-headed coneflower)

statewide. Leaves are alternate and finely divided. Flowers are yellow, in cone-shaped, rayless heads, producing a distinct pineapple aroma when bruised. Flowers appear in late April.

Native Americans used a leaf infusion for stomach gas pains and as a laxative. The plant decoction was regarded as tonic and was used for fever, indigestion, colds, "the heart," and for infant convulsions. The leaf and flower decoction was taken for diarrhea. A dried–seed head decoction was taken for colds and indigestion, and the plant was used for fragrance in the steambath.

Prenanthes alba (rattlesnake root, white lettuce) is a 2- to 5-foot native perennial found in well-drained, dry or moist areas of northern and southern New Jersey. Leaves are alternate, triangular, lobed and toothed. Leaves and purplish stems have a whitish bloom. Flowers, appearing in early September, are white, with deep red brown hairs beneath the bracts.

Native Americans added the powdered, dried root to food to stimulate postpartum lactation. A root poultice was applied for dog and rattlesnake bites; the root was also used as a "female remedy." "Milk" of the plant was used as a diuretic and in female diseases.

Rudbeckia hirta (*R. serotina*) (black-eyed Susan, coneflower, yellow daisy) is a 1- to 3-foot native biennial or short-lived perennial found in well-drained, open areas statewide, including the pinelands. Leaves are alternate, lanceolate, hairy, and slightly toothed to entire. Flowers are yellow and daisylike, with a deep brown globose center, appearing in mid-June.

Native Americans used coneflower as a wash for snakebite and "swelling caused by worms" (intestinal?); a root infusion was given to children for worms, taken for colds, and used as a wash for sores. A plant decoction was taken for heart problems and sore eyes. The expressed root juice was used for earache, and the tea was taken for dropsy.

Rudbeckia laciniata (coneflower, green-headed coneflower, tall coneflower) is a 3- to 12-foot branched, native perennial found in moist, rich-soiled, low grounds of shaded woods, swamps, fields, roadsides, and waste areas throughout the state, including the pinelands. Leaves are alternate, with the lower leaves deeply divided into three to seven toothed lobes. Daisylike yellow flowers (partial doubling is not rare) with a green disk appear in late July.

Native Americans cooked young leaves to eat as a preventive medicine to "keep well."

Senecio aureus (golden ragwort, swamp squaw weed) is a 6-inch to 4-foot native perennial found in wet or moist areas of woods or meadows statewide. The leaves are alternate, with basal leaves heart-shaped, egg-shaped, or rounded, and upper leaves lanceolate. Yellow, daisylike flower heads in flat-topped clusters are $1/2$ to $3/4$ inches wide, on at least $1/2$-inch stalks, appearing in late April. *Senecio* is probably the largest genus of plants.

Native Americans used golden ragwort infusion for heart trouble and as a contraceptive. The plant decoction was also taken for kidneys and broken bones. A flower infusion was given to children for fever. The root was used as a diaphoretic. Species of *Senecio* are today regarded as poisonous.

Senecio vulgaris (common groundsel) is a 4-inch to 2-foot naturalized annual weed found statewide. Leaves are soft, somewhat fleshy, toothed and lobed. Rayless flowers with black-tipped bracts appear in early May. This is one of the most successful weeds, reseeding itself as long as it is growing.

Native Americans apparently did not use this ragwort for medicinal purposes. The entire plant is an official drug, used to improve blood, and although known to contain toxic alkaloids, it is available today as a

Compositae

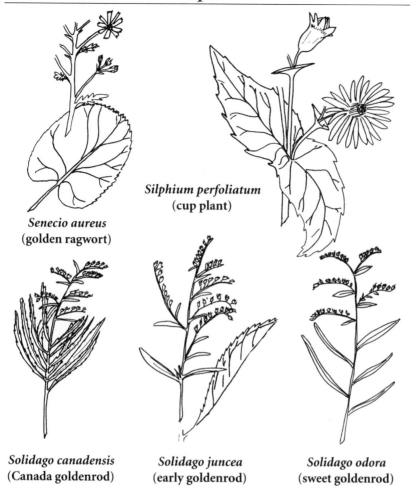

Senecio aureus
(golden ragwort)

Silphium perfoliatum
(cup plant)

Solidago canadensis
(Canada goldenrod)

Solidago juncea
(early goldenrod)

Solidago odora
(sweet goldenrod)

dried, cut plant preparation or a crude extract. Most if not all species of *Senecio* should be added to a growing number of plants previously regarded as safe for consumption but now known to contain hepato-toxic pyrrolizidine alkaloids such as heliosupine, found in species of *Heliotropium* (Boraginaceae).

Silphium perfoliatum (cup plant, Indian cup) is a 3- to 8-foot native perennial found in well-drained, rich-soiled, moist areas of northern New Jersey and naturalized elsewhere. Leaves are opposite and egg-shaped, with the upper pair fused at the base to form a cup. The stem is square and smooth. The flowers are 2 to 3 inches wide, yellow with many rays, and appear in late July.

Native Americans used the root decoction as an abortifacient ("stoppage of periods"), for lung hemorrhage, back and chest pains, and as a face wash for paralysis. The root was also used to reduce menses and prevent premature childbirth, and as an antiemetic during pregnancy. A poultice of moistened, dry root was applied as a styptic.

Solidago canadensis (Canada goldenrod) is a 1- to 5-foot native perennial found in moist or dry, open areas of northern and southern New Jersey. This is the most common goldenrod. Leaves are alternate, narrowly lance-shaped, three-veined, and sharply toothed. The stem is smooth at the base and hairy below the lower flower branches. Flower heads are less than $1/8$ inch long, in broad, triangular panicles, appearing in late August.

Native Americans used a plant infusion to prepare a bath for the mother at childbirth. A flower infusion was used to treat fever and relieve body pain, and as an emetic. Crushed flowers were chewed for sore throat.

Solidago juncea (early goldenrod) is a 1- to 4-foot native perennial found in dry, open, sandy or rocky areas of northern and southern New Jersey. Leaves are alternate and lance-shaped, with the basal leaves sharply toothed. The midstem leaves are essentially entire, and the stem is smooth and green. Goldenrod-type flowers appear in late June.

Native Americans chewed leaves or used a leaf infusion for diarrhea and fever. A root decoction was taken for convulsions and fever. A plant infusion was taken for nausea and jaundice. A flower decoction was taken as an emetic and for gaseous upset stomach.

Solidago odora (blue mountain tea, fragrant goldenrod, goldenrod, sweet goldenrod) is a 2- to 5-foot native perennial found in dry, sandy, open areas statewide but particularly abundant in the pinelands. Leaves are 2 to 4 inches long, lance-shaped, and entire, with prickles along the leaf edges that can be felt by rubbing backward along the leaf edges. Leaves are anise or licorice-scented when bruised. Flowers are goldenrod-type, appearing in mid-July.

Native Americans used the infusion for bloody diarrhea, fever, coughs, nerves, and measles, and as a diaphoretic. The leaf infusion was taken for tuberculosis, and a root infusion was held in the mouth for neuralgia. The root was chewed for a sore mouth.

Bigelow described goldenrod as having an "extremely pleasant odour and taste" and as stimulant, carminative, and diaphoretic.

Sonchus arvensis (field sow thistle) is a $1^1/2$- to 4-foot naturalized perennial weed found in open areas, along gravelly shores, and in salt marshes of northern and southern New Jersey. The leaves are alternate, clasping, and divided dandelionlike. Dandelionlike flowers appear in late June.

Native Americans used sow thistle infusion to calm nerves and a leaf infusion for caked breasts.

Tanacetum vulgare (golden buttons, tansy) is a 1- to 4-foot naturalized perennial weed found in waste areas of northern and southern New Jersey. Leaves are alternate; fernlike (i.e., deeply cut into fine divisions);

Compositae

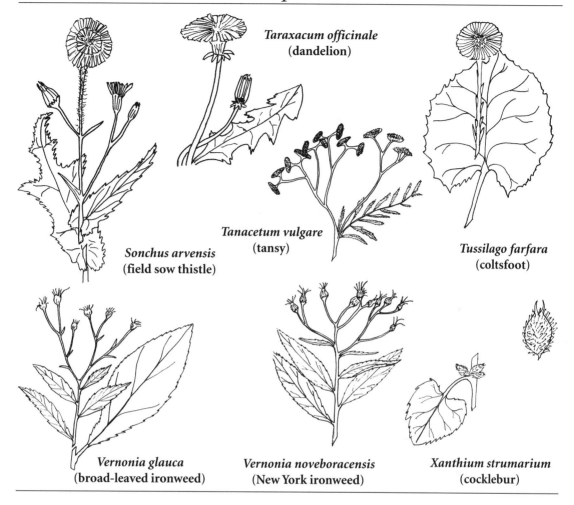

Taraxacum officinale
(dandelion)

Sonchus arvensis
(field sow thistle)

Tanacetum vulgare
(tansy)

Tussilago farfara
(coltsfoot)

Vernonia glauca
(broad-leaved ironweed)

Vernonia noveboracensis
(New York ironweed)

Xanthium strumarium
(cocklebur)

and strongly aromatic. Flowers are yellow and buttonlike in flat terminal clusters, appearing in early August.

Native Americans used tansy as a treatment for worms in children and as a medicine for stomach disorders. The leaf decoction was used as an abortifacient ("stoppage of periods") in young girls, an emetic, and an antiseptic wash and for bloody diarrhea and kidney trouble. The plant was used as a contraceptive, for fevers, as a sudorific, and to treat cuts and bruises. A leaf poultice was applied to the head for headache and to the body for pains.

Bigelow described tansy as tonic and anthelmintic and as having been used in "obstructed catamenia and hysteric affections."

Taraxacum officinale (dandelion) is a 2- to 18-inch naturalized, common perennial weed found in all environments statewide. Leaves are basal and toothed. Yellow flowers appear in late March on hollow stalks with milky juice.

Native Americans applied a poultice of steamed leaves to indolent ulcers, stomachache, and sore throat. A poultice for swollen testicles was prepared from crushed flowers. Leaves were chewed for toothache, and the plant was used to make a laxative tonic, a blood builder in anemia, and a wash for crushed testicles. A decoction prepared from young leaves was taken by women for menstrual cramps. A root infusion was taken for stomach pain, chest pain, nervousness, and heartburn, and as an emetic. The flower stem was chewed for "worms" in the teeth, and a flower infusion was taken for menstrual cramps. Dandelion wine was taken as a tonic. Young leaves were and are today eaten in salads.

Tussilago farfara (coltsfoot, coughwort) is a 4- to 8-inch naturalized perennial found in moist, lightly shaded areas of northern and occasionally southern New Jersey. The leaves are rounded, slightly lobed, toothed, and heart-shaped (some say colt's foot–shaped). Yellow, dandelionlike flowers appear in early April, before the leaves.

Coltsfoot root was used for coughs and as an ingredient in a compound cough medicine.

Vernonia glauca (broad-leaved ironweed, ironweed) is a 2- to 5-foot rare native perennial found in rich-soiled, wooded areas of southern New Jersey. The leaves are alternate, lance-shaped, and toothed. Plants are blue-green, with yellowish flowers appearing in July.

Native Americans used ironweed (usually the root) to prepare infusions for anemia, "monthly periods," and to prevent menstruation (menses regulator). The root infusion was also taken for bleeding stomach ulcers, for loose teeth, and to relieve pain after childbirth.

Vernonia noveboracensis (ironweed, New York ironweed) is a 3- to 7-foot common native perennial found in moist areas and along streams statewide, excluding the pinelands. Leaves are alternate, lance-shaped, finely toothed, and 3 to 10 inches long. Each head is composed of 30 to 50 purple flowers, which appear in late July.

Native Americans used New York ironweed as they did *V. glauca*. Although not included in this list or most herbals, *V. altissima* grows very well in New Jersey and should be expected to show similar medicinal properties.

Xanthium strumarium (cocklebur) is a native, weedy annual of up to 5 feet tall and found in open areas of the state. Leaves are alternate, oval to heart-shaped, and lobed or toothed on long petioles. Green, inconspicuous flowers form in September and produce oval fruit with hooked spikes described as being the model for the development of Velcro fasteners.

Native Americans used a seed decoction for bladder problems.

030 *Convolvulaceae*

The morning glory family of herbs, shrubs, and trees, with the herbs usually twining. The family is primarily tropical and subtropical but extends into the temperate regions. *Ipomoea violacea* (morning glory) is native to Mexico. Morning glory seeds contain ergot alkaloids including ergine (D-lysergic acid amide), a potent hallucinogen similar to LSD.

Convolvulus arvensis (field bindweed, hedge bindweed) is a naturalized creeping vine, a weed found in waste areas and along roadsides of northern and southern New Jersey. Leaves are entire and arrow-shaped at the base. Flowers are $3/4$ inches long, white or pink, and appear in early June.

Native Americans used a plant decoction to control menses. A cold infusion of the plant was applied as a lotion for spider bites and was taken with food after swallowing a spider.

Convolvulus sepium (great bindweed, hedge bindweed, wild morning glory) is a native trailing vine, a weed found in moist areas and fields statewide. Leaves are entire and arrow-shaped, with square lobes at the

Convolvulaceae

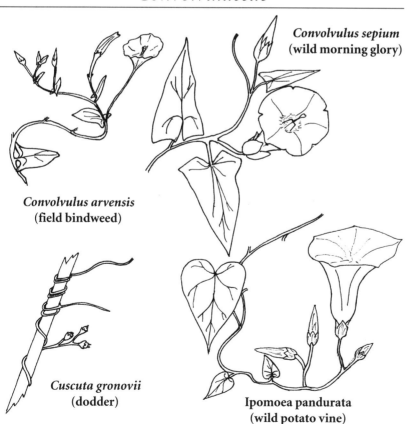

Convolvulus sepium
(wild morning glory)

Convolvulus arvensis
(field bindweed)

Cuscuta gronovii
(dodder)

Ipomoea pandurata
(wild potato vine)

base. Flowers are showy, 1^1/$_2$ to 3 inches long, white or pink, and appear in early June.

The root tea was used by European settlers for jaundice and as a purgative.

Cuscuta gronovii (dodder, love vine) is a native annual, parasitic vine found on many woody and herbaceous plants growing in moist, low areas of northern and southern New Jersey. Plants are without chlorophyll and leafless. Stems are yellow or orange. Small, dense clusters of bell-shaped white flowers appear in late July.

Native Americans used dodder as a poultice for bruises.

Ipomoea pandurata (man-of-the-earth, wild potato vine) is a native twining or climbing vine found in open, dry and sandy areas of northern and southern New Jersey. Leaves are heart-shaped, and stems are often purple. The tuberous root is 1 to 3 feet in length, growing straight down. Flowers are funnel-shaped, white with pink or purple stripes in the throat, and appear in early July.

Native Americans used a root poultice for rheumatism and hard tumors. A cold infusion of the root was taken for headache, coughs, asthma, and tuberculosis, and as a laxative and diuretic.

031 *Cornaceae*

The dogwood family of perennial herbs, shrubs, woody vines, and trees. Leaves are simple, usually opposite, and deciduous. The family is distributed throughout the tropical and temperate regions.

Cornus alternifolia (dogwood, green osier, pagoda dogwood) is a shrub or small tree found in dry, rich-soiled areas and rocky slopes of northern and southern New Jersey. Leaves are alternate and entire, on nearly horizontal, greenish branches. Flowers are white, in flat clusters, appearing in early May and giving rise to bluish black fruit in July.

Native Americans chewed dogwood bark for headache and prepared an astringent infusion for "woman's backache," as a wash for granulation of the eyelids, and as an enema for piles and diarrhea; a bark poultice was applied to the anus. A beaten bark infusion was used as a bath after poisoning of any kind. The expressed bark juice was used to poultice ulcers, and a poultice of powdered bark was applied to blisters and to heal the navel at childbirth. The inner-bark infusion was used as an emetic and as a cough and laryngitis remedy. The root bark was used as a tonic, stimulant, antiseptic, astringent, and febrifuge. The flower infusion was taken for colic and as a sudorific in influenza. The scraped-root infusion was used as a wash or compress for sore eyes.

Cornus canadensis (bunchberry, dwarf cornel, pudding berry) is a 3-

Cornaceae

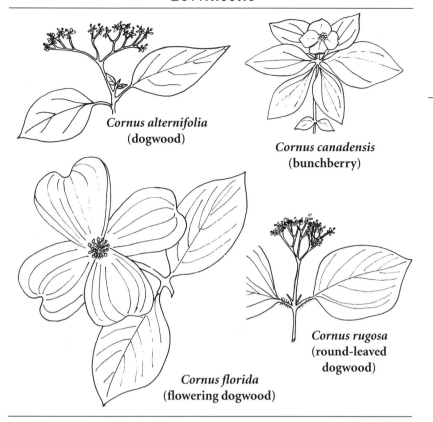

Cornus alternifolia
(dogwood)

Cornus canadensis
(bunchberry)

Cornus rugosa
(round-leaved
dogwood)

Cornus florida
(flowering dogwood)

to 8-inch native perennial found in cold, wet, acidic areas of woods and shaded edges of northern New Jersey. Leaves are entire and in a single whorl of six. The "flower" is 1 inch wide, white, and appears solitary; it is actually composed of four petallike bracts surrounding a dense cluster of whitish, four-petaled flowers. Flowers appear in May and give rise to clusters of bright red berries in late July.

Native Americans used a whole-plant decoction for coughs, fevers, and tuberculosis, and an infusion to treat paralysis. The berries, roots, and leaves were used to treat epilepsy, and a strong decoction, without the berries, was used for an eyewash. Leaf ash or toasted leaf powder was sprinkled on sores.

Cornus florida (flowering dogwood) is a 10- to 30-foot native tree or shrub found in wooded areas in light shade among other trees statewide. Leaves are opposite, oval, and entire. Flowers are greenish white and clustered at the center of four large, showy, white bracts. Flowers appear in late April and give rise to clusters of bright red fruit in September.

Native Americans used this dogwood as they did *C. alternifolia*; in addition, the bark infusion was used as a bath for children with worms.

Bigelow described the bark of dogwood as bitter, astringent, and aromatic, useful in intermittent fevers and other cases where tonics are indicated. The fresh bark was described as causing diarrhea and stomach upset but losing this side effect as it aged.

Cornus rugosa (*C. circinata*)(round-leaved dogwood) is a native shrub, found in dry or moist, rocky, woody areas and shaded edges of northern New Jersey. The leaves are paired and rounded, on green, purple-spotted branches. Flowers are white in flat clusters, appearing in mid-May and giving rise to light blue fruit in August.

Native Americans used the bark decoction as an emetic and cathartic.

Bigelow described round-leaved dogwood as exceeding any other in bitterness and astringency. It was highly valued as a tonic and stomachic. In Connecticut, it was official and a substitute for cinchona. Officinals were kept in stock by apothecaries among other drugs that did not require special preparation or compounding.

Crassulaceae

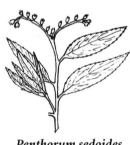

**Penthorum sedoides
(ditch stonecrop)**

032 *Crassulaceae (Sedaceae)*

The stonecrop or orpine family of annual or perennial herbs with succulent stems. They are readily distinguished from the Cactaceae by their lack of spines. The family is large and very widely distributed. The ditch stonecrop is often placed in the Saxifrage family.

Penthorum sedoides (ditch stonecrop) is a 6-inch to 3-foot native perennial found in moist and swampy areas of northern and southern New Jersey. Leaves are 2 to 4 inches long, alternate, broadly lance-shaped or elliptical, and finely toothed. Flowers, appearing in late June, are yellowish green, in branching, spiked clusters.

Native Americans used the seeds to prepare a cough syrup.

033 *Cruciferae (Brassicaceae)*

The mustard family of annual or perennial herbs and small shrubs with a characteristic pungent taste. The leaves are simple or pinnate, alternate or opposite. The family is large and widely distributed but concentrated in the temperate and arctic regions of the Northern Hemisphere.

Armoracia rusticana (*A. lapathifolia*) (horseradish) is a 2- to 3-foot escaped perennial found in moist or dry, open areas statewide. Stem leaves are alternate and toothed, and basal leaves are long-stalked and up to a foot in length. Flowers are small and white in upright racemes appearing in May.

Cruciferae

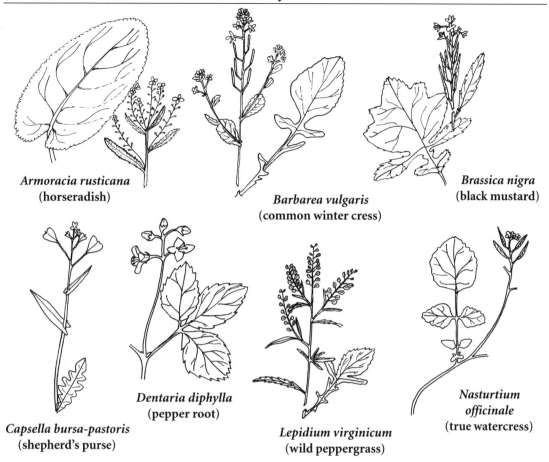

Armoracia rusticana
(horseradish)

Barbarea vulgaris
(common winter cress)

Brassica nigra
(black mustard)

Capsella bursa-pastoris
(shepherd's purse)

Dentaria diphylla
(pepper root)

Lepidium virginicum
(wild peppergrass)

Nasturtium officinale
(true watercress)

Native Americans used horseradish for gravel, rheumatism, asthma, colds, and "obstructed menses." It was also taken as a diuretic and tonic, and to increase appetite and aid digestion. The root was chewed for diseases of the tongue and mouth, and a crushed-root infusion was taken for the blood. A leaf poultice was applied for neuralgia and was bound to the face for toothache.

Bigelow described horseradish as primarily a condiment with food. The medicinal action was described as diuretic and, in large quantity, emetic. The fresh, green leaves are rubefacient.

Horseradish, black mustard, and several other brassicas can kill livestock and cause diarrhea and intestinal bleeding in humans. They contain high levels of toxic isothiocyanates. Dried sinagrin produces an irritant mustard oil when hydrated. It is converted to allylisothiocyanate which can serve as a precursor to mustard gas.

Barbarea vulgaris (common winter cress, creases, Indian posey, yellow rocket) is a 1- to 2-foot naturalized annual weed found in moist meadows and waste areas statewide. Leaves are alternate, with basal leaves showing four to eight lateral, earlike lobes. Upper leaves are rounded, coarsely toothed, and clasping. Flowers are yellow and appear in early April.

Native Americans cooked leaves to eat as a "blood purifier." Indian posey leaf infusion was taken every half hour to cure coughs.

Brassica nigra (black mustard; wild mustard) is a 1- to 7-foot naturalized annual weed found in fields and waste areas statewide. Leaves are alternate; the lower being bristly and coarsely lobed, and the upper, lance-shaped and entire or toothed. Flowers are yellow, appearing in late May and giving rise to narrow, erect seedpods in June.

Native Americans used black mustard to increase appetite, and as a stimulant and a tonic. It was taken for fever, dropsy, palsy, tuberculosis, asthma, and as a poultice for croup, headache, toothache, and body pains. A snuff of ground seed was used for head colds and when mixed with flour and water was used as an emetic to make "insides come up."

Bigelow described mustard as stimulant, diuretic, and emetic, but primarily used externally as a rubefacient.

Capsella bursa-pastoris (pepper grass, pick-pocket, shepherd's purse) is a 6- to 20-inch native annual weed found in fields and waste areas throughout the state. Basal leaves are lobed and in a rosette, while stem leaves are alternate, arrow-shaped, small, and clasping. Small, white flowers appear in late April and give rise to heart-shaped or triangular seedpods in May.

Native Americans used a cold stem-and-leaf infusion for headache. A whole-plant decoction was used for diarrhea and dysentery and an infusion as a wash for poison ivy. A seedpod infusion was used for stomachache and internal worms.

Dentaria diphylla (crinkle-root, pepper root, toothwort, two-leaved toothwort) is a 6-inch to 1-foot native perennial found in well-drained, moist, wooded areas of northern New Jersey. Stem leaves, usually two, are opposite and divided into three toothed leaflets. Basal leaves are similar to the stem leaves. Flowers are white or pink, four-petaled, in small, terminal clusters, appearing in late April.

Native Americans used toothwort root as a tonic and sedative as well as to clear the throat and treat hoarseness.

Lepidium virginicum (peppergrass, poor man's pepper, wild peppergrass) is a 6-inch to 2-foot native annual or biennial weed found in dry, open fields and waste areas statewide. Stem leaves are alternate, lance-shaped, and toothed. Basal leaves, if present, are lobed. Flowers are small, inconspicuous, and white, appearing in late April. Seedpods are nearly round and slightly winged at the tip, appearing in late July.

Native Americans used the crushed plant or plant infusion to treat poison ivy. It was poulticed for croup, and the crushed root was used as a poultice to "draw" blisters. The infusion was also given to sick chickens and mixed with feed for egg laying.

Nasturtium officinale (true watercress) is a 4-inch to 3-foot creeping or floating, naturalized perennial found in cool, clear, running water of northern and southern New Jersey. Leaves are alternate and divided into three to nine essentially entire leaflets. Flowers are small and white, appearing in early May.

Native Americans used a cold infusion of plants for fevers and a decoction for kidney and liver diseases.

034 *Cucurbitaceae*

The gourd family of annual or perennial herbs, shrubs, and small trees. The herbs are usually prostrate or climbing vines. The leaves are simple, lobed, and alternate. The family is concentrated in the tropics, but extends into the temperate regions.

Echinocystis lobata (balsam-apple, wild cucumber) is a native climbing vine with forked tendrils found in rich-soiled, moist areas, especially along streams throughout the state. Leaves are maplelike, with five deep lobes. Flowers are greenish white in axillary clusters, appearing in late July. The pistillate flowers give rise to spiny, green, bladderlike fruit in early September.

Native Americans used wild cucumber for chills and fevers, kidneys, and rheumatism, and as an abortifacient in "obstructed menses." The root decoction or infusion was taken as a bitter tonic for the stomach, and a poultice of crushed root was applied for headache.

Cucurbitaceae

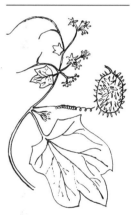

**Echinocystis lobata
(wild cucumber)**

035 *Cupressaceae*

The cypress family of gymnosperms. They range from small trees to prostrate shrubs. Leaves are not needles, but scalelike and usually triangular. The largest trees in the family occur in the northwestern United States.

Juniperus communis (common dwarf juniper, ground juniper) is a native shrub or small tree found in sterile, dry, rocky areas of northern New Jersey. The bark is reddish brown and peels off in papery sheets. Leaves are striped green and white in whorls of three, and tapering to sharp tips. The fruit is bluish black and three-seeded.

Native Americans regarded juniper as a "hot" medicine and therefore

Cupressaceae

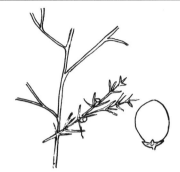

Juniperus communis
(ground juniper)

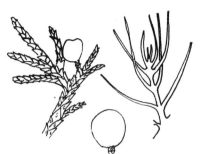

Juniperus virginiana
(eastern red cedar)

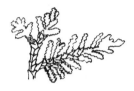

Thuja occidentalis
(northern white cedar)

used it to treat "cold" conditions. A decoction of roots, leaves, branches, and bark was taken for stomachache and deep coughs. A branch or cone infusion was taken for high fever and coughs and as a sedative. Cones were chewed, and branches and cones were steamed for colds. A twig-and-leaf decoction was used for asthma, as an emetic and purgative, and a wash for sore eyes, and was taken for venereal disease. A bark poultice was applied to wounds as an antiseptic. Berries were eaten for kidney disorder, and leaves were burned at childbirth to promote delivery.

Bigelow described juniper berries as the officinal part of the plant, but found the American berries "far inferior" to the European berries in stimulating the kidneys and neighboring organs and complained that most of the berries sold in America were the "refuse of gin distilleries."

Juniperus virginiana (eastern red cedar) is a 10- to 50-foot native spire-shaped tree found in dry, sterile areas throughout the state, including the pinelands. The bark is reddish brown and easily shredded. Leaves are dark green needles on young branches, but scalelike and overlapping on older branches. The fruit is a small cone, blue or bluish black, and covered with a grayish bloom. The fruit has juicy, resinous flesh and may contain one or two seeds.

Native Americans use red cedar as a diaphoretic; for colds, rheumatism, and measles; and as an abortifacient in "female obstruction." The leaf decoction was used as a wash for cholera and as a diuretic. A berry decoction was used for worms, and berries were chewed for canker sores.

Bigelow described the red cedar as resembling the European savin botanically and medicinally. The leaves were described as stimulant, diuretic, and emmenagogue, with uses in rheumatism, dropsy, and catamenial obstructions.

Thuja occidentalis (eastern arborvitae, northern white cedar) is a rare native tree of up to 60 feet in height found in swamps and cool, rocky, wooded areas of northern New Jersey. Leaves are small, appressed, and overlapping in flattened sprays. Cones are bell-shaped with loose scales.

Native Americans used arborvitae as a deodorant, and twigs were burned as a disinfectant to fumigate for smallpox. The steam from boiling leaves was inhaled for colds, and the decoction was used as a wash or poultice for cuts, bruises, and sores. An infusion prepared from dried inner bark was taken during a cold to stimulate menses.

036 *Cyperaceae*

The sedge family of annual but more usually perennial grasslike plants of bogs, marshes, and meadows. They may also be found along streams and in dry areas including lawns and gardens. The main stem is a rhizome with a triangular, usually unbranched flowering stalk. Flowers are unisexual and in spikes; monoecious or rarely dioecious; the staminate naked and subtended by a bract or scale, the pistillate comprising a single pistil enclosed in a thin sac (perigynium). The leaves are alternate, grasslike, and essentially basal. The family is found worldwide but is concentrated in the cooler regions of both hemispheres. The largest genus is *Carex*, with hundreds of species.

Carex brevior (shorter fescue sedge) is native and found in dry, open areas of inner-coastal northern and southern New Jersey. Staminate and pistillate flowers appearing in late May are mingled in uniform ovoid heads clustered or usually separate at the end of the stalk, each composed of a number of closely overlapped flat perigynia (sacs that enclose the ovaries) and scales. The perigynia are orbicular or broadly ovate in a brown head. The achenes are not stalked.

Native Americans used sedge in a compound infusion taken to aid in placental expulsion.

Carex pensylvanica (Pennsylvania sedge) is native and found in open, dry, sandy areas statewide. Pistillate spikes are in one to three small clusters at the base of the stalkless, staminate spike. The inflorescence is pink and less than 1 inch long, appearing in early April. The perigynia are dense-woolly, with long, flat beaks.

Native Americans used a cold infusion of sedge for indigestion and "eagle infection."

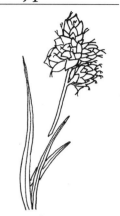

**Carex brevior
(shorter fescue sedge)**

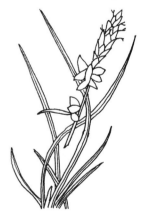

**Carex pensylvanica
(Pennsylvania sedge)**

The tree fern family, also called the Cyatheaceae. Plants are treelike, with stems aboveground or growing as rhizomes underground. When the family is given as Cyatheaceae, one of the genera is *Dennstaetia*.

Pteridium aquilinum (bracken, bracken fern, brake) is a 3- to 6-foot native fern found in open, dry, sandy areas throughout the state. It is the most common of the area ferns, forming large colonies. Leaves and first-division leaflets are triangular. The third-division leaflets are blunt, with some cut to the midrib.

Native Americans used the root as a tonic, antiemetic, and antisep-

Dennstaedticeae

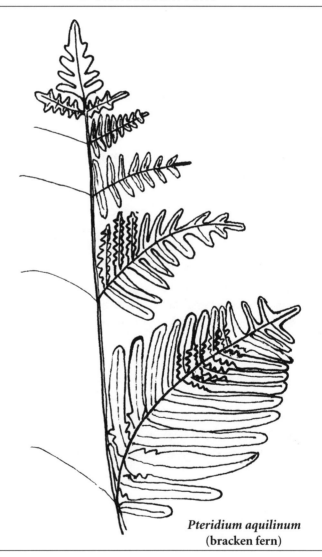

Pteridium aquilinum
(bracken fern)

tic, and for "cholera-morbus." The root decoction was taken for stomach cramps, "after-birth complaints" (anemia), diarrhea, rheumatism, liver diseases, tuberculosis, and caked breasts; it was also used as a hair rinse. Roots were rubbed on the scalp for hair growth. The ground-root decoction was taken for chest pain. A heated, crushed-root poultice was applied to burns. Smoke from dried leaves was inhaled for headache.

Bracken contains the enzyme thiaminase and at least three carcinogens. Thiaminase causes vitamin B1 deficiency and is particularly hazardous to grazing horses and cattle. The toxins may accumulate in the milk of grazing cows.

038 *Dioscoreaceae*

The yam family of monocotyledonous, herbaceous or woody vines with an underground stem that is either a rhizome or a caudex. The roots are often tuberous. Leaves are entire, and alternate or opposite. The family is primarily tropical and subtropical, with few in the temperate regions.

Dioscorea villosa (colic root, wild yam) is a native perennial, twining vine found in moist, open-wooded areas throughout the state. Lower leaves are entire, in whorls of three to eight, while the upper ones are alternate, heart-shaped, and hairy underneath, on a smooth stem.

Native Americans used wild yam root to relieve childbirth pains.

039 *Droseraceae*

The sundew family of annual or perennial herbs and somewhat shrubby plants. The leaves are simple and basal, and covered with stalked glands that capture insects. Distribution is nearly global for the largest genus, *Drosera*.

Drosera rotundifolia (round-leaved sundew) is a 4- to 9-inch native perennial found in wet, peaty, boggy areas of cedar swamps throughout New Jersey, including the pinelands. Leaves are basal, rounded, and covered with reddish, glandular hairs. Flowers are in racemes, white or pinkish, opening one at a time beginning in June.

Native Americans used sundew for corns, warts, and bunions.

Dioscoreaceae

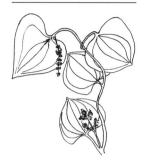

**Dioscorea villosa
(wild yam)**

Droseraceae

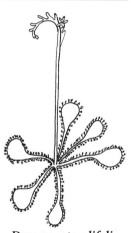

**Drosera rotundifolia
(round-leaved sundew)**

040 *Ebenaceae*

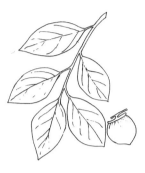

Ebenaceae

Diospyros virginiana
(**wild persimmon**)

The ebony family of shrubs and trees with milky juice. Leathery leaves are simple, entire, and alternate. The fruit is a berry. The family is widely distributed, but only one species of persimmon is native to the northeastern United States, south of Canada. The heartwood of most genera is black, red, or brown.

Diospyros virginiana (wild persimmon) is a 15- to 50-foot native tree found in dry, open areas of old fields throughout New Jersey, with the exception of the area designated as the central pine barrens. Leaves are alternate, entire, shiny, and elliptic. Yellow flowers appear in May and produce at first astringent then sweet, edible, orange, plumlike fruit.

Native Americans used persimmon for liver ailments, venereal diseases, and piles; a syrup was used for bloody diarrhea, thrush, and sore throat. The bark was chewed for heartburn. An infusion prepared from the bark on the north side was taken for sore throat.

041 *Equisetaceae*

The horsetail family of flowerless plants in a single genus, occurring on all continents except Australia. About 15 species are native to America north of Mexico, and at least 8 species are native to New Jersey.

Equisetum arvense (devil's guts, field horsetail, horsetail grass) is a leafless native herb of up to 1 foot, found in open, moist, sterile areas. Stems are stiff, with elongated internodes showing eight to ten distinct teeth (leaves) and whorled branchlets. Fertile stems are unbranched, appearing in spring only and followed by senescence.

Native Americans used a horsetail infusion for kidney and bladder problems, constipation (strong infusion), headache, rheumatism, dropsy, and lumbago. Plants were poulticed for cuts and sores, and raw stems were chewed by teething babies.

Equisetum hyemale (greater horsetail, scouring rush) is a leafless native, evergreen herb of up to 5 feet found in moist, shady areas such as roadside ditches and along sandy stream- and riversides statewide. It is similar in appearance to field horsetail but lacks branchlets.

Native Americans used scouring rush as they did field horsetail, and in addition as an insecticide, disinfectant, eye medicine, hair wash, contraceptive, and abortifacient.

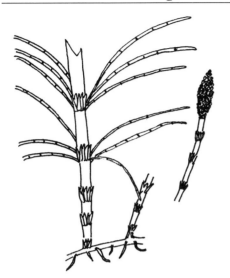

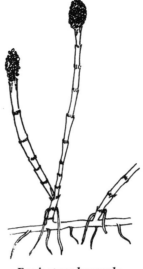

Equisetum arvense
(field horsetail)

Equisetum hyemale
(scouring rush)

042 *Ericaceae*

The heath family of perennial herbs, shrubs, and trees. Leaves are simple, usually alternate but sometimes opposite, leathery and usually evergreen. Among the plants included in this family are wintergreen, pipsissewa, Indian pipe, rhododendrons (azaleas), laurel, bearberries, huckleberries, and blueberries. The family is distributed throughout the temperate regions of the globe and at higher elevations in the tropics.

Arctostaphylos uva-ursi (bearberry, kinnikinnick) is a 6- to 12-inch native perennial trailing shrub found in dry, sandy or rocky areas of northern New Jersey and especially the pinelands. Leaves are evergreen, shiny, leathery, entire, and spatula-shaped. Stems are fine-hairy with a thin, reddish bark. Compact clusters of nodding, bell-shaped, white or pinkish flowers appear in April, giving rise to dull red berries.

Native Americans smoked dried leaves as an intoxicating narcotic often diluted with tobacco. In Canada, the mixture was called sagack-homi, and in the United States, kinnikinnick or larb. The plant infusion was used as a diuretic and for dropsy. Stems, leaves, and berries were used in decoction or rubbed for back pain and sprain. The powdered dry leaves were sprinkled on sores, and the whole-plant infusion was used as a hair wash for dandruff and scalp diseases and to promote hair growth for young girls.

Uva-ursi has been known from ancient times as an astringent and

Ericaceae

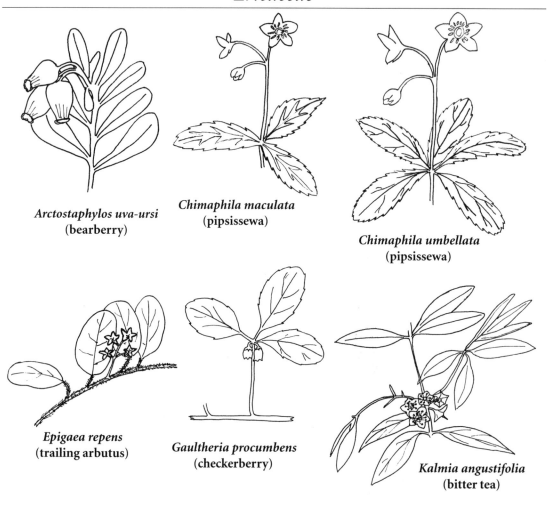

Arctostaphylos uva-ursi
(bearberry)

Chimaphila maculata
(pipsissewa)

Chimaphila umbellata
(pipsissewa)

Epigaea repens
(trailing arbutus)

Gaultheria procumbens
(checkerberry)

Kalmia angustifolia
(bitter tea)

was described in 1601 by Clusius as the hemostat of Galen. Its use in kidney disorders dates to the mid-eighteenth century, and it was admitted to the London Pharmacopoeia in 1763. The urinary diuretic and antiinfective compound arbutin was first isolated in the pure state from this plant in 1853. Leaves also contain gallic acid and tannins.

Bigelow described *Arbutus uva ursi* (upland cranberry) leaves as astringent and tonic; he used them in the treatment of nephritis and "strangury."

Chimaphila maculata (pipsissewa, spotted wintergreen) is a 6- to 10-inch native perennial found in dry, well-drained areas statewide, including the pinelands. Leaves are lance-shaped, toothed, in whorls, and variegated, with white tissue along the veins. Flowers are pinkish white, waxy, and nodding, appearing in late June and giving rise to fruit from July through October.

Native Americans used a root poultice for pain, and the leaf infusion for colds and fever. Tops and roots were used for rheumatism and urinary problems. The infusion was given as an emetic for babies. The plant was also used as a wash for scrofula, cancer, ulcers, and ringworm, and as a poison to kill rats.

Chimaphila umbellata (pipsissewa, prince's pine, ratbane) is a 6- to 12-inch native perennial found in dry, wooded areas statewide. Leaves are evergreen in whorls, dark green, shiny, lance-shaped, and toothed; they appear in late June, with fruit from July through October.

Native Americans used the dried leaves of pipsissewa as a favorite smoking tobacco. A root decoction was used as drops for sore eyes and as a blood medicine. A dried-root decoction was taken for pimples and sores on the face and neck. The plant was also used for rheumatism, kidney trouble, backache, gonorrhea, and consumption. A plant decoction was taken to induce sweating, and an infusion was given to babies for worms. The plant was chewed or a leaf infusion was taken before, during, and after childbirth. A stalk-and-root decoction was taken for stomach cancer.

Epigaea repens (ground laurel, mayflower, trailing arbutus) is a 6- to 12-inch prostrate, trailing native perennial found in moist to dry, acid to peaty areas throughout the state, but most abundant in the pinelands. Leaves are evergreen, hairy, 1 to 3 inches long, alternate, leathery, and entire. Flowers are white to pinkish white, in clusters appearing in early April.

Native Americans used a plant decoction as an emetic for abdominal pains, as a digestive aid, and to control diarrhea in children. It was also used for kidney and chest ailments.

Millspaugh described trailing arbutus as of greater value than uva-ursi or buchu as a treatment for kidney disorders and as a urinary tract sterilant.

Gaultheria procumbens (checkerberry, Jersey tea, partridgeberry, teaberry, wintergreen) is a 2- to 8-inch creeping native perennial found in dry, acidic hardwood areas throughout the state, but most abundant in the pinelands. Leaves are aromatic, alternate, shiny, oval, and entire. Flowers appear in late June and give rise to dry, red, berry-type fruit.

Native Americans chewed the leaves for dysentery and tender gums. Dried leaves were used as a substitute for chewing tobacco. A leaf decoction was taken for colds, fever, rheumatism, and lumbago. The tea was also taken as a spring and fall tonic.

Bigelow described partridgeberry as astringent and aromatic, exactly

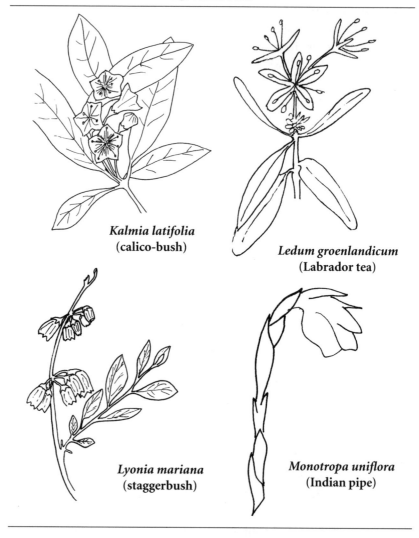

Kalmia latifolia
(calico-bush)

Ledum groenlandicum
(Labrador tea)

Lyonia mariana
(staggerbush)

Monotropa uniflora
(Indian pipe)

resembling black birch (*Betula lenta*). Medicinally, he described it as similar to "cinnamon, being a warm, aromatic astringent, particularly useful in the secondary stage of diarrhea" and "popularly considered an emmenagogue."

Chemically, wintergreen is similar to uva-ursi with the addition of methyl salicilate, also found in the bark of black birch.

Kalmia angustifolia (bitter tea, lambkill, sheep laurel) is a 6-inch to 3-foot native shrub found in dry or wet but usually acid areas throughout the state, including the pinelands. Leaves are opposite, often in whorls, evergreen, entire, elliptical to lance-shaped, but not shiny. Flowers, appearing in late May, are pale to crimson-pink and clustered around the stem.

Native Americans used a leaf-and-twig decoction for bowel complaints. A decoction of leaves, twigs, and flowers was taken as a tonic. A leaf infusion was taken for colds and backache. A crushed-leaf poultice was applied for headache, and the plant was used for pain, swelling, and sprains. The plant was also known to be very poisonous.

Kalmia latifolia (calico-bush, mountain laurel, spoonwood) is a 3- to 30-foot large, native shrub found statewide in rocky woods and clearings, but most abundant in the pinelands. Leaves are evergreen, entire, leathery, pointed at both ends, dark green, and shiny. Flowers, appearing in late May, are pink or waxy white in showy terminal clusters.

Native Americans used a leaf decoction for diarrhea. An infusion was used as a rub for pain and a disinfectant wash for pests. Crushed leaves were used for brier scratches and rheumatism. The plant was known to be poisonous to humans and most animals; however, deer feed on laurel leaves regularly with immunity. Leaves and honey contain toxic diterpenoids known as grayanotoxins. Mountain laurel was used by the Delaware Indians to commit suicide.

Ledum groenlandicum (Labrador tea) is a 1- to 3-foot native shrub found in peaty areas and bogs of northern New Jersey. Leaves are evergreen, entire with rolled-in edges, leathery, oblong, brown-woolly beneath, and fragrant when bruised. Flowers, appearing in late April, are pink, rose, or white in terminal clusters.

Native Americans used a leaf decoction as a diuretic; for stomach pain, asthma, colds, scurvy, kidney problems, rheumatism, and poison ivy; and as a beverage. The leaves are narcotic. A plant poultice was applied or an infusion taken for fever and for jaundice in children. A poultice of fresh-chewed leaves was applied to wounds. The powdered root was used for burns and ulcers, and the boiled and powdered wood was applied to chafed skin. The flower infusion was used for insect sting pain and rheumatism.

Other species of *Ledum*, Pacific Labrador tea and western Labrador tea, are poisonous and similar to *Kalmia*.

Lyonia mariana (staggerbush) is a 1- to 7-foot native shrub, found in sandy or peaty pine thickets of northern and southern New Jersey, including the pinelands. Leaves are oval to oblong, entire, and deciduous. Flowers appear in late May in clusters on leafless branches. Flowers are white or pinkish, bell-shaped, and nodding.

Native Americans used staggerbush infusion for "toe itch," "ground itch," and ulcers.

Monotropa uniflora (corpse plant, Indian pipe) is a 6- to 8-inch, saprophytic (living on dead and decaying plant matter) native perennial found statewide in rich-soiled, moist, wooded areas. Leaves are scale-like, and the entire plant is white or pinkish and waxy. Flowers, appearing in early June, are at first nodding, then upright at fruiting in August.

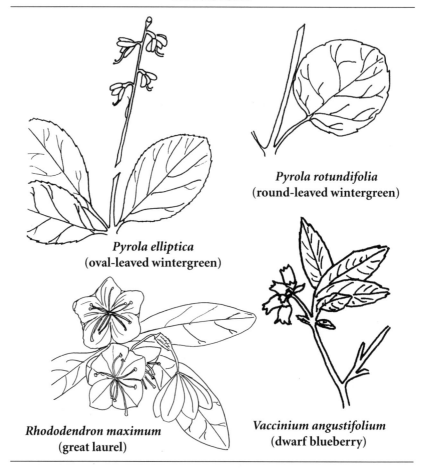

Pyrola rotundifolia
(round-leaved wintergreen)

Pyrola elliptica
(oval-leaved wintergreen)

Rhododendron maximum
(great laurel)

Vaccinium angustifolium
(dwarf blueberry)

Native Americans used the crushed plant as a rub for bunions and warts and the expressed juice as an eyewash. The pulverized root is given for epilepsy and convulsions, and the root infusion is taken for fever and pain associated with colds, and also for "female problems."

Pyrola elliptica (canker lettuce, oval-leaved wintergreen, shinleaf) is a 4-inch to 1-foot native perennial found in dry, rich-soiled, wooded areas of northern and southern New Jersey. Leaves are thin and elliptical, and in a basal rosette. Flowers are white or greenish white, appearing in June.

Native Americans used shinleaf to heal cuts and sores; a root and leaf decoction was given to babies with fits or epileptic seizures. A leaf infusion was used as a gargle for sores or cankers, and a plant decoction was used as drops for inflamed eyelids, sore eyes, and sties. A crushed-plant poultice was applied to tumors.

Pyrola rotundifolia (round-leaved wintergreen, shinleaf) is a 4-inch to 1-foot native perennial found in moist or dry, wooded areas of northern and southern New Jersey. Leaves are in a basal rosette but are more leathery, thicker, larger, and shinier than those of *P. elliptica*, with similar flowers.

Native Americans used shinleaf to heal cuts and sores.

Rhododendron maximum (great laurel, rose bay, white laurel) is a 10- to 14-foot native shrub or tree that forms thickets and is found in moist, wooded areas and swamps of northern and occasionally southern New Jersey. Leaves are evergreen, large and leathery, fine-woolly beneath, with edges rolled under. Flowers are white and spotted or rose-pink, appearing in showy clusters in June.

Native Americans used a leaf infusion for heart trouble and as an external analgesic for pain.

Vaccinium angustifolium (dwarf blueberry, low sweet blueberry, narrow-leaved blueberry) is a 3-inch to 2-foot native perennial shrub found in dry, open, sandy areas statewide. Leaves are lance-shaped, finely toothed, green, and hairless on both sides. Flowers are small, bell-shaped, solitary, or in small clusters, appearing in late April, with edible fruit in late June.

Native Americans used a leaf infusion to "purify the blood" and placed dried flowers on hot rocks to produce an inhalant as a psychological aid for "crazyness."

Vaccinium oxycoccos (*Oxycoccus microcarpus*) (European cranberry, small cranberry) is a 4- to 10-inch rare native, evergreen, creeping perennial found in wet boggy or peaty soils of northern New Jersey. Leaves are small and ovate or triangular. Flowers appear from April through July, giving rise to small berries becoming red or white when ripe. The specific name, *oxycoccos*, means "sour berry."

Native Americans took a whole-plant infusion to relieve mild nausea.

043 *Euphorbiaceae*

The spurge family of herbs, shrubs, and trees, usually with milky sap that is often acrid. Leaves are simple or compound; alternate, opposite, or whorled. This is one of the largest families of flowering plants and includes poinsettias, castor bean, croton, cassava, Mexican jumping beans, and *Hevea*, the chief rubber tree of commerce. Distribution is worldwide, but concentrated in the tropics. *Ricinus communis* (castor bean) seeds contain the protein ricin, which causes serious poisoning or death when the seeds are ingested. The seasonally popular poinsettias (*Euphorbia pulcherrima*) may cause temporary blindness due to toxic terpenes in the latex.

Euphorbia corollata (flowering spurge, milkweed, tramp's spurge, wild

Euphorbiaceae

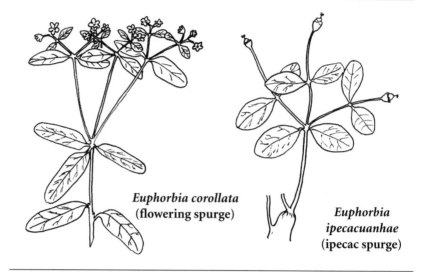

**Euphorbia corollata
(flowering spurge)**

**Euphorbia
ipecacuanhae
(ipecac spurge)**

hippo) is a 1- to 3-foot native perennial found in dry fields and along roadsides of southern New Jersey and the southern portion of northern New Jersey. Leaves are alternate, entire, oval to linear without stalks, and in a whorl at the top of the stem. The plant is deep-rooted and smooth-stemmed, with a milky juice. Flowers are white, arising in early June from the whorled leaves in an open cluster.

Native Americans used a decoction prepared with other herbs for cancer and venereal diseases, as a purgative, and to stop bleeding after childbirth. The milk was used as an ointment for sores, especially on children's heads, and sore nipples. The root decoction was taken for rheumatism, urinary diseases, and as an emetic. A crushed-root infusion was taken as a physic before eating. Bigelow described flowering spurge as a very active cathartic, and in large doses emetic.

Flowering spurge honey can cause vomiting and purging. The milky juice can cause severe skin irritation similar to poison ivy. "Burns" caused by skin contact are sufficiently permanent to make the juice useful as a branding agent for cattle.

Euphorbia ipecacuanhae (ipecac spurge, wild spurge) is a 6-inch to 1-foot perennial found in dry, sandy areas of the pinelands. The root is large, giving rise to several smooth, succulent, underground stems with milky juice. The leaves are green to red-purple, opposite or in small rosettes, entire, and fleshy. Flowers are solitary on long stalks, yellow-green, without petals, and appear in late April, before the leaves.

Native Americans used ipecac spurge as an emetic, diaphoretic, and expectorant. In small doses it was used to "stop violent hemorrhaging from the lungs and womb."

Bigelow described the effects of ipecac spurge as differing from the violent catharsis and emesis associated with other members of the genus *Euphorbia* in that the plant is "milder in its operation" and described a number of "experiments on its action . . . at the Boston Dispensary and Almshouse" to establish the proper dosages.

044 *Fagaceae*

The beech family of trees and shrubs. The best known are the oaks. The family is primarily distributed in the temperate regions.

Fagus grandifolia (American beech) is an 80- to 120-foot large native tree found in well-drained, moist, rich-soiled, wooded areas throughout the state. Leaves are alternate, oval, sharp-toothed, dark bluish green above and yellowish green beneath, and persisting through the winter. Leaf veins, 9 to 14 pairs, are silky underneath, and the bark is smooth and gray. Flowers appear in late April, producing edible triangular nuts in the fall.

Native Americans used leaves to treat chancre and a leaf decoction for burns or scalds and frostbite. The bark was used for abortions and pulmonary troubles. The nut was chewed for worms.

Quercus alba (white oak) is a 60- to 120-foot native tree found in dry, wooded areas statewide, including the pinelands. Leaves are without sharp tips, but with 4 to 10 evenly rounded lobes. They are whitish

Fagaceae

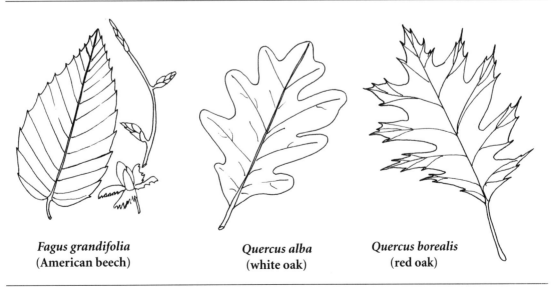

Fagus grandifolia
(American beech)

Quercus alba
(white oak)

Quercus borealis
(red oak)

beneath when mature. Acorns are $^3/_4$ inch long and light brown, with a bowl-shaped crown covering $^1/_4$ to $^1/_3$ of its length.

Native Americans used the astringent bark for indigestion, diarrhea, chronic dysentery, asthma, laryngitis, coughs, chills and fevers, sore throat, and bleeding piles, and as an expectorant, douche, tonic, antiseptic, emetic, and a liniment for muscular pains in humans and horses. The bark was chewed for mouth sores.

Bigelow described white oak bark as a poor substitute for cinchona, useful as an external astringent and antiseptic. A strong tea was used as a gargle for cynanche (serious sore throat), as a lotion for gangrenous ulcers, and for "offensive discharges."

Quercus borealis (*Q. rubra*) (gray oak, northern red oak) is a 60- to 120-foot native tree found in dry or moist, swampy areas statewide. Leaves are thin and dull, with 7 to 10 sharply tipped lobes. Acorns are $^1/_3$ covered by the cap.

Native Americans used the astringent bark decoction for indigestion, chronic dysentery, sore throat, lung troubles, and chapped skin, and as a tonic, antiseptic, and emetic. A bark infusion was given to children "old enough to walk but too weak to do so" and was used as a wash for "bad smelling sores of the head or feet." A poultice of powdered bark was applied to ruptured or improperly healed navels. The bark was chewed for mouth sores, and a root bark infusion was taken for gonorrhea.

045 *Fumariaceae*

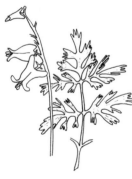

**Dicentra cucullaria
(dutchman's breeches)**

The fumitory family of herbs and vines; sometimes included in the poppy (Papaveraceae) family. Leaves are usually alternate, dissected, and divided into narrow segments. Flowers are in racemes, and fruits are capsules or nutlets. The family is essentially limited to the Northern Hemisphere.

Dicentra cucullaria (dutchman's breeches) is a 5- to 9-inch native perennial found in well-drained, moist, wooded areas of northern and occasionally southern New Jersey. Leaves are highly divided and basal. Flowers are white with yellow tips. They appear in early April and look like upside-down pairs of inflated pantaloons.

Native Americans used the leaf infusion as a component in a liniment for muscle ache.

046 *Gentianaceae*

The gentian family of herbaceous and, rarely, woody plants. Leaves are simple or trifoliate. Leaf venation may suggest a monocot, but this is a dicotyledonous, large family distributed globally though concentrated in temperate regions.

Gentiana crinita (fringed gentian) is a 1- to 3-foot native perennial found in wet or moist, open areas throughout northern New Jersey and in a few areas of southern New Jersey. Leaves are opposite, clasping, lance-shaped, and entire. Violet-blue flowers with fringed lobes appear in September.

Native Americans used a root infusion as a "stomach strengthener" and "blood purifier."

Gentiana quinquefolia (agueweed, stiff gentian) is a 2- to 2^1/$_2$-inch native perennial found in rich-soiled, wooded, moist or dry areas of northern New Jersey. The stem has four distinct ridges. Leaves are opposite, clasping, pointed-oval, and entire. Pale-violet, toothed clusters of flowers appear in September.

Native Americans used stiff gentian as a remedy for dyspepsia and for "weak stomach and hysterical affections," worms, and stomachache. A plant infusion was taken for diarrhea or "sore chest," and a root infusion was used as a tonic, stimulant, laxative, and cathartic. Expressed root juice was used to stop hemorrhage.

Menyanthes trifoliata (bogbean, buckbean, marsh buckbean, pondweed) was classified in the Menyanthaceae, a widely distributed family of aquatic or bog plants, formally distinguished from the Gentianaceae by their basal or alternate leaves. The genus *Menyanthes*, now placed in the Gentianaceae, has the bogbean as its only native species, found in shallow water of bogs and swamps in northern and occasionally southern New Jersey. Leaves are cloverlike, with three oval leaflets, and arise from the root. Flowers, appearing in late April, are pinkish white and hairy in a raceme on a naked stem.

Native Americans used a root infusion for gas pains, constipation, and rheumatism. A root or leaf decoction was taken as an antiemetic for a sick stomach and to gain weight during influenza. A decoction of ground stems and roots was taken as an antihemorrhagic for "spitting of blood and other internal diseases."

Bigelow described buckbean as a good tonic in small doses. In large doses it was diaphoretic, emetic, and purgative, and had been used in intermittent fevers, skin diseases, rheumatism, dropsy, and worms.

Sabatia angularis (bitter bloom, rose-pink, square-stemmed centaury) is a 1- to 3-foot native perennial found in well-drained, rich-soiled, moist

Gentianaceae

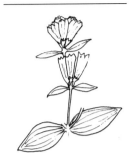

**Gentiana quinquefolia
(stiff gentian)**

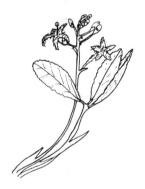

**Menyanthes trifoliata
(bogbean)**

areas statewide. The stem is sharply four-square with opposite, clasping, pointed-oval leaves. Flowers are pink, five-petaled, and appear in July.

Native Americans used rose-pink to prepare an analgesic infusion as a gynecologic aid for menstrual pains.

Geraniaceae

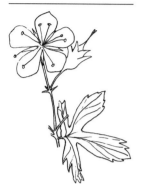

Geranium maculatum
(wild geranium)

047 *Geraniaceae*

The geranium family of herbs. The leaves are simple or compound. The family occurs in temperate and subtropical regions.

Erodium cicutarium (alfilaria, alfileria, filaree, pin-clover) is a 3-inch to 1-foot naturalized annual or biennial weed found in waste areas of northern and southern New Jersey. Leaves are opposite or in a basal rosette and pinnately divided. Flowers arise from leaf axils in April. Flowers are pink to purple, $1/2$ inch in diameter, and in long-stalked umbels.

Native Americans used pin-clover for wildcat, bobcat, and mountain lion bites and as a disinfectant. A leaf infusion was used for typhoid fever.

Geranium maculatum (cranesbill, spotted geranium, wild geranium) is a 1- to 2-foot native perennial found in well-drained, wooded areas of northern and southern New Jersey. Leaves are broad and deeply cleft into three to five toothed lobes. Flowers are pink, rose-purple, or white, 1 to $1^1/2$ inches wide, appearing in late April.

Native Americans used wild geranium as a styptic and to remove canker sores, close open wounds, and "clean out the innards." Combined with fox grapes it was used as a children's mouthwash for thrush. The dried, pulverized root was put in the mouth to treat sores. The root infusion is a powerful astringent and was used to treat diarrhea, "the venereal," pyorrhea, sore gums, toothache, heart trouble and neuralgia. A root decoction was also used as a wash for sores on the face or parts infected with "itch." The root decoction poultice was applied to burns, and a crushed-root poultice was applied to piles. A poultice of chewed or powdered root was applied to the severed umbilical cord or one that would not heal.

Bigelow described cranesbill as a very useful astringent especially for diarrhea and mouth and throat ulcers, for which the tea was used as a gargle.

048 *Graminea (Poaceae)*

The grass family of annual or perennial herbs and giant, woody reeds or bamboos. Stems are often rhizomes with leaves basal or alternate. The fruit is a caryopsis.

Agropyron repens (crouch grass, quick wheatgrass, witch wheatgrass) is a 3-foot native grass that spreads by means of a yellow rhizome and is found in sandy waterside areas and in fields and gardens throughout the state, differing from other *Agropyron* species in that the flower spike is not square.

Native Americans used crouch grass infusion for bedwetting and gravel, and in decoction, externally as a wash for swollen legs.

Andropogon gerardi (big bluestem, forked beardgrass) is a 4- to 7-foot coarse native grass found in dry areas and meadows statewide. Plants are in large clumps, with bluish stems and purplish or bronze-green flowers in racemes.

Native Americans used bluestem root decoction as an analgesic for stomach pain and as a diuretic. The blade decoction was a febrifuge used as a wash for fevers and was also taken as a stimulant.

Arundinaria gigantea (*A. tecta*) (cane, cane-brake, giant cane) is a 10-foot woody-stemmed, bamboolike, rare native grass found in moist or shallow-water areas of Cape May County. The leaves are lance-shaped and in fan-shaped clusters. Flowers, seen in states to the south, appear in racemes on leafy branches in April. Cane does not flower in New Jersey.

Native Americans used the root decoction as a kidney stimulant and for breast pain.

Hierochloe odorata (holy grass, sweet grass. vanilla grass) is a 1- to 2-foot spreading native grass on a slender rhizome. It is found in brackish areas along the eastern coast of northern and southern New Jersey. Leaves are vanilla-scented and in clumps arising from dead foliage of the previous growing season. Flowers, in pyramidal clusters, appear in April.

Native Americans used sweet grass as a ceremonial medicine (incense) and in a wash for the hair and body.

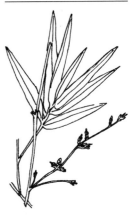

Graminea

Arundinaria gigantea (cane-brake)

049 *Hamamelidaceae*

The witch-hazel family of shrubs and trees. The leaves are simple, toothed or lobed, and alternate. The family is primarily East Asian, with genera in Africa, Australia, and eastern North America.

Hamamelis virginiana (devil's tea, witch hazel) is a 5- to 15-foot native shrub or small tree, found in rich, well-drained wooded areas of northern and southern New Jersey. Leaves are 2 to 5 inches long, oval, and wavy-toothed. Flowers are in axillary clusters, yellow, with long, slender petals, appearing in late fall, often after leaf drop.

Native Americans used witch hazel for toothache, an infusion for sore

Hamamelidaceae

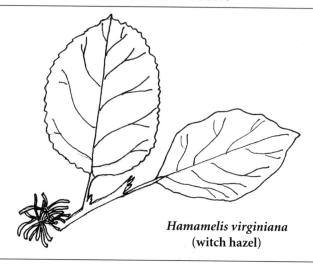

Hamamelis virginiana
(witch hazel)

throat and menstrual pain, for colds, and as a wash for sores and abrasions. The bark infusion was taken for tuberculosis, to stimulate appetite, as an emetic, and as an astringent. The inner-bark infusion was used as a skin lotion and as a wash for sore eyes. Twig bark infusion was taken for bloody dysentery and cholera, and twigs were used as a steam for sore muscles. Twig decoctions were used to regulate kidneys, and bark poultices were applied to bruises.

Liquidamber styraciflua (bilsted, sweet gum) is a 20- to 125-foot native tree found in rich-soiled, wet, wooded areas of northern and southern New Jersey. Leaves are maplelike, with five to seven toothed, pointed lobes. Leaves are pine-scented when bruised. Fruit is spherical and prickly.

Native Americans used sweet gum rosin or inner bark for diarrhea and dysentery. The bark and inner-bark infusion were taken as a gynecological aid for nervousness and for night sickness. A plant decoction was used as a poultice for cuts and bruises, and a root tea was applied to skin sores thought to be caused by worms. The gum was used as a "drawing plaster" and was placed in the dog's nose for distemper.

050 *Hippocastanaceae*

The buckeye family of shrubs and trees. The leaves are deciduous, opposite, and palmate, with three to nine serrate leaflets. Most species are found in the northern temperate zone, and approximately 25 species are native to North America.

Aesculus hippocastanum (buckeye, horse chestnut) is a tree growing

Hippocastanaceae

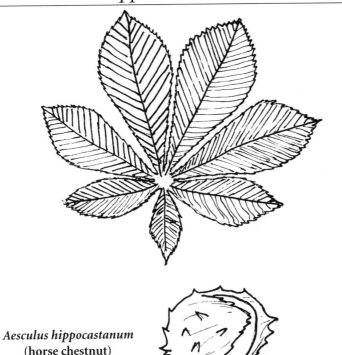

Aesculus hippocastanum
(horse chestnut)

to 100 feet and is naturalized in northern New Jersey. Leaves are divided into seven toothed leaflets. Fruit is spherical with a prickly husk.

Native Americans considered horse chestnuts a sure cure for rheumatism and hemorrhoids. They were prepared either as a decoction or as a salve prepared in lard. The boiled and washed seeds were used as livestock food. The bitter taste is also reduced and converted to a somewhat sweet taste by germination, and the nuts then become edible.

Leaves, bark, flowers, twigs, and seeds contain esculin (6,7–dihydroxycoumarin-6–glucoside), which probably accounts for the reported poisonings of children and livestock. Hydrolysis of esculin during germination may account for the reported development of a sweet taste in the seeds.

051 *Hydrophyllaceae*

The waterleaf family of herbs and shrubs. The leaves are simple, entire to pinnate, or palmately divided. The family is distributed globally, with the exception of Australia.

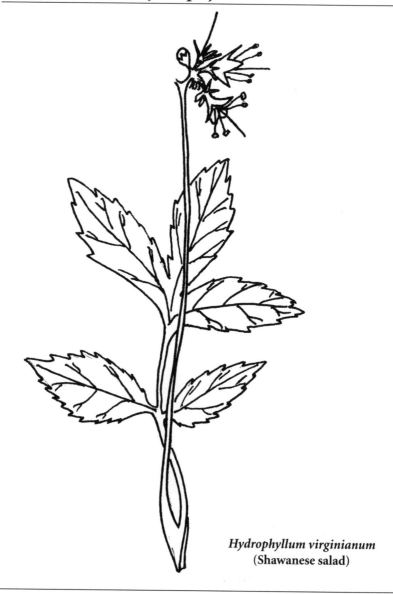

Hydrophyllum virginianum
(Shawanese salad)

Hydrophyllum virginianum (John's cabbage, Shawanese salad, Virginia waterleaf) is a 1- to 3-foot native perennial found in rich-soiled, moist areas of northern and southern New Jersey. Leaves are alternate, deeply divided into five to seven toothed lobes, and edible. Flowers are white to lavender, bell-shaped, and nodding, with protruding stamens. Flowers appear in May.

Native Americans used Virginia waterleaf root as an antidiarrheal "good for man, woman, or child." A chewed-root decoction was used as a wash for cracked lips and mouth sores.

052 *Hypericaceae (Clusiaceae, Guttiferae)*

The St.-John's-wort family of herbs, shrubs, trees, and woody vines. The leaves are opposite, simple, entire, and dotted with resinous glands. The flowers are regular, with many stamens and berry or capsular fruit. The family is primarily tropical, but extends into the temperate regions.

Hypericum perforatum (common St.-John's-wort) is a 1- to 3-foot naturalized perennial weed found in waste areas statewide. Leaves are opposite, narrowly oblong, entire, and dotted with translucent glands. Flowers, appearing in late June, are golden-yellow with petals black-dotted along the margins.

Native Americans used a plant infusion for bloody diarrhea, bowel complaints, fever, and as a cough medicine. The crushed plant was sniffed for nosebleed. The root was chewed, swallowed, or poulticed for snakebite. The root infusion was used as a wash for infants.

St.-John's-wort is an antidepressive in humans while causing poisoning in animals (shedding of wool and blindness) and photosensitivity in livestock and humans.

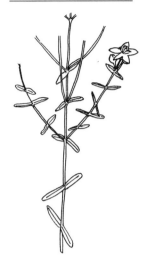

Hypericum perforatum
(**common St.-John's-wort**)

053 *Iridaceae*

The iris family of monocotyledonous perennial herbs with underground stems as bulbs, corms, or rhizomes, producing leaflets or leafy flower stems. Family distribution is global, but concentrated in Africa.

Iris versicolor (larger blue flag) is a 1- to 2-foot native perennial found in shallow water and other wet areas of northern and southern New Jersey. Leaves are alternate, swordlike, entire and $1/2$ to 1 inch wide. Blue flowers, 4 inches wide, appear in late May.

Native Americans used blue flag to treat sore throat and as a powerful cathartic. The root poultice was applied to swellings, scrofulous sores, burns, and earache. A crushed-root infusion was taken to induce paralysis, as an emetic, and at menses to induce conception. The root was also used for liver and kidney problems, colds, lung problems, and rheumatism.

Bigelow described blue flag root as emetic and cathartic, and in small doses diuretic.

Sisyrinchium angustifolium (blue star flower grass, northern blue-eyed-grass, pointed blue-eyed-grass) is a 4- to 18-inch native perennial found in moist, open areas statewide. Leaves are basal, $1/4$ inch wide, entire, and deep green. The lower stem is flattened or winged. Flowers are pale blue at the end of a long, flat stalk and appear in May.

Native Americans used the cooked greens as food for "regular

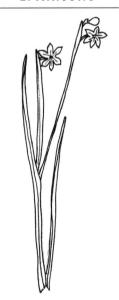

Sisyrinchium angustifolium
(**blue-eyed-grass**)

bowels." A root infusion was given to children for diarrhea, and the whole-plant infusion was taken for stomach troubles and worms. A decoction was taken before morning meals for constipation.

054 *Juglandaceae*

The walnut family of trees, cultivated mainly for their edible seeds and hard wood. Leaves are pinnate, and staminate flowers are in catkins. The fruit is a nut. The family occurs in Europe, Asia, and North America.

Juglans cinerea (butternut, white walnut) is a native tree of up to 80 feet found in rich-soiled, hardwood areas of northern and southern New Jersey. Leaves are pinnate, with 7 to 17 opposite, toothed leaflets. Fruit is egg-shaped and sticky on the surface. The nut is rough and furrowed.

Native Americans used a bark infusion as an antidiarrheal, and the infusion or chewed bark was applied to wounds to stop bleeding. Syrup prepared from the sap or pills prepared from the inner bark were used as cathartics. The expressed juice was used for toothache, and a shoot decoction was taken for venereal disease and as a laxative.

Bigelow described butternut bark as laxative and of use in dysentery. The most medicinally active bark was the inner bark of the root.

Juglans nigra (black walnut) is a native tree of up to 120 feet found in moist, rich- and deep-soiled areas of northern and southern New Jersey. Leaves are pinnate, with 12 to 23 almost alternate, toothed leaflets. Fruit is spherical.

Native Americans regarded black walnut bark as poisonous but chewed it for toothache and used an infusion to wash sores and as an emetic or cathartic. The bark poultice was applied to the head for headache, and an inner-bark infusion was taken for smallpox. A root bark

Juglandaceae

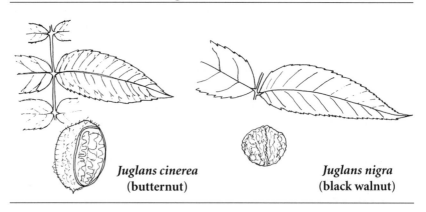

Juglans cinerea
(butternut)

Juglans nigra
(black walnut)

decoction was used to kill intestinal worms and prevent dysentery. A leaf infusion was taken for goiter, and a crushed-leaf decoction was taken for "blood pressure." Crushed leaves or juice from the hull of green fruit was used as a rub for ringworm. The sap was applied to any inflammation, and the nutshell infusion was used as a wash for "the itch." The leaves were scattered about the house to repel fleas.

055 *Labiatae (Lamiaceae)*

The mint family of aromatic herbs, shrubs, trees, and woody vines. Leaves may be simple or pinnate. Distribution of the family is global.

Agastache nepetoides (catnip giant-hyssop, yellow giant-hyssop) is a 2- to 5-foot native perennial found in rich-soiled, open areas and wood edges of northern and southern New Jersey. Leaves are opposite, pointed-ovate, and toothed, on a square stem. Pale green flowers in dense spikes appear in late July.

Native Americans used yellow giant-hyssop as a component in a wash for poison ivy and itch.

Collinsonia canadensis (horse balm, rich weed, stoneroot) is a 2- to 5-foot native perennial found in rich-soiled, moist areas of northern and southern New Jersey. Leaves are opposite, pointed-oval, and toothed, and produce a citronella fragrance when bruised. Loose-clustered flowers are light yellow and lemon-scented with protruding stamens; they appear in August.

Native Americans used a plant decoction as an emetic and as a treatment for swollen breasts. A poultice of powdered leaves was applied to the head for headache. The root decoction was used as a soak for rheumatic pains of the foot, back, or leg and was taken for heart or kidney trouble. A crushed-root infusion was given to children for listlessness and was used as a wash for weak babies.

Cunila origanoides (common dittany, stone mint) is a 6-inch to 2-foot native perennial found in dry or rocky, open-wooded areas of northern and southern New Jersey. Stems are stiff and branched, with leaves pointed-oval and toothed. Loose clusters of purplish flowers appear in August on stem tips and in upper axils.

Native Americans used the infusion as a tonic and stimulant; for colds, headache, and fever; and to induce perspiration.

Glecoma hederacea (gill-over-the-ground, ground ivy) is a creeping, ivylike, naturalized perennial weed found in moist, shaded waste areas statewide. Leaves are opposite and roundish, with scalloped margins, some with a purple tinge. Whorls of axillary, blue-violet, two-lipped flowers appear in April.

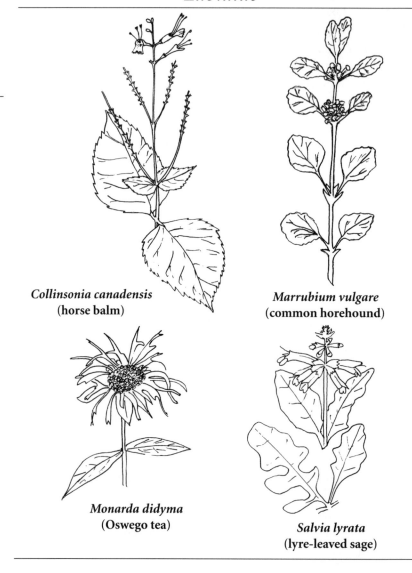

Collinsonia canadensis
(horse balm)

Marrubium vulgare
(common horehound)

Monarda didyma
(Oswego tea)

Salvia lyrata
(lyre-leaved sage)

Native Americans used a ground ivy infusion for measles, colds, and babies' hives.

In Chinese medicine, the dried or fresh whole plant is used to prepare a decoction for internal or external use. It is used to treat influenza, infantile marasmus (progressive emaciation), urinary tract stones, bruises, sores, and rheumatoid arthritis.

Hedeoma pulegioides (American pennyroyal, false pennyroyal, pudding-grass) is a 4- to 18-inch native annual weed found in dry, open areas statewide. Leaves are opposite, small, lance-shaped, and entire or toothed on a soft-hairy stem. Bluish white flowers are whorled in the leaf axils and appear in late July.

Native Americans used a root decoction for colds and a cold infusion for application to the forehead for itching eyes. The plant infusion was taken for "obstructed menses," fever, diarrhea, kidney and liver problems, and menstrual pain, and as a stimulant, diaphoretic, and expectorant. A leaf infusion was taken for stomach pains. Crushed leaves were held in the mouth for toothache, a leaf poultice was applied for headache, and leaves were rubbed on the body to repel insects.

Bigelow described American pennyroyal as a warm aromatic that is heating, carminative, diaphoretic, and an emmenagogue.

The essential oil is highly toxic. When ingested it may cause liver damage and abortion.

Leonurus cardiaca (motherwort) is a 2- to 5-foot naturalized perennial weed found in open areas and roadsides throughout the state. Leaves are opposite, with three toothed lobes. Lilac or purple flowers are in axillary whorls and appear in June.

Native Americans used motherwort as a stimulant against fainting, "nervous and hysterical affections," "diseases of the stomach," and "ills peculiar to women."

Lycopus americanus (cut-leaved water horehound, water horehound) is a 1- to 2-foot native perennial found in wet or moist areas statewide. Leaves are opposite, with upper leaves toothed and lower leaves lobed oaklike. White flowers in axillary whorls appear in July.

Native Americans used the whole plant in a compound medication for stomach cramps.

Lycopus virginicus (purple water-horehound, Virginia bugleweed, wild horehound) is a 1- to 3-foot native perennial found in wet or moist areas statewide. Leaves are opposite, lance-shaped, toothed, and dark green or purple. Flowers are white in axillary whorls, appearing in July.

Native Americans used the chewed root to treat snakebite and gave the chewed root to infants to improve speech. The plant infusion was taken at the "green corn ceremony." The roots and leaves were regarded as poisonous.

Marrubium vulgare (American horehound, common horehound, water horehound, white horehound) is a 1- to 2-foot escaped perennial weed found scattered throughout the state in waste places and along roadsides. Leaves are opposite, round-oval, deeply veined (wrinkled), and toothed. The entire plant is white-woolly. Flowers are white and inconspicuous in axillary whorls, appearing in early summer.

Native Americans used common horehound infusion for "breast complaints." It was taken for hoarseness, colds, whooping cough, stomachache, diarrhea, and influenza. The infusion or decoction was mixed with sugar to make a cough syrup, and a heated leaf salve was used on boils. The root was used before and after childbirth, and branches were used to whip aching body parts as a circulatory stimulant.

Bigelow described horehound as tonic, diuretic, and laxative, and a remedy for coughs, catarrh, and catamenial irregularities.

Melissa officinalis (balm, garden balm, lemon balm) is a 1- to 2-foot escaped perennial weed found in open areas and shaded edges of woods statewide. Leaves are opposite, pointed-oval, and toothed. Flowers are whitish in axillary whorls and appear in July.

Native Americans used a balm plant decoction for colic in infants, typhus fever, and colds, and as a stimulant and tonic.

Mentha aquatica (water mint) is a 1- to 2-foot escaped weed found in scattered moist or wet, open areas of northern and southern New Jersey. Leaves are opposite, rounded-oval, and toothed. Flowers are pale purple in terminal clusters, appearing in August.

Native Americans used water mint leaf infusion or decoction for colds and stomach troubles.

Mentha arvensis (*M. canadensis*) (corn mint, mint, wild mint) is a 6-inch to 2-foot native perennial found in moist or wet, open areas statewide, but concentrated in the northern part of the state. Leaves are opposite, pointed-oblong, and toothed. Flowers are lilac in axillary whorls, appearing in July.

Native Americans used the sweetened infusion as a beverage. The whole-plant decoction was taken for stomach pain, fever, coughs, colds, headache, croup, and pleurisy, and as an antidiarrheal, sedative, and hair oil. Ground leaves and stems were taken as an antiemetic and to strengthen heart muscle and other vital organs. They were applied as a poultice for pain and swelling. A leaf-and-plant-tip infusion was given to children with colic. The plant was chewed or a plant infusion (without the root) was taken to "keep cool." Leaves and tops were used as an herbal sweatbath for cold and rheumatic pains.

Mentha piperita (peppermint) is a 1- to 3-foot naturalized perennial found in moist and wet areas statewide. Stems are purple, with the leaves opposite, pointed-oblong, and toothed. Flowers are pale purple in interrupted terminal spikes, appearing in June.

Native Americans used peppermint infusion for fevers, colds, and colic; as an antiemetic; and to relieve hysterics and to flavor foods and other medicines. It was taken for gravel and suppressed urine, bowel problems, and infant cholera, and to treat adults and children for worms. A tincture was applied externally to piles.

Bigelow described peppermint as a valued carminative.

Mentha spicata (spearmint) is a 6-inch to 3-foot naturalized, spreading perennial found in moist or wet, open areas statewide. Leaves are opposite, essentially stalkless, lance-shaped, and toothed. Flowers are pale pink on slender, interrupted spikes, appearing in June.

Native Americans used spearmint as they did peppermint and also snuffed the dried, powdered plant or applied a cold infusion to the head for headache. The infusion was also used as a sedative and as an emetic for children.

Bigelow described spearmint as used for the same purposes as peppermint, but less pleasant in taste.

Monarda didyma (bee balm, horsemint, Oswego tea) is a 2- to 5-foot native perennial found in rich-soiled, moist, wooded areas and along streams of northern and southern New Jersey. Leaves are opposite, pointed, and toothed. Flowers are scarlet in dense heads and with protruding stamens. Bracts of the flower head are reddish. This is a colorful wildflower, extensively cultivated in gardens, and although native, it has also escaped. Flowers appear in July.

Native Americans used horsemint for "female obstructions," as a carminative for colic and flatulence, as a sedative, as a diuretic for heart trouble, to "bring out measles," and as a diaphoretic to "sweat off flu." A leaf poultice was used for headaches and colds.

Bigelow described horsemint as a warm diaphoretic, antiemetic, and carminative used in flatulent colic, rheumatism, and so on.

Monarda fistulosa (horsemint, wild bergamot) is a 2- to 3-foot native perennial found in moist or dry, open areas of northern and southern New Jersey. Leaves are opposite, pointed, toothed, and grayish in color. Flowers are lavender or pink in dense heads with protruding stamens. Bracts of the flower heads are tinged with pink. Flowers appear in July.

Native Americans used wild bergamot as they did *M. didyma* and also placed chewed leaves in the nostrils for headache. A blossom-and-root decoction was used for worms. A blossom-and-leaf infusion or decoction was used as a wash for pimples and taken for abdominal pains. A leaf tea was taken as a cathartic, as a bath for chills, and as a lotion for gunshot or arrow wounds. A poultice of moistened dry flowers and leaves was applied to burns and scalds, and the steam from boiling plants was inhaled for catarrh and pulmonary problems.

Monarda punctata (dotted monarda, horsemint, spotted horsemint) is a 1- to 4-foot native perennial found in dry, open areas of central and southern New Jersey. Leaves are opposite, lance-shaped, and toothed. Flowers are yellowish and purple-spotted, with protruding stamens, in mintlike, axillary, dense whorls.

Native Americans used spotted horsemint infusion as a face wash for fever, and it was taken or applied as a poultice for colds, headache, coughs, fever, and stomach and bowel problems.

Nepeta cataria (catmint, catnip) is a 1- to 3-foot naturalized perennial found in open areas statewide. Stems are grayish with opposite, heart-shaped, toothed leaves. Flowers are whitish with purple dots; in short, tight spikes; and appearing in June.

Native Americans used catnip infusion for "female obstruction" hysterics, worms, colic, spasms, babies' colds, and hives, and as a stimulant and tonic, a laxative and astringent for diarrhea, an antiemetic in fever, a diaphoretic and sedative, and a wash to raise the body temperature. It was used with honey to prepare a cough syrup for colds, and a leaf poultice was used for boils and swellings. Dried leaves were smoked in a pipe for rheumatism.

Perilla frutescens (beefsteak plant, yellow perilla) is a 1- to 3-foot naturalized annual weed found in moist, open areas of northern New Jersey. Leaves are opposite, oval, and toothed, with wavy margins. Flowers are whitish in axillary and terminal clusters, appearing in July.

Native Americans used yellow perilla as an ingredient in a "blood medicine."

In Chinese medicine, a decoction of the whole plant is used as a prophylactic for epidemic influenza, colds, and malaria; to control vomiting especially associated with seafood poisoning; as a digestive aid in flatulence; and to calm a restless fetus.

Prunella vulgaris (carpenter weed, heal-all, selfheal) is a native perennial weed of less than 1 foot found in waste and other well-drained, open areas statewide. This is a very common weed of lawns. Leaves are opposite, lance-shaped, and entire. Flowers are purple in a compact terminal head and appear in June.

Native Americans used a weak root, leaf, and blossom decoction for the heart; as a wash for burns, colds, coughs, and diarrhea; as an antiemetic and emetic; for backache, boils, stomach cramps, and gas; and to strengthen the womb. A stalk infusion was used for dysentery, especially in babies.

Pycnanthemum incanum (hoary mountain mint, mint) is a 1- to 3-foot native perennial found in dry, open or wooded areas statewide. Leaves are opposite, oval to lance-shaped, toothed, and pale greenish white. Flowers are pale lilac in axillary whorls, appearing in July.

Native Americans used a leaf poultice or infusion for headache, fevers, cold, heart trouble, upset stomach, and as a stimulating bath particularly useful for an inflamed penis. Soaked plants were inserted in the nose for bleeding, and an infusion taken with green corn was used to prevent diarrhea.

Pycnanthemum virginianum (Virginia mountain mint) is a 2- to 4-foot native perennial found in moist areas of northern New Jersey. Leaves are opposite, lance-shaped, and entire. Flowers are pale lilac in compact terminal clusters, appearing in July.

Native Americans used an infusion prepared from plant tops for chills and fever and a powdered-root decoction for "stoppage of periods."

Salvia lyrata (blue sage, cancer weed, lyre-leaved sage) is a 1- to 2-foot native perennial found in well-drained sandy areas of central and southern New Jersey. Leaves are mostly basal and lobed, and form a rosette. Stem leaves are opposite and mostly entire. Flowers are violet in interrupted whorls on a spike appearing in May.

Native Americans used a blue sage infusion as an antidiarrheal and as a laxative as well as for colds, coughs, and nervous debility. A root salve was applied to sores, and a syrup of leaves and honey was taken for asthma. The syrup was also mildly diaphoretic.

Scutellaria elliptica (hairy skullcap) is a 1- to 2-foot native perennial found in dry, open or wooded areas statewide. The stem is hairy, with leaves opposite, oval, and toothed. Flowers are blue, growing in paired axillary racemes, appearing in June.

Native Americans used the root infusion for monthly periods and diarrhea. A decoction was taken for "nerves."

Scutellaria lateriflora (mad dog skullcap) is a 1- to 3-foot native perennial found in rich-soiled woods and wet, shaded areas statewide. Leaves are opposite, pointed-oval, and toothed. Flowers are blue or violet, growing in paired axillary racemes, and appearing in June.

Native Americans used mad dog skullcap as they used hairy skullcap but also used a powdered-root infusion to prevent smallpox and to "keep the throat clean."

Teucrium canadense (American germander, wood sage) is a 1- to 4-foot native perennial found in moist areas and thickets statewide. Leaves are opposite, pointed-oval, toothed, and white-hairy beneath. Flowers are purplish in spikes with upward-protruding stamens; they appear in June.

Native Americans apparently did not use wood sage for medicinal purposes. The leaf infusion is diuretic and diaphoretic, and has been described as abortifacient.

Thymus serpyllum (creeping thyme, wild thyme) is a prostrate, naturalized perennial weed found in dry, open areas of northern New Jersey. Leaves are small, opposite, oblong, and entire. Flowers are purple in dense terminal clusters, appearing in July.

Native Americans used wild thyme in a compound preparation taken for chills and fever.

056 *Lauraceae*

The laurel family of trees and shrubs, usually aromatic. The leaves are simple, usually entire, usually leathery, and usually evergreen. The family

Lauraceae

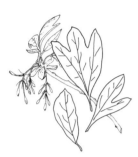

Sassafras albidum
(white sassafras)

is largely tropical, but there are North American representatives. In the East, the most widespread are sassafras and *Lindera* (wild allspice). In California and Florida, the major laurel is avocado. Although wild allspice is in the laurel family, "true" allspice is obtained commercially from *Pimenta dioica*, in the myrtle family. *Laurus nobilis*, the source of culinary bay leaves, and *Cinnanomum zeylanicum*, the bark of which is used to produce cinnamon, are also Lauraceae. Before camphor was produced synthetically, *Cinnanomum camphora* was the only commercial source.

Lindera benzoin (benjamin bush, spicebush, spicewood) is a 3- to 15-foot native shrub found in moist woods and along streams statewide. Leaves are alternate, pointed-oval, entire, and aromatic. Flowers are small, without petals, and appear in early April, before the leaves.

Native Americans used spicewood for colds, coughs, phthisis, and croup; as a tonic and emetic; and for "female obstructions" and painful or delayed menses. A bark infusion was taken to "break out" measles and for "bold hives." A leaf-and-branch infusion was used as an herbal steam for aches and pains and to induce perspiration.

Sassafras albidum (white sassafras) is a 10- to 100-foot native tree found in dry or moist, rich or poor soils of wooded areas statewide. Leaves are alternate, pointed-oval, bi- or trilobed, entire, and aromatic. Flowers are yellow, in clusters, and appear in April, before the leaves.

Native Americans used a bark infusion as a wash for skin diseases and rheumatism and to poultice wounds and sores. The infusion was also given to children with worms, for "overfatness," and as a tonic. The root bark was taken for colds, diarrhea, fever after childbirth, the rash and fever associated with measles and scarlet fever, and heart trouble. Raw buds were chewed to "increase vigor in males."

Bigelow described sassafras as a warm stimulant and diaphoretic. The twig pith was described as "highly mucilaginous, and a minute quantity renders water viscid and ropy." The mucilage was taken for dysentery and catarrh and particularly as a lotion for eye inflammation.

Sassafras oil is 80 percent safrole, which is suspected of causing contact dermatitis. Safrole has also been shown to cause liver cancer in rats.

057 *Leguminosae*

The bean family of herbs, shrubs, and trees. Leaves are usually pinnate, but sometimes palmate or simple. The fruit are typically leguminous and sometimes indehiscent. This is the pea family with about 13,000 species, second only to the Compositae in number, and distributed globally. This family contains many interesting poisons that should be avoided.

Leguminosae

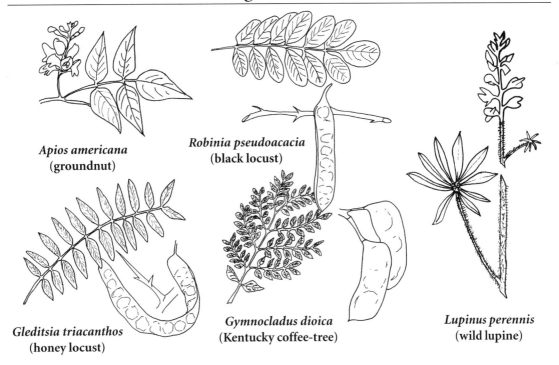

Apios americana
(groundnut)

Robinia pseudoacacia
(black locust)

Gleditsia triacanthos
(honey locust)

Gymnocladus dioica
(Kentucky coffee-tree)

Lupinus perennis
(wild lupine)

Abrus precatorius (rosary pea) grows as a weed in the tropics. The small peas are shiny and bicolored red and black. The seeds are used in artworks and sold to tourists as beads. Rosary peas contain abrin, a glycoprotein inhibitor of protein synthesis, which causes serious poisoning and death. *Lathrus odoratus* (sweet pea) is called the "sweet" pea for its fragrant flowers. Seeds contain a nonprotein amino acid, gamma-L-glutamyl-beta-aminopropionitrile, that causes lathyrism, a paralytic syndrome not usually fatal but difficult to diagnose. Long-term ingestion causes osteolathyrism, a bone and mesenchymal disease. Other species of *Lathrus* cause neurolathyrism in humans and most animals. *Wisteria* seeds contain poisonous compounds that cause mild to severe gastroenteritis.

Apios americana (groundnut) is a native vine found in rich-soiled, moist areas throughout the state, including the pinelands. Leaves are divided into five to seven sharp, pointed-oval leaflets. Pealike flowers are fragrant and brownish purple, in axillary, short racemes, appearing in late July.

Native Americans use groundnut as a high-protein food that can be eaten raw, boiled, or roasted, or dried and ground into a flour for breadmaking. A poultice of boiled and crushed nuts was applied to a sore "to eat out proud flesh." Groundnut has great potential in the developing food/medicine industry.

Baptisia tinctoria (black root, horsefly weed, rattleweed, wild indigo) is a 1- to 3-foot native perennial found in dry, open areas throughout the state, including the pinelands. Stems are smooth and bushy, with leaves divided into three cloverlike leaflets. Pealike flowers are yellow, in few-flowered racemes on upper branches. Plants are bluish, becoming black on drying.

Native Americans used wild indigo as an emetic, antiemetic, and purgative. A root decoction was used as a wash for cuts and ulcers; as a douche; to treat gonorrhea and kidney disorders; and as a rub for cramps in the arms, legs, or stomach. A hot root infusion or crushed root was held against a tooth for toothache.

Cassia fasciculata (golden cassia, partridge pea) is a 6-inch to 3-foot native perennial found in dry, open areas statewide. Leaves are alternate and divided into 8 to 15 pairs of leaflets. Flowers are large (1 to $1^1/2$ inches), yellow, and axillary, appearing in July.

Native Americans used partridge pea root as a stimulant during play or exercise.

Cassia hebecarpa (wild senna) and *Cassia marilandica* (wild senna) are similar; however, there is some question regarding the occurrence of the latter in New Jersey and whether the species are separable. Since the medicinal uses are similar and the species *hebecarpa* is native, only *hebecarpa* will be described. The plant is a 3- to 6-foot perennial found in moist or dry, open areas statewide, but less frequently in southern New Jersey. Leaves are alternate and divided into five to nine pairs of elliptical, entire leaflets. Stipules are sharp and pointed. Flowers are yellow, with $3/4$-inch chocolate-brown stamens, in axillary racemes, appearing in July. The major difference between the two species is said to be the appearance of the pods. The pods of *C. hebecarpa* are composed of roughly square units, while those of *C. marilandica* have units twice as wide as they are long. Fruits appear in late September. The young leaves and pods are eaten for food, and the roasted seeds are ground to make a coffeelike beverage.

Native Americans used wild senna infusion as a purgative, a worm remedy, for fevers, and for "blacks" (a condition in which the hands and eye sockets turn black). The seeds were soaked until mucilaginous, then swallowed for sore throat.

Cassia nictitans (sensitive pea, wild sensitive plant) is a 6-inch to 1-foot native perennial found in dry, open, areas statewide. Leaves are alternate and divided into 8 to 15 pairs of leaflets. Flowers are axillary, showy, and yellow, with yellow or purple anthers, appearing in mid-July.

This plant differs from *C. fasciculata* (partridge pea) only in being smaller and having leaves sensitive to touch.

Native Americans used wild sensitive plant root as a stimulant during exercise or play.

Cercis canadensis (Judas tree, redbud) is a naturalized perennial shrub or tree of up to 40 feet found in moist, rich-soiled, wooded areas statewide. Leaves are heart-shaped and entire. Flowers are purple, appearing in small clusters in April, before the leaves.

Native Americans used a bark infusion as an antiemetic and febrifuge, and to treat whooping cough. A cold inner-bark-and-root infusion was taken for congestion and fever.

Cytisus scoparius (Scotch broom) is a 3- to 5-foot shrub of western Europe that has escaped from cultivation. It is found in dry, sandy, open coastal areas of southern New Jersey. Lower leaves are divided into three small leaflets, and upper leaves are often reduced to a single leaflet. This is a stiffly branched shrub with large, yellow flowers in racemes, appearing in May.

Native Americans apparently did not use Scotch broom as a medicinal plant. In India, an infusion of green twigs, collected before flowering, is used as a diuretic in dropsy and as a heart tonic. In larger doses it is emetic and purgative.

Scotch broom contains several alkaloids, including hydroxytyramine, isosparteine, and sparteine. Plants are toxic to sheep, and sparteine is abortifacient.

Desmodium nudiflorum (smooth small-leaved tick-trefoil) is a 1- to 3-foot native perennial found in rich-soiled, dry, wooded areas statewide. Leaves are basal and divided into three entire leaflets. The flower stalk is separate, usually leafless, with rose-purple flowers in a loose raceme. Flowers appear in July and give rise to jointed pods that adhere to clothing.

Native Americans chewed tick-trefoil seed for pyorrhea and sore mouth or gums. The root infusion was used as a wash for cramps.

Gleditsia triacanthos (honey locust, honeyshuck) is a native or escaped tree of up to 80 feet found in rich-soiled, moist or dry, wooded areas statewide. Leaves are compound, with oblong, barely toothed leaflets. The trunk and branches are armed with large, triple-tapering (three-pointed) thorns. There is a thornless form. Dense clusters of greenish flowers appear in May, giving rise to thin, flat, apple-paring-like pods.

Native Americans used the pods to sweeten worm medicine (probably wormseed), and a pod infusion was taken for measles. A twig bark infusion was taken for colds, and a root-and-bark infusion was taken for coughs and colds. A bark infusion was taken and used as a bath for dyspepsia, measles, fevers, and smallpox.

Gymnocladus dioica (Kentucky coffee-tree) is a 50- to 60-foot escaped tree with rough bark found in rich-soiled, wooded areas, but more likely under cultivation in New Jersey. Leaves are alternate, 3 feet in length, and pinnately compound, with ovate, entire leaflets. Flowers are whitish, in terminal racemes, appearing in June. The fruit is a large (6 to 10 inches) flat bean pod with four to seven large, flat seeds.

Native Americans used a root infusion enema as an "infallible" remedy for constipation. The powdered root was used as a snuff to cause sneezing in the comatose, and when mixed with water was given to women in difficult labor. The root bark was used for hemorrhage, especially nosebleed, and the pods were powdered and sniffed to cause sneezing as a cure for headache.

Lespedeza capitata (rabbit foot, round-headed bush clover) is a 2- to 5-foot native perennial found in dry, open areas statewide. Leaves are alternate and divided cloverlike into three lance-shaped leaflets with silvery undersides. Flowers are creamy white and purple-spotted, in dense, bristly, terminal or upper-axillary clusters, appearing in mid-August.

Native Americans used the root as a poison antidote, and a moxa of stems was used for neuralgia and rheumatism.

Lupinus perennis (wild lupine) is an 8-inch to 2-foot native perennial found in dry or moist, open areas statewide. Leaves are alternate and divided whorllike into 7 to 11 lance-shaped leaflets. Flowers are blue and pealike, in showy, 4- to 10-inch racemes, appearing in May.

Native Americans used a lupine infusion internally "to check hemorrhage and vomiting" and externally as a wash.

Lupines contain many alkaloids; those of the quinolizidine type are poisonous.

Medicago sativa (alfalfa, lucerne) is a 1- to 3-foot naturalized and escaped perennial weed found in open waste areas statewide. This is a deep-rooted, bushy plant with leaves alternate and divided cloverlike into three elongated, toothed leaflets. The middle leaflet is turned upward. Flowers, in short racemes, are blue-violet and appear in June.

Native Americans applied a heated leaf poultice to the ear for earache.

Melilotus officinalis (yellow sweet clover) is a 2- to 8-foot naturalized perennial weed found in waste and other open areas statewide. Leaves are alternate and divided cloverlike into three elongated, toothed leaflets. Leaves are fragrant when crushed or dried. Flowers are yellow, in 2- to 4-inch racemes or spikes, appearing in May.

Native Americans used a cold infusion of sweet clover internally for colds and applied externally as a lotion.

Robinia pseudoacacia (black locust, false acacia) is a 70- to 90-foot native tree found in moist, rich-soiled, open areas statewide. The stem is straight and coarse-barked. Branches have paired spines below the leaf base. Leaves are alternate and divided into 7 to 21 oval leaflets. Flowers are white and fragrant, in showy, drooping racemes, appearing in May.

Native Americans used the bark as a flavoring for other medicines, and the root bark was chewed as an emetic. Crushed root bark was held on a tooth for toothache.

All parts of the black locust tree contain robin, a phenol, and robitin, a glycoside. Both are lectins that interfere with protein synthesis in the small intestine, leading to anorexia, vomiting, and even death.

Tephrosia virginiana (catgut, devil's shoestring, goat's rue, rabbit's pea) is a 1- to 2-foot native perennial found in dry, open areas throughout the state, including the pinelands. The plant is silky-hairy with leaves alternate and divided into 17 to 25 finely toothed leaflets. Flowers are yellow and pink with purple markings, in one or more clusters, appearing in June.

Native Americans used a cold root infusion to regain potency in men and a decoction as a shampoo for women to prevent hair loss. A cold crushed-root infusion was taken for bladder problems. The plant was also used to treat pulmonary tuberculosis.

Trifolium pratense (red clover) is a 6-inch to 2-foot naturalized perennial common weed found statewide. Leaves are composed of three oval leaflets with distinct V shaped white markings. Flowers are reddish, magenta, or purple and present for essentially the entire growing season from May to November.

Red clover infusion has been used by native Americans for fevers and Bright's disease. A cold infusion of the blossoms was taken by women for the change of life. A flower decoction was taken as a blood medicine, and a teaspoonful of powdered flowers was mixed in boiling water and taken for cancer. This native American reference to cancer is of great interest in that, for those who read the introduction, Thomson's Guide gives the following recipe:

Cancer Plaster

Take the heads of red clover, and fill a brass kettle, and boil them in water for one hour; then take them out, and fill the kettle again with fresh ones, and boil them again as before in the same liquor. Strain it off, then press the heads to get out all the juice; then simmer it over slow fire until it is about the consistency of tar, when it will be fit for use. Be careful not to let it burn. When used, it should be spread on a piece of bladder, split and made soft. It is good to cure cancers, sore lips, and all old sores.

Today, we know that clover has estrogenic activity, that consumption of large quantities by sheep can lead to infertility, and that this activity is perhaps due to the presence of a group of compounds known as isoflavonoids. Two of these compounds, genistein and daidzein, may have a role in hormone-dependent breast cancer. The "cancer doctor" used a "cancer plaster" and the reader should speculate!

Trifolium repens (white clover) is a creeping naturalized weed found statewide. This is a very common weed of nitrogen-poor areas, with three leaflets and dense flower heads of white or pink. Flowers are present throughout the flowering season from spring through fall.

Native Americans and others use white clover flower infusions as a febrifuge, a gynecological aid for leucorrhea, a kidney aid for Bright's disease, a remedy for coughs and colds, and a poultice applied to eyes for "paralysis."

058 *Lentibulariaceae*

The bladderwort family of herbs of moist and aquatic areas. Many are insectivorous, with highly specialized leaves or leaflets forming insect traps. This is a global family, dominated by the genus *Utricularia*. Ponds and lakes of the glaciated area of the northern and southern United States are rich in this genus. As the common name suggests, the insectivorous organs are bladderlike and open by a trap door, through which insects enter.

Utricularia sp. (bladderwort) is native and found throughout the state, wherever shallow, quiet water is found. The species are difficult to distinguish and at least 5 species are found in the pinelands and perhaps 16 species statewide. Flowering begins in May, June, or July.

Native Americans apparently did not use bladderwort as a medicinal plant. In Europe and India, the whole plant is used as a diuretic in urinary diseases and in wound healing (vulnerary).

059 *Liliaceae*

The lily family; a less-than-clearly-defined family of monocotyledonous plants. They are herbs or occasionally woody plants with rhizomes, corms, bulbs, or other fleshy structures. Leaves, somewhat similar to those of the Graminae, may be alternate, whorled, or, rarely, opposite. Family distribution is worldwide. Many of the Liliaceae are poisonous, including *Bowiea volubilis* (sea or climbing onion), which is native to eastern and southern Africa and contains cardioactive glycosides and the toxic alkaloid bowieine. *Colchicum autumnale* (fall crocus) contains colchicine as its major toxic alkaloid. *Hyacinthus orientalis* (hyacinth)

Liliaceae

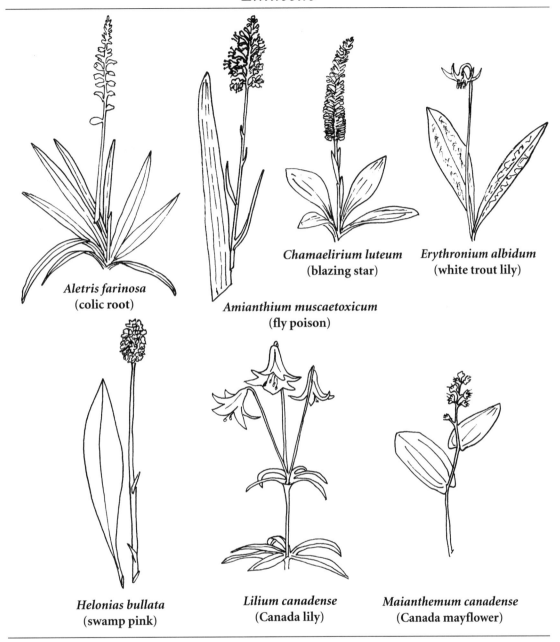

Aletris farinosa
(colic root)

Amianthium muscaetoxicum
(fly poison)

Chamaelirium luteum
(blazing star)

Erythronium albidum
(white trout lily)

Helonias bullata
(swamp pink)

Lilium canadense
(Canada lily)

Maianthemum canadense
(Canada mayflower)

bulbs are highly toxic when ingested. Digestive upset can lead to convulsions and death.

Aletris farinosa (ague root, colic root, star-grass) is a 1- to 3-foot native perennial found statewide but usually in dry, open areas and especially in the pinelands. Leaves are lance-shaped in a basal rosette. The flowering stem, with a few small bracts, produces small, white, tubular flowers in June.

Native Americans used a leaf infusion for bloody dysentery, colic, and stomach disorders. A plant infusion was taken by girls and women for "female troubles," and the root was used as a stomachic, tonic, and emmenagogue. It was used for restricted urine flow, rheumatism, jaundice, coughs, consumption, and diseases of the lungs. It was also used to "strengthen the womb" and prevent abortions.

Bigelow described star-grass as tonic and stomachic in small doses and narcotic in large doses.

Allium canadense (meadow garlic, tree onion, wild garlic) is a 6- to 18-inch native perennial found in moist, shaded areas of northern and southern New Jersey. Leaves are grasslike and very narrow. Flowers are whitish or pink, occurring in erect clusters of small bulbs in late May.

Native Americans used wild garlic as a stimulant, carminative, diuretic, expectorant and mild cathartic. It was also used for scurvy, dropsy, asthma, and "to remove deafness." The plant was rubbed on the body to repel insects.

Bigelow described garlic as stimulant, expectorant, and diuretic. Externally, the crushed-bulb poultice was used as a rubefacient. As a syrup, it was used for chronic coughs and pneumonia.

Allium cernuum (nodding wild onion) is a 1- to 2-foot native perennial found in dry, rocky areas of northern New Jersey. Leaves are grasslike and very narrow. Flowers are pink or white, in nodding clusters without bulbs, on two-ridged stalks.

Native Americans used nodding wild onion juice for colds, sore throat, phthisic, and liver complaints, and it was given to children for hives and croup. A poultice of soaked bulbs was applied to sores and swellings. A poultice of chewed plants was applied to the chest for pleurisy. A whole-plant infusion was taken for colic, and a poultice of the dried plant was applied to the chest for croup. A whole-plant poultice was also applied to the feet in "nervous fever."

Allium tricoccum (ramps, wild leek) is a 6- to 18-inch native perennial found in rich-soiled, moist, wooded areas of northern and southern New Jersey. Leaves are large, lily-of-the-valley-like, and strongly onion- or leek-scented. Flower stalks bearing clusters of small, creamy white flowers appear during leaf senescence in summer.

Native Americans ate ramps for croup, colds, and a spring tonic that "cleans you out." The decoction was given to children for worms, and a root decoction was used as a quick-acting emetic. The warmed juice was used for earache.

Allium vineale (field garlic, scallions) is a 1- to 3-foot naturalized perennial weed found in open areas statewide. Leaves are similar to those of *A. canadense* but differ in being tubular and somewhat higher up on the stalk. Flowers are greenish or purplish in umbels, appearing in June.

Native Americans used field garlic as they did wild garlic and also chewed the raw bulbs for shortness of breath and high blood pressure.

Amianthium muscaetoxicum (crow poison, fly poison, staggergrass) is a 1- to 2-foot native perennial found in open, sandy, wooded areas of northern and southern New Jersey. Leaves are basal, entire, grasslike, and blunt at the tip. Flowers appear in a raceme, initially white, then becoming bronze-green with age. The flowering stem is smooth, appearing in June.

Native Americans used fly poison root to poison crows and as a sure, but severe, cure for "itch."

Staggergrass contains poisonous alkaloids that have caused death in grazing animals.

Chamaelirium luteum (blazing star, devil's bit, fairy wand) is a 1- to 3-foot native perennial found in rich-soiled, moist meadows of northern New Jersey and the inner-coastal areas to the south. Leaves are basal, oblong, smooth, and entire in a rosette. Plants are male or female, with the female being somewhat more leafy. Flowers are small and whitish yellow, in crowded, slender, spikelike racemes, appearing in late May.

Native Americans apparently did not use blazing star as a medicinal plant. The root was used by others for many medical disorders associated with male and female reproductive organs. A root infusion or decoction is diuretic and emetic, and regarded as tonic for reproductive organs, also as a stomachic and vermifuge. The effect on the uterus is such that it should not be consumed during pregnancy.

Clintonia borealis (blue bead lily, corn lily, heal-all, yellow clintonia) is a 6-inch to 1-foot native perennial found in rich-soiled, moist, cool woods of northern New Jersey. Leaves are basal, pointed-oval, shiny, and entire. Flowers are greenish-yellow, bell-shaped, and nodding on a smooth stem. Flowers appear in late April and produce dark blue berries.

Native Americans used a fresh leaf poultice as a burn dressing, and a leaf decoction was applied externally to scrofulous sores. The root infusion was used as an aid in childbirth, and a plant decoction was taken for the heart.

Convallaria majalis (lily-of-the-valley) is a 4- to 10-inch introduced and escaped perennial found in wooded areas of northern New Jersey. Leaves are basal, pointed-oval, and entire. Flowers are white, bell-shaped, and nodding, in one-sided racemes, appearing in May and producing red berries.

Native Americans apparently did not use lily-of-the-valley for medicinal purposes. The plant is native to Europe and was used as a milder-acting substitute for digitalis. The flower and root preparations were used as a heart tonic, sedative, diuretic, and emetic.

Lily-of-the-valley contains 20 or more cardiac glycosides, mainly convallatoxin. The effect on the heart is similar to that produced by digitalis.

Erythronium albidum (white trout lily) is a 6-inch to 1-foot native perennial found in cool, moist, wooded areas of northern New Jersey. Leaves are basal, lance-shaped, and entire. They may occasionally be slightly mottled. Flowers are solitary, white, and lilylike, with their petals curved backward; they appear in early April.

Native Americans either did not use the white trout lily for medicinal purposes or did not separate the species from *E. americanum.*

Erythronium americanum (trout lily, yellow adder's tongue) is described the same as *E. albidum* except that the leaves are brown-mottled and the flowers are yellow. Both species are usually found in colonies. The curved petals of the flower account for another common name, dogtooth violet.

Native Americans used the warm, crushed leaves and juice for wounds difficult to heal and a poultice of crushed roots for swellings and drawing splinters. A root infusion was used for fever, and the raw plant, excluding the root, was taken by young girls as a contraceptive.

Bigelow described *E. americanum* as emetic in its "recent" state, but inactivated by drying. It is suggested that the bulb be harvested when the leaves first appear, before flowering.

Helonias bullata (swamp pink) is a 1- to 3-foot endangered native perennial found in swamps and bogs throughout the state and especially the pinelands. Leaves are evergreen and spatulate or lance-shaped, in a basal rosette. Flowers are brilliant pink or purple, in an egg-shaped cluster on a hollow stem, appearing in early April.

Native Americans apparently did not use swamp pink for medicinal purposes. Others use the plant for the same disorders as given for *Chamaelirium luteum.*

Hemerocallis fulva (common orange day-lily) is a 3- to 6-foot native of eastern Asia. Having escaped from cultivation, it is now a naturalized perennial found in many areas, especially roadsides throughout the state. Leaves are basal, swordlike, and entire, forming large clumps. Large, showy flowers are orange and lilylike, fading after one day, thus the common name.

Native Americans apparently did not use the day-lily for medicinal or food purposes. Others have used a root preparation as a diuretic for restricted urine flow, jaundice, and hemorrhage, and as a poultice for mastitis.

Lilium canadense (Canada lily, wild lily, yellow lily) is a 2- to 5-foot native perennial found in moist or wet areas throughout the state, but concentrated in the northern regions. Leaves are lance-shaped and usually in whorls. Flowers vary in color and may be solitary or in nodding clusters of two or three, appearing in mid-June.

Native Americans used a wild lily root infusion for diarrhea, rheumatism, and irregular menses. The boiled tuber decoction was given "to make child fleshy and fat."

Lilium philadelphicum (Philadelphia lily, red lily, wood lily) is a 1- to 3-foot rare native perennial found in dry, open areas of northern New Jersey. Leaves are lance-shaped and in whorls. Flowers are erect, bright orange, and spotted, appearing in early June.

Native Americans used a poultice of boiled bulbs for sores and wounds, especially dog bites. The root was used to treat coughs, consumption, and fevers. A whole-plant decoction was used to expel the placenta after childbirth.

Maianthemum canadense (beadruby, Canada mayflower, false lily-of-the-valley) is a 2- to 6-inch native perennial found in moist, wooded or cleared areas statewide. Leaves are alternate and heart-shaped at the base. Flowers are white, in a small raceme, appearing in May and producing speckled red berries.

Native Americans used a plant infusion for headache, sore throat, and "to keep the kidneys open during pregnancy."

Medeola virginiana (Indian cucumber-root) is a 1- to 3-foot native perennial found in rich-soiled, moist, wooded areas statewide. Leaves are lance-shaped in two whorls, the upper whorl consisting of three to five leaves and the lower of five to nine leaves. The spiderlike flowers are greenish yellow, appearing in May and hanging below the upper whorl. The fruit is a dark purple berry.

Native Americans used an infusion prepared from crushed, dried berries and leaves as an anticonvulsive for babies.

Polygonatum biflorum (Solomon's seal) is a 1- to 3-foot native perennial found in dry or moist, wooded areas statewide. Leaves are alternate, pointed-elliptical, smooth, and entire. Flowers are white and tubular, growing in pairs from leaf axils, appearing in May.

Native Americans used Solomon's seal as an antidiarrheal for dysentery, for diseases of the breast and lungs, for "white or profuse menstruation," and as a sedative. A roasted-root infusion was taken for stomach trouble, and fumes from the heated root were used to revive the unconscious. The root decoction was taken as a mild tonic, a cathartic, and a cough medicine, and was applied to cuts, bruises, and sores.

Smilacina racemosa (false Solomon's seal, false spikenard) is a 1- to 3-foot native perennial found in rich-soiled, moist, wooded areas statewide. Leaves are alternate, pointed-oval, smooth, and entire. Flowers are small and white, clustered in terminal racemes, and appear in May.

Native Americans inhaled the root smudge for headaches and pain,

Liliaceae

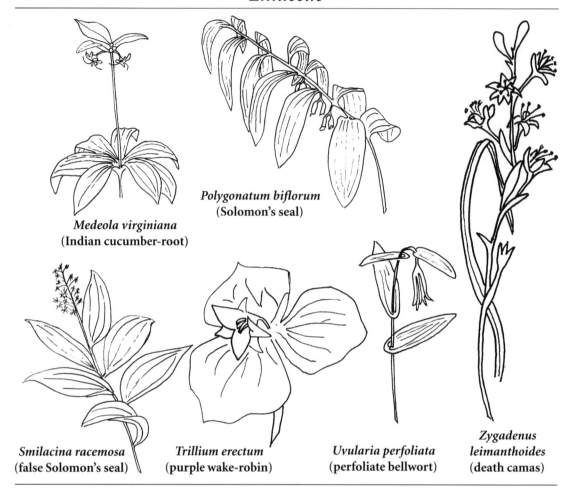

Medeola virginiana
(Indian cucumber-root)

Polygonatum biflorum
(Solomon's seal)

Smilacina racemosa
(false Solomon's seal)

Trillium erectum
(purple wake-robin)

Uvularia perfoliata
(perfoliate bellwort)

Zygadenus leimanthoides
(death camas)

in fits of insanity, to "hush a crying child," and to revive the unconscious. A cold root infusion was used as an eyewash, for rheumatism, for sore back and kidney trouble, as a purgative, and in an herbal steam for catarrh. A root poultice was applied to the cut umbilical cord. The leaf decoction was used as a contraceptive, a cough remedy, and by "lying-in" women. Leaves and stems were used to treat rashes and itch, and a poultice of fresh leaves was applied to cuts to stop bleeding. A rhizome infusion was used as a stomach medicine and was taken during the menstrual period. The root decoction was considered a "strong medicine."

Smilax glauca (glaucous greenbrier, sawbrier, wild sarsaparilla) is a native, prickly, climbing, viny, woody shrub found in dry, wooded areas and thickets of southern and decreasingly toward northern New Jersey. Leaves are oval, heart-shaped, entire, and whitish on the undersurface. Flowers are inconspicuous, green, and in umbels, giving rise to blue-black berries.

Native Americans used sawbrier thorns to scratch areas of pain, and for muscular cramps, twitching, and rheumatism. An infusion was taken for stomach trouble, and a root decoction was taken to expel the afterbirth. Wilted leaves were applied to boils, and dried, powdered leaves were used for scalds.

Bigelow described sarsaparilla as a mild demulcent, alterative, and subtonic.

Smilax rotundifolia (bull brier, cat brier, common greenbrier, horse greenbrier) is a native, green, thorned, climbing, viny, woody shrub found in moist to dry, open-wooded areas statewide. Leaves are heart-shaped, pointed-oval, leathery, shiny, and green on both sides. Flowers are inconspicuous, appearing in late June and giving rise to blue-black fruit.

Native Americans used common greenbrier as they did sawbrier, adding the use of "plant splints" to scratch the back for headache.

Trillium erectum (birthroot, purple wake-robin, stinking benjamin) is a 6- to 20-inch native perennial found in moist, rich-soiled, wooded areas of northern New Jersey. Leaves are diamond-shaped and entire, in a single whorl of three. Flowers are maroon to purple and malodorous, or white and odorless, appearing in April.

Native Americans used red trillium as a cancer poultice for "putrid ulcers, tumors and inflamed parts." It was also taken for coughs, asthma, bowel complaints, excessive menstruation, and "change of life."

Uvularia perfoliata (merry bells, perfoliate bellwort) is a 6- to 18-inch colonial native perennial found in moist, open-wooded areas of northern and decreasingly toward southern New Jersey. Leaves are alternate, long-oval, with a perforating stem. Flowers are yellow-orange and bell-shaped, appearing in May.

Native Americans used a root infusion as a cough medicine for children. A crushed-root infusion was used as an eyewash, and the plant was also used as an internal and external treatment for broken bones.

Uvularia sessilifolia (sessile-leaved bellwort, wild oats) is a 6-inch to 1-foot native perennial found in moist, wooded areas statewide. Leaves are alternate, clasping (not perforated), and pale on the underside. The stem is forked, with small, straw-yellow, bell-shaped flowers appearing in April.

The root infusion was taken for diarrhea, as a "blood purifier," and as a poultice for boils. The root infusion was taken internally, and roots were poulticed for broken bones.

Veratrum viride (false hellebore, Indian poke, white hellebore) is a 2- to 8-foot native perennial found in wet, swampy, wooded areas of northern and decreasingly toward southern New Jersey. Leaves are large, alternate, broad, pointed-oval, strongly ribbed lengthwise, and clasping.

Flowers are small, yellow-green, and star-shaped, in large, branching, multiflowered clusters, appearing in late May.

Native Americans were aware that false hellebore was poisonous and that overdoses could be fatal. The bulb decoction was taken for chronic cough, constipation, and gonorrhea, and as an emetic for stomach pain. The root infusion was used as a rub on leg scratches for rheumatism, as a scalp rub for dandruff, and to "make hair grow on a bald head." The fresh root was held in the mouth as a laxative and a dried, burned-root decoction was taken for blood disorders. The dried plants or powdered roots were snuffed for catarrh, headaches, colds, and tuberculosis. A leaf poultice was applied for pain, and the juice was taken to induce abortion.

Bigelow described American hellebore as an acrid emetic and a powerful stimulant, followed by sedative effects. It was used in gout and rheumatism, but to be taken with caution.

False hellebore contains alkaloids that produce major effects on the cardiovascular system, lowering blood pressure and depressing heart activity.

Yucca filamentosa (Adam's needle, bear grass, devil's shoestring, silkgrass, Spanish bayonet) is a 5- to 10-foot native perennial found in dry, sandy areas throughout the state, especially in the pinelands. Leaves are basal, lance-shaped, stiff, and spine-tipped, with curled threads on the margins. Flowers are creamy white and nodding, in a panicle several feet long, on a smooth, polelike, branchless stem.

Native Americans used bear grass as a rub for skin diseases and in an infusion for skin disease and diabetes, and as a soporific. The beaten root was used as a salve for sores and a poultice for sprains, and was placed in water to "intoxicate fishes." Bear grass was also used as an ingredient in green corn medicine with broom sedge and amaranth.

Zygadenus leimanthoides (black snakeroot, death camas, oceanorus, zigadenus) is a 2- to 3-foot native perennial found in swampy areas of central and southern New Jersey. Leaves are basal and grasslike, approximately $1/4$ inch in width. The stem is leafy, terminating in a creamy white raceme or panicle of flowers in late June.

Native Americans used species of death camas with full knowledge that it was a poisonous plant. A root decoction was taken as an emetic, but it was more usually applied as a poultice for burns, bruises, sprains, lameness, neuralgia, toothache, rheumatism, or swellings.

Death camas contains alkaloids similar to those found in *Amianthium muscaetoxicum* and *Veratrum viride*, and the effects are similar. The poisons are concentrated in the bulb, but children and livestock have been killed by the ingestion of flowers, leaves, or bulbs.

060 *Linaceae*

The flax family of woody or herbaceous plants, with leaves simple and entire, and alternate, opposite, or, rarely, whorled. There are 9 genera and 120 species, 90 of which are in the genus *Linum*. *Linum* is the Latin word for "flax," from the Celtic word for "thread." The family is global, but concentrated in the temperate regions.

Linum usitatissimum (common flax) is a 1- to 2-foot rare, escaped annual weed found in waste areas statewide. Leaves are alternate, lance-shaped, narrow, three-veined and 1 to $1^1/2$ inches long. Flowers are $^3/4$ inch, blue, with five broad, slightly overlapping petals, appearing in June.

Native Americans used flax for violent colds, coughs, and diseases of the lungs. A tea was poured over the body for fever, and the seed was used for gravel or burning during urination.

Bigelow described flaxseed decoction as demulcent and useful in catarrh and pneumonia, in dysentery, and particularly in strangury and other inflammations of the urinary tract.

Linaceae

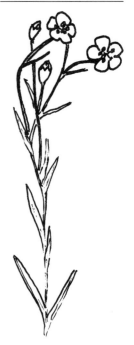

Linum usitatissimum
(**common flax**)

061 *Loganiaceae*

The logania family of herbs, shrubs, trees, and woody vines. Leaves are simple and usually opposite, but may be alternate in some species of *Buddleia*. The family occurs throughout the warmer and tropical regions of the globe, with butterfly bush common in cultivation, and very popular in New Jersey.

Buddleia davidi (butterfly bush) is a 6- to 10-foot escaped, woody, perennial shrub found in dry, open areas of northern New Jersey. Leaves are opposite, lance-shaped, and fine-toothed. Flowers may be white, blue, or purple, in terminal and axillary racemes, appearing in June.

Native Americans apparently did not use butterfly bush as a medicinal plant. Roots, bark, and leaves of several species of *Buddleia* have been used for their diuretic properties and as healing agents. *B. asiactica* is used in the Philippines for skin complaints and as an abortifacient.

062 *Loranthaceae*

The mistletoe family of small parasitic shrubs, usually on the branches of trees, including conifers. The family is primarily tropical but there are two genera in North America, *Phoradendron* and *Arceuthobium*.

Phoradendron includes the common green mistletoe, which is partially parasitic on oaks and softwood trees along streamsides.

Phoradendron flavescens (American mistletoe) is a rare, native, parasitic perennial found in southern New Jersey. Branches are thick, and spatula-shaped leaves are partially evergreen. Flowers are inconspicuous, appearing in September and giving rise to white, translucent fruit 14 months later.

Native Americans used the plant or root infusion to induce abortions. A plant decoction was used for debility, paralytic weakness, and as a panacea for general sickness, including as a wash for rheumatism. The plant was regarded as poisonous, but the root was chewed for toothache.

Berries contain beta-phenylethylamine, tyramine, and toxic lectins. Poisoning can occur from as few as 1 to 3 berries, and death can result from drinking tea prepared from the berries.

063 *Lycopodiaceae*

The club moss family of existing Carboniferous period plants composed of one genus. About 20 species occur in North America, concentrated

Lycopodiaceae

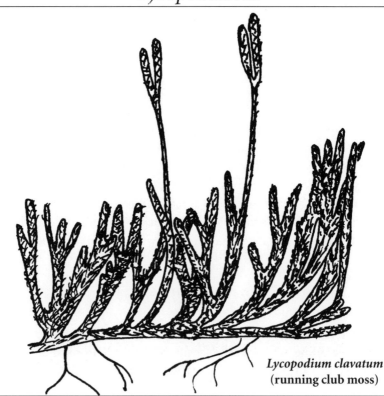

Lycopodium clavatum
(running club moss)

in the Northeast. The plants of *Lycopodium* are usually only 1 or 2 inches high.

Lycopodium clavatum (running club moss, trailing club moss) is a native, mosslike, 3- to 15-inch evergreen perennial found in dry, open areas of primarily northern but also southern New Jersey. Leaves are very small and tipped with soft, hairlike bristles. Spores form in terminal, elongated strobili in June.

Native Americans used a plant infusion for weakness, fever, and postpartum pain. The spores of the fruiting spikes were used as a styptic and coagulant, and the moss was inserted in the nose to cause bleeding as a headache cure.

064 *Lythraceae*

The lythrum family of herbs, shrubs, or trees, with leaves usually simple and entire, and opposite or whorled. The North American species are herbaceous, and shrubs and trees of the family are particularly abundant in the tropical regions of South America. A tree, Lagerstroemia, is an Asiatic species called "crepe myrtle," cultivated in the southern United States and container-grown in New Jersey.

Lythrum salicaria (purple loosestrife, spiked loosestrife) is a naturalized 2- to 4-foot downy perennial found in wet areas statewide. Leaves are opposite or whorled, lance-shaped, and clasping. Flowers are purple in dense spikes, appearing in June.

Native Americans used spiked loosestrife as an ingredient in a compound preparation taken for fever and "sickness caused by the dead."

065 *Magnoliaceae*

The magnolia family of trees and shrubs, with simple leaves, usually entire and alternate. Large flowers are characteristic. The family is limited to the temperate areas of the Northern Hemisphere.

Liriodendron tulipifera (tulip tree, whitewood, yellow poplar) is a native 75- to 100-foot tree found in moist, well-drained areas statewide, including the pinelands, where it has been introduced. Leaves are alternate, with four pointed lobes. Flowers are greenish to yellow-orange and tuliplike, appearing in May.

Native Americans used tulip tree for infant cholera, and a bark tea was taken for pinworms, dyspepsia, dysentery, rheumatism, and fevers. The raw green bark was chewed as a stimulant and aphrodisiac. The root bark infusion was taken for fever, and a leaf poultice was bound to the head for neuralgic pain.

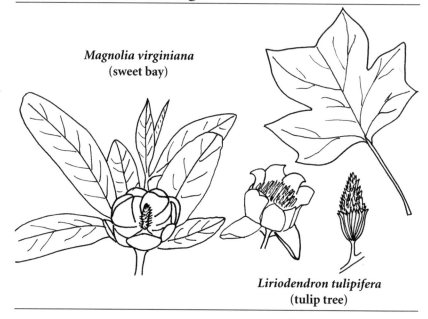

Magnolia virginiana
(sweet bay)

Liriodendron tulipifera
(tulip tree)

Bigelow described tulip tree bark as a stimulating tonic and dia-phoretic as useful as cinchona bark in intermittent fevers and also taken as a warm sudorific in rheumatism.

Magnolia acuminata (cucumber tree) is a naturalized 50- to 80-foot tree found in rich-soiled, moist, shaded areas of southwestern New Jersey. Leaves are large and pointed-oblong. Flowers are greenish and cup-shaped, appearing in April before the leaves.

Native Americans used a bark infusion for stomachache and cramps and as a hot snuff for sinus. The inner bark was chewed for toothache. Known as the "great-leaved magnolia," it was also used in the steam bath for indigestion.

Magnolia virginiana (beaver tree, laurel magnolia, sweet bay) is an 8- to 30-foot native shrub or tree found in swamps and other wet areas of southern New Jersey. Those found in the northern parts of the state are probably escapes. Leaves are dark green above and white on the un-derside, leathery, entire, and blunt-tipped. In the southern part of the state, they are also evergreen. The flowers are white, cup-shaped, and very fragrant, and appear in May. The fruit is dark red and conelike.

Native Americans used a decoction prepared from leaves and twigs for colds, chills, and to "warm the blood." Leaves and bark were sniffed as a mild dope (narcotic).

The mallow family of herbs and, rarely, shrubs and trees. The leaves are usually palmately lobed, veined, and entire, to lobed and parted. The family is global and best known by the flowers. Perhaps the best known are the hibiscus, hollyhock, and cotton.

Abutilon theophrasti (American jute, butter print, velvet leaf) is a 3- to 6-foot naturalized annual weed found in open areas such as farmland in northern New Jersey. The entire aboveground plant is velvety. Leaves are alternate, heart-shaped, and blunt-toothed. Yellow flowers in leaf axils appear in July.

Native Americans apparently did not use velvet leaf as a medicinal plant. In India and China, a leaf tea is used for dysentery, fevers, and in a poultice for ulcers. The seeds are laxative, demulcent, and diuretic. The

Malvaceae

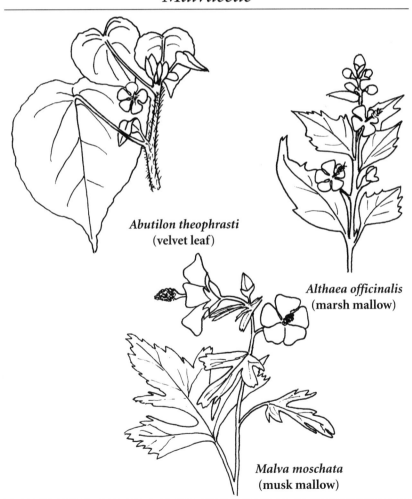

Abutilon theophrasti
(**velvet leaf**)

Althaea officinalis
(**marsh mallow**)

Malva moschata
(**musk mallow**)

bark is astringent and diuretic, and the root tea is used for fever and dysentery, and to control bedwetting.

Althaea officinalis (marsh mallow) is a 2- to 4-foot naturalized perennial found in fresh- or saltwater marshes of southern New Jersey. The entire plant is velvety and gray-green. Leaves are alternate, pointed-oval, and coarsely toothed. Flowers are 1 to 1$^1/_2$ inches with five large, pale rose petals, appearing in July. The roots are the original source of marshmallow.

Native Americans apparently did not use the marsh mallow as a medicinal plant. In India, the leaves and flowers are applied to burns, and a leaf-and-flower tea is taken for catarrh and bronchitis. The root is demulcent and emollient.

Hibiscus palustris (*H. moscheutos*) (mallow rose, swamp rose, wild cotton) is a 5- to 7-foot native perennial found in shallow, fresh- or saltwater marshes and along streams statewide. The stems and leaf undersides are white-velvety. Leaves are alternate, pointed-oval or three-lobed, and toothed. Flowers are 8 inches, pink, or white, and five-petaled, with a red center, appearing in July.

Native Americans applied an infusion of dried stalks for inflammation of the bladder.

Malva moschata (musk mallow) is a 1- to 3-foot naturalized perennial weed found in waste areas primarily of northern New Jersey. Leaves are alternate and deeply divided into geraniumlike narrow segments. Flowers are large, white or pink, and mallowlike, and appear in June.

Native Americans used a plant infusion for chills and lassitude.

Malva neglecta (cheeses, dwarf mallow) is a 4-inch to 1-foot naturalized perennial weed found in waste areas statewide. This is a deeprooted, prostrate plant, with alternate, oval, slightly lobed, toothed leaves. Flowers are axillary, pale lilac or white, and appear in May.

Native Americans used a crushed-plant infusion as an emetic. A cold plant infusion was taken and applied as a lotion for injury or swelling.

Malva sylvestris (high mallow) is a 1- to 3-foot escaped biennial found in waste areas statewide. It is not common. This is an erect, hairy plant, with alternate, rounded, five- to seven-lobed, toothed leaves. Flowers are showy, rose-purple with red veins, and appear in June.

Native Americans apparently did not use high mallow as a medicinal plant. The plant is mucilaginous, demulcent, emollient, and cooling. In China and India, it is used as a febrifuge, as well as for diseases of the urinary bladder and mucous membranes of the pulmonary tract. A poultice is applied externally for inflammation. The leaves are edible, containing a stimulant for uterine and intestinal muscles.

Menispermaceae

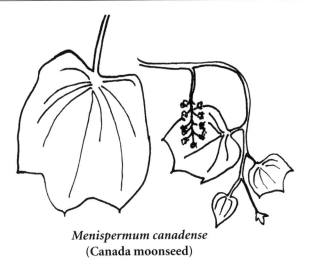

Menispermum canadense
(Canada moonseed)

067 *Menispermaceae*

The moonseed family of woody vines and, rarely, shrubs and trees. Leaves are alternate, simple, in three leaflets, and may be palmately lobed. The fruit is an achene or drupe. The family is tropical, extending into the temperate areas. The family also contains members that are sources of potent neurotoxins such as curare, a crude extract of species of *Chondodendron* and *Strychnos*, used as arrow poison by Indians of the Amazon and Orinoco valleys.

Menispermum canadense (Canada moonseed, yellow parilla, yellow sarsaparilla) is an 8- to 12-foot native, climbing, woody vine without tendrils found in moist, rich-soiled, wooded areas of northern and decreasingly toward southern New Jersey. Leaves are somewhat grapelike and entire, with three to seven angular, shallow lobes. Flowers appear in June. They are small and whitish, in loose, separately sexed clusters. The fruits are black, in grapelike clusters.

Native Americans used yellow sarsaparilla as an antidiarrheal and for "weak stomach and bowels." The root was taken for venereal disease, as a laxative, and for skin diseases.

Moonseed seeds and rhizomes are hallucinogenic. The plant is a vine with leaves similar to those of wild grape, and children have died from eating the fruit. The toxins are isoquinoline alkaloids, including dauricine, with a curarelike action.

068 *Moraceae*

The mulberry family of shrubs, trees, and, rarely, herbs, with milky sap. The family is tropical and subtropical, with the mulberry and fig trees typical of the family in temperate areas.

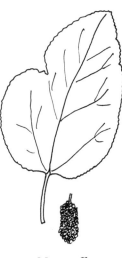

Moraceae

Morus alba
(white mulberry)

Maclura pomifera (hedge-apple, Osage orange) is a 30- to 60-foot naturalized tree found in rich-soiled, moist, open areas of northern and southern New Jersey. The branches are spiny, with the leaves shiny, and pointed-oval to lance-shaped. The fruit is large and green, with a brainlike wrinkled surface.

Native Americans used a root decoction as an eyewash.

Morus alba (white mulberry) is a 20- to 60-foot naturalized tree found in moist, open areas statewide. Leaves are variable, from simple to lobed, and toothed. The fruit is white, with a slight purple tinge.

Native Americans used white mulberry bark as a laxative and purgative, for worms, and to "check dysentery."

Morus rubra (red mulberry) is a 20- to 60-foot native tree found in moist, open areas statewide. Leaves are variable, from simple to lobed, and toothed. The fruit is purple to black.

Native Americans used red mulberry bark as a laxative, purgative, cathartic, and emetic, for worms, to "check dysentery," and as a liver medicine "to remove bile from the intestines." The root decoction was used as an emetic, for weakness, and for urinary problems. The tree sap was rubbed on the skin for ringworm.

069 *Myricaceae*

The sweet gale or wax myrtle family of shrubs and trees, with leaves alternate, usually simple, and resinous. The family is composed of two genera, *Myrica* and *Comptonia*, occurring in the cool areas of the northern temperate zone and in South Africa.

Myrica asplenifolia (*Comptonia peregrina*)(sweet fern) is a 1- to 3-foot native shrub found in dry areas statewide, especially in the pinelands. This is a highly branched, strongly aromatic, deciduous shrub with long, narrow, fernlike leaves. Flowers are inconspicuous in catkins, appearing in April.

Native Americans used a plant infusion for roundworms, fevers, stomach cramps; as a wash for poison ivy; and to cure flux, treat scrofula, and remove mucus from the lungs. A plant decoction was also described as "a potent medicine in childbirth." Berries, bark, and leaves were used to prepare an "exhilarant" and a beverage.

Myrica cerifera (candleberry, wax myrtle) is a 15- to 25-foot native

Myricaceae

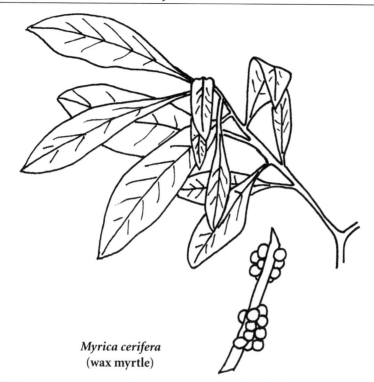

Myrica cerifera
(wax myrtle)

shrub or small tree found in moist or wet areas of southern New Jersey. Leaves are evergreen, leathery, lance-shaped, and toothed, with waxy globules. Flowers appear in May, giving rise to waxy berries that persist through the winter.

Native Americans used a leaf-and-stem decoction for fevers, and a leaf decoction was taken as a vermifuge. A root decoction was used as a gargle for tonsillitis and was given to children for stomachache. Roots were also used to treat headache and inflammation. Berries, bark, and leaves were used to prepare an "exhilarant" and a beverage.

Myrica gale (meadow fern; sweet gale) is a 2- to 6-foot native shrub found in wet areas of northern New Jersey. This is an aromatic, deciduous shrub with gray, lance-shaped, toothed leaves. Flowers are in clusters at the tips of old wood and appear in April.

Native Americans used a decoction prepared from crushed branches for gonorrhea and as a diuretic.

Myrica pensylvanica (bayberry, candleberry) is a 3- to 12-foot native shrub found in wet, sandy areas statewide, especially along the coasts. Branches are grayish white, with leaves toothed, oblong and expanded at the tip. Flowers are clustered below the branch tips and appear in May.

Native Americans used bayberry as they did *M. cerifera* and *M. gale.*

In addition, a bark preparation was taken for kidney trouble, and a leaf preparation was emetic.

070 *Nyctaginaceae*

Nyctaginaceae

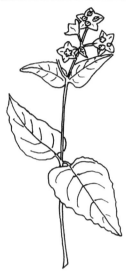

**Oxybaphus nyctagineus
(wild four-o'clock)**

From a generic name meaning "night" or "nocturnal flowering," the four-o'clock family of primarily herbs, but also shrubs and trees. The leaves are usually opposite, simple, and entire, without stipules. The family is tropical and subtropical, extending into the temperate regions.

Oxybaphus nyctagineus (*Mirabilis nyctaginea*) (heart-leaved umbrella-wort, wild four-o'clock) is a 1- to 5-foot native perennial found in rich, dry, open areas of central New Jersey. Leaves are opposite, heart-shaped, and entire. Flowers are pink or purple in clusters of two to five on a star-shaped, green, veiny cup. Flowers appear in May.

Native Americans used the root decoction or poulticed root for application to sprained or strained muscles. The root decoction was also taken for fever, as a vermifuge, and for swelling after childbirth. The root or whole plant was used for bladder troubles and externally to treat broken bones. The dried, ground root was applied to babies' mouths for soreness, and the chewed root was used to treat wounds. The beaten root was used to poultice boils. Milk poured over the leaves is described as a fly poison.

071 *Nymphaeaceae*

Nymphaeaceae

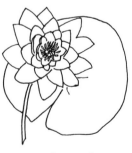

**Nymphaea odorata
(fragrant water lily)**

The water lily family of usually perennial, aquatic herbs, sometimes with milky juice. Leaves, simple or peltate, float or are above water. The family is distributed globally.

Nuphar advena (*N. luteum*) (marsh collard, upright spatterdock, yellow water lily) is a native, aquatic perennial found in fresh waters of ponds, swamps, and slow streams statewide. Leaves are basal and round-oval, with a wide notch and round leaf stalk; most are held above the water. Flowers are $1^1/2$ to 3 inches, yellow, and cuplike, appearing in May.

Native Americans used a poultice of the dried, powdered root; fresh or dried leaves; or dried, powdered rhizome to treat cuts, wounds, sores, and swellings. Poulticed fresh roots and leaves were also used for swellings, boils, and "many inflammatory diseases." A stem or cold root decoction was taken for internal pains.

Nymphaea odorata (fragrant water lily, sweet white water lily, white water lily) is a native, aquatic perennial found in fresh waters of ponds, swamps, bogs, and slow streams statewide. Leaves are floating, basal, and round, with a purplish undersurface. There is a V-shaped notch at the base. Flowers are white, 3 to 5 inches, with a sweet fragrance, and appear in June.

Native Americans used the dried, powdered root to treat mouth sores, a boiled-root poultice for swellings, and the fresh root as a cough medicine for colds and tuberculosis and to treat suppurating glands. The leaves were used to treat colds and grippe.

072 *Oleaceae*

The olive family of trees and shrubs. Leaves are opposite, simple, or pinnate. The family occurs primarily in the warm regions and tropics of the Eastern Hemisphere.

Chionanthus virginicus (fringe tree, old man's beard) is a 6- to 20-foot native shrub or small tree found in rich-soiled, dry or moist, low areas of southern New Jersey. Leaves are opposite, entire, pointed-oval, and 6 to 8 inches in length. Flowers are white, with long, narrow petals in drooping clusters; they appear in May.

Native Americans used a bark decoction as a wash or poultice for infected sores and wounds. A crushed-bark poultice was also applied to cuts and bruises.

Fraxinus americana (American ash, white ash) is a 100-foot common native tree found in well-drained, moist, rich-soiled, wooded areas of northern New Jersey and western regions of southern New Jersey. Leaves are opposite and divided into five to nine pointed-oval, slightly toothed leaflets with whitish undersides. Flowers appear in April, giving rise to clusters of winged fruit.

Oleaceae

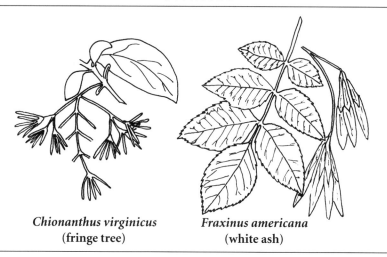

Chionanthus virginicus
(fringe tree)

Fraxinus americana
(white ash)

Native Americans used an inner-bark tonic for liver and stomach ailments. A bark decoction was taken as an emetic or cathartic. A bark infusion was used as a wash for sores, to cure itch, and for parasites on the scalp. A root decoction was taken and applied as a poultice for snakebite, and a flower decoction was taken for snakebite. A strong leaf decoction was taken for "cleansing" after childbirth.

Ligustrum vulgare (common privet) is a 6-inch to 2-foot naturalized shrub found along roadsides and in well-drained, open areas statewide. Leaves are opposite, lance-shaped, and entire. Flowers are white, in dense panicles, appearing in June.

Native Americans apparently did not use privet for medicinal purposes. In Europe, a bark tea was used as a stomachic. The leaf tea or poultice is used externally as a vulnerary (for healing wounds) and as a detergent. The berries and leaves are poisonous. The leaves have caused fatal poisoning in horses and sheep, and the purplish black berries contain glycosides that cause severe gastrointestinal upset in children.

073 *Onagraceae*

The evening primrose family of herbs and, rarely, shrubs and trees. Stipules are rare, and leaves may be alternate or opposite. The family is

Onagraceae

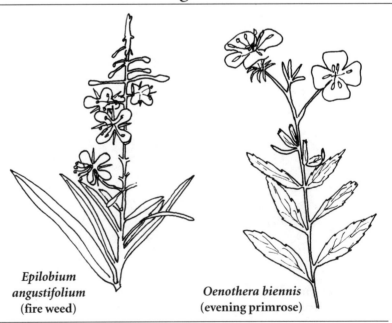

Epilobium
angustifolium
(fire weed)

Oenothera biennis
(evening primrose)

distributed globally, but is most abundant in the Western Hemisphere. The major genera are *Oenothera* and *Epilobium.*

Epilobium angustifolium (fire weed, great willow-herb, wickup) is a 1- to 7-foot native perennial found statewide in clear, high-humus areas, especially after fires. Leaves are alternate, lance-shaped, entire or fine-toothed, with a whitish undersurface. Flowers are $^3/_4$ to 1-inch and magenta, in a long spikelike raceme, appearing in June.

Native Americans used a poultice of roasted, crushed root for boils. A fresh-root poultice was applied to swollen knees, and a moistened fresh- or dried-leaf poultice was applied to bruises and to remove splinters. A bark infusion was applied as a poultice for pain, and the dried-leaf or root infusion was taken for bowel hemorrhage. The root decoction was taken for sore throat, tuberculosis, gastritis, and internal injuries from lifting, and an infusion was taken for urinary tract problems. As a cancer treatment, a poultice of seeds, down, and oil was applied to the wound when a tumor was cut open.

Oenothera biennis (evening primrose) is a 1- to 8-foot native biennial weed found in dry, open areas statewide. Leaves are alternate, lance-shaped, wavy-edged, and toothed. Flowers are 1 to 2 inches and yellow, with four petals; they open at sunset. Flowering begins in June.

Native Americans applied a whole-plant poultice to bruises and rubbed the chewed root on muscles to increase strength. The hot root poultice was applied to piles, and an infusion was taken as a dietary aid in weight control.

074 *Ophioglossaceae*

The adder's-tongue family of ferns. The name is descriptive of the fruiting spike. Family affiliation may be disputed, but identification is not difficult. Family distribution is global.

Botrychium virginianum (rattlesnake grape fern, Virginia grape fern) is a 1- to 2-foot native common fern found in rich-soiled, wooded areas of northern New Jersey and decreasingly southward. This is the most fernlike of the genus, with delicate, lacy, broadly triangular sterile fronds and taller fertile fronds bearing bright yellow spores in late May.

Native Americans used the root decoction as an emetic, a diaphoretic, and an expectorant for the cough of consumption. The root decoction was also reduced by boiling to a syrup and used as a rub for snake bite.

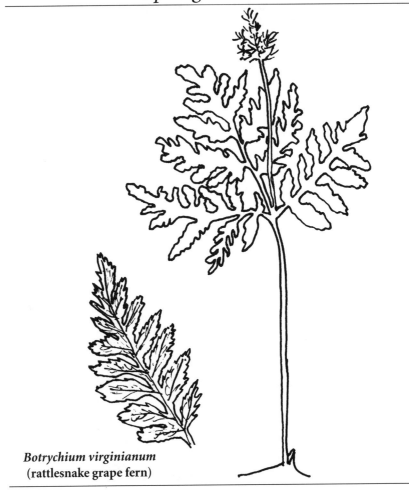

**Botrychium virginianum
(rattlesnake grape fern)**

075 *Orchidaceae*

The orchid family of herbaceous plants of many habitats and structures. They are primarily tropical, terrestrial, epiphytic or saprophytic (especially those of the forest floor), and sometimes climbing. Most of the orchids of the colder regions live in moist habitats of meadows or forested areas.

Aplectrum hyemale (adam-and-eve, putty-root) is a 10- to 16-inch native perennial found in rich-soiled, wet swamps and wooded areas of northern New Jersey. Tuberous roots produce an oval, wrinkled, single leaf with distinct folds and white lines in the fall. The leaf is not present when purplish brown or yellowish brown flowers appear in May.

Native Americans applied a poultice of beaten roots to boils and for head pain.

Corallorhiza maculata (dragon's claw, large coralroot, spotted coralroot)

Orchidaceae

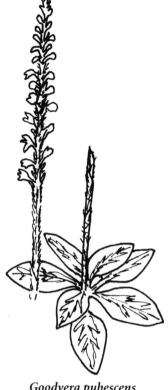

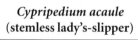

Cypripedium acaule
(stemless lady's-slipper)

Goodyera pubescens
(downy rattlesnake-plantain)

is an 8- to 20-inch native perennial found in dry, wooded areas of northern New Jersey. The plant is a leafless, nongreen saprophyte with purplish, brownish, or yellowish stems and purple-spotted, yellowish flowers appearing in June.

Native Americans applied a plant infusion for ringworm and other skin diseases. An infusion prepared from fresh or dried stalks was taken to "build up the blood" of pneumonia patients.

Cypripedium acaule (squirrel's shoe, stemless lady's-slipper, two-leaved lady's-slipper) is a 6- to 15-inch native perennial found in moist to dry, acidic, wooded areas statewide, including the pinelands. The plant has two basal leaves and a pink or, rarely, white, orchidlike flower, appearing in May.

Native Americans used the root for neuralgia and other pains, spasms, fits, hysterical affections, nervousness, and male disorders. A root infusion was taken for colds, influenza, and worms, and a plant infusion was taken for diabetes, nervousness, "female trouble," and rupture pain.

Cypripedium calceolus (yellow lady's-slipper) is a 1- to 3-foot native perennial found in moist, rich-soiled, wooded areas of northern New Jersey. This is a hairy plant with alternate, broadly lance-shaped leaves. Large-flowered and small-flowered varieties are recognized. Flowers are yellow, appearing in May.

Native Americans used yellow lady's-slipper to treat the same disorders as listed for *C. acaule.*

Goodyera pubescens (downy rattlesnake-plantain, networt) is a 6-inch to 2-foot native perennial found in rich-soiled, dry, wooded areas of northern and southern New Jersey. Leaves are in a basal rosette, with distinctively white-veined, pointed-oval, and entire leaves. Flowers are whitish, in a dense cylindrical spike, appearing in July.

Native Americans used a cold leaf infusion for colds and kidney problems, a wilted-leaf poultice for burns, and a crushed-leaf wipe or poultice for sore mouth in babies. The expressed juice was used for eye drops, and a plant infusion was held in the mouth for toothache. The root was used as a remedy for rheumatism and pleurisy and was given to women after childbirth. The plant was taken in whiskey to improve the appetite and as an emetic.

Spiranthes cernua (nodding ladies' tresses, screw auger) is a 4-inch to 2-foot native perennial found in wet, open-wooded areas statewide. Leaves are basal, long, narrow, and entire. Flowers are small, white, and slightly nodding, appearing in late August.

Native Americans used a root infusion as a diuretic and for venereal disease. A warm plant infusion was used as a stimulating wash for babies.

Spiranthes lucida (early ladies' tresses, pearl twist, wide-leaved ladies' tresses) is a 4-inch to 1-foot native perennial found in wet, open-wooded areas of northwestern New Jersey. Leaves are basal, shining, lance-shaped, and entire. Flowers are white and appear in spring and early summer.

Native Americans used early ladies' tresses for the same medicinal purposes as *S. cernua.*

076 *Orobanchaceae*

The broomrape family of succulent, root-parasitic, achlorophyllous herbs, with alternate, scalelike, simple leaves. The major genus in North America is *Orobanche,* with several species known as cancerroot.

Epifagus virginiana (beech drops, cancerroot) is a nongreen, parasitic plant found in rich-soiled, moist, beechwood areas of northern New Jersey. Leaves are scalelike on brown, yellowish, or reddish plants; the stem branches from the base. The flowers are whitish with purple-brown spots and appear in early September.

Native Americans used a plant infusion as an antidiarrheal.

077 *Oxalidaceae*

The wood sorrel family of herbs, occasionally shrubby. The name refers to the sour taste of the foliage, which is characteristic. The leaves are palmate with usually three leaflets. The family is primarily tropical and includes perhaps 1000 species, mostly of the genus *Oxalis*.

Oxalis corniculata (creeping lady's sorrel, yellow wood sorrel) is a 6- to 10-inch native, creeping perennial weed found in waste areas of northern New Jersey. Leaves are alternate and divided cloverlike. Flowers are yellow, appearing in April, and giving rise to seed pods with stalks bent downward.

Native Americans used yellow wood sorrel for hookworms in children. It was chewed for sore throat and used to treat cancer "when it is first started." The cold leaf infusion was taken as an antiemetic.

In Chinese medicine, the whole plant is used internally, or externally as a crushed poultice. It is used to treat influenza, urinary tract infections, diarrhea, injuries, and snakebites.

Oxalis stricta (yellow sheep sorrel) is a 3- to 15-inch native, erect perennial weed found in open waste areas of northern and southern New Jersey. Leaves are alternate and divided cloverlike. Flowers are yellow, appearing in late April, and giving rise to seed pods that are horizontal or bent sharply downward.

Native Americans applied a poultice of the plant to swellings.

Oxalidaceae

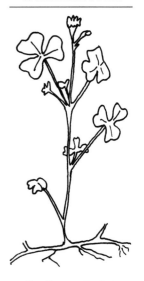

**Oxalis corniculata
(creeping lady's sorrel)**

078 *Papaveraceae*

The poppy family of annual or perennial herbs, and, rarely, shrubs and trees. They usually have milky or colored sap. Leaves are alternate or whorled and if not entire, then pinnately, palmately, or ternately dissected. Flowers are usually single, large, and showy.

Chelidonium majus (celandine, swallow-wort) is a 1- to 2-foot naturalized perennial weed found in rich-soiled, moist, shaded areas statewide. Leaves are alternate and divided into several irregularly lobed leaflets. Flowers are yellow, $^1/_2$ to $^3/_4$ inches, and in small umbels. Flowering begins in April.

Native Americans apparently did not use celandine as a medicinal plant. Celandine is native to Europe and has been used to treat warts, eczema, ringworm, corns, and cancer. The plant sap is yellow and extremely acrid, making it unlikely to cause accidental poisoning; however, it has been taken internally.

Sanguinaria canadensis (bloodroot, dill, red puccoon) is a 3-inch to 1-foot native perennial found in rich-soiled, open, wooded areas of northern New Jersey. The leaf is large and deeply lobed, having appeared first wrapped around the flower stalk. Showy, white flowers appear in late March or early April.

Native Americans used bloodroot as a wash for ulcers and sores and as a snuff for catarrh. The plant was chewed for colds and sore throat, and a plant poultice was applied for drawing thorns and splinters. A poultice of cooked plants was applied to cuts and wounds. A plant or root decoction was taken for fevers and as a spring emetic or tonic. The powdered-root infusion was used as an eyewash and antiemetic, and the fresh-root infusion was used as a wash for burns, and as a treatment for asthma, tuberculosis, gonorrhea, syphilis, and piles.

Bigelow described bloodroot as an acrid narcotic, causing heartburn, nausea and emesis, faintness, vertigo, and diminished vision. In smaller doses, it has a digitalislike effect on the pulse and accelerates circulation. In still-smaller doses it was considered tonic and taken for phthisis, catarrh, "typhoid pneumonia," dyspepsia, and other complaints.

The underground stem of bloodroot contains sanguinarine and other alkaloids that cause irritation of the mucous membranes of the mouth, throat, and stomach, producing burning with nausea and emesis. Ingestion also affects the nervous and cardiovascular systems. In modern medicine, bloodroot has also been used in a cancer treatment.

Stylophorum diphyllum (celandine poppy) is a 1- to 2-foot naturalized perennial found in rich-soiled, moist, shaded areas statewide. Leaves are opposite, deeply lobed, and divided. Flowers are bright yellow, appearing in April, and giving rise to poppylike fruit in May.

Native Americans apparently did not use the celandine poppy for medicinal purposes. Uses are similar to those described for *Chelidonium majus*, and the effects of the alkaloids on the heart require a similar caution.

Papaveraceae

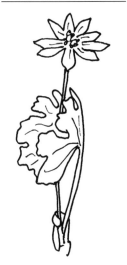

*Sanguinaria
canadensis*
(**bloodroot**)

079 *Phytolaccaceae*

The pokeweed family of herbs, shrubs, trees, and, rarely, woody vines. Leaves are simple, entire, and alternate. The family occurs primarily in tropical America.

Phytolacca americana (pigeonberry, pokeberry, pokeweed) is a 4- to 10-foot native perennial weed found in well-drained, moist areas statewide. The stem is stout, succulent, and branching with large, pointed-oval, entire, alternate leaves. White or pinkish flowers in racemes appear in June and give rise to dark purple berries.

Native Americans used a berry infusion for dysentery and arthritis. A berry wine and a fermented leaf infusion were taken for rheumatism.

A poultice of crushed berries was applied to breast sores. The cooked greens were eaten, and the root infusion taken to "build blood." The cold powdered-root infusion was taken for kidneys, and steam from the root decoction was used for piles. A crushed-root poultice was applied to warts, cuts, and bruises. A strong, whole-plant infusion was used in herbal steam for rheumatism. The plant was used as an expectorant, emetic, and cathartic, and a stem decoction was taken for chest colds. Leaves were used to treat bleeding wounds, for skin diseases, and to remove pimples and blackheads.

Bigelow described poke as a certain emetic and cathartic producing occasional narcotic symptoms. Externally, it produced a burning sensation and was useful in psora and other skin diseases.

Pokeweed seeds and roots are especially toxic. The leaves and stems cause less acute toxicity, but are still regarded as dangerous because of their mitogenic properties. The roots and seeds are also mitogenic, but their acute toxicity is associated with the action of triterpene saponins such as phytolaccigenin. Roots, leaves, and unripe berries contain phytolaccatoxin and other toxic triterpenes. Ingestion can lead to death within 24 hours.

080 *Pinaceae*

The pine family of small and large trees. The best known of the living genera are the 80 to 90 species of *Pinus*, about 40 species of *Abies* (fir), about 40 species of *Picea* (spruce), 7 species of *Pseudotsuga* (includes Douglas fir), 14 species of *Tsuga* (hemlock), and about 10 species of *Larix* (larch, tamarack), all of which, with the exception of *Pseudotsuga*, can be found in New Jersey.

Larix laricina (black larch, eastern larch, tamarack larch) is an 80- to 100-foot native coniferous tree found in wet, boggy forest areas of northern New Jersey. Needles are 1 inch long, in deciduous, circular clusters. Cones are oval, $3/4$ inches long, with rounded scales. Pollen is shed in March and April.

Native Americans used dried leaves of tamarack as an inhalant and fumigant. A bud-and-bark infusion was taken as an expectorant. A fresh inner-bark poultice was applied to burns, wounds, and inflammations. A bark infusion was taken for anemia, colds, tuberculosis, and gonorrhea. The bark was also used to treat suppurating wounds, and it is said that it "drives out inflammation and generates heat."

Picea mariana (black spruce) is a 20- to 30-foot or occasionally 100-foot native coniferous tree found in cool, wet sphagnum bogs of northern New Jersey. Leaves are evergreen on slender, often pendulous

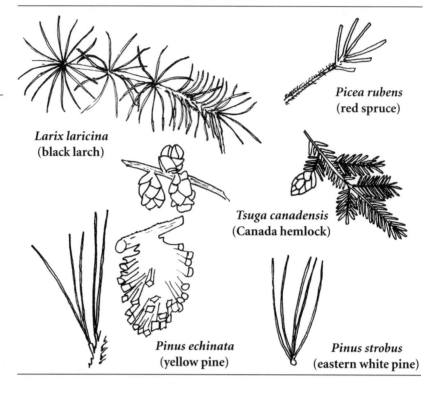

Larix laricina
(black larch)

Picea rubens
(red spruce)

Tsuga canadensis
(Canada hemlock)

Pinus echinata
(yellow pine)

Pinus strobus
(eastern white pine)

branches, forming a narrow, irregular head. The bark is gray-brown, with the young branches brown or yellowish brown. Leaves are $^1/_4$ to $^3/_4$ inch, quadrangular, and dull, dark to bluish green. Flowers and young cones are purple. Mature cones are dull grayish brown, $^1/_2$ to $1^1/_2$ inches long, with rounded scales.

Native Americans used black spruce twig decoction for coughs and the leaves as a stimulant. The bark was used as a "medicinal salt," and the inner-bark poultice was applied to inflammations associated with infection.

Picea rubens (*P. rubra*) (he-balsam, red spruce) is an 80- to 100-foot native coniferous tree found in wet, rocky areas of northern New Jersey. Leaves are evergreen on short, slender branches, forming a narrow, pyramidal head. The bark is red-brown, with the young branches reddish brown. Leaves are $^1/_2$ inch, pointed, quadrangular, dark or bright green, and shiny. Flowers are purple, and young cones are green. Mature cones are light reddish brown, glossy, $1^1/_4$ to 2 inches long, with rounded scales.

Native Americans used a branch infusion for colds and to "break out measles."

Pinus echinata (shortleaf pine, spruce pine, yellow pine) is an 80- to 120-foot native coniferous tree found in dry, sandy areas of southern

New Jersey, including the pinelands. Leaves are evergreen, on slender, pendulous branches in regular whorls, forming a rounded head. Leaves are 3 to 5 inches long, pointed, dark bluish green, and in groups of three. Cones are nearly stalkless, dull brown, $1^1/2$ to 2 inches long, with a soft prickle on each scale.

Native Americans used a cold bud infusion for worms. Pellets of tar were used as a cathartic and were considered "beneficial for soreness of the back."

Pinus strobus (eastern white pine) is a 100- to 150-foot native and escaped coniferous tree found in moist areas statewide. Leaves are evergreen on horizontal branches in regular whorls, forming a symmetrical, open pyramid. Needles are 2 to 5 inches long, soft, and bluish green. Cones, on $1/2$- to 1-inch stalks, are 2 to 4 inches long, cylindrical, slender, and curved.

Native Americans used a poultice of pitch to draw boils, thorns, and splinters and to reduce pain and inflammation. A poultice of crushed leaves was applied for a headache, and dried leaves were inhaled as a stimulant. A twig infusion was taken for kidney disorders and scrofula, and as an emetic. A bark infusion was an "important medicine" taken for chest pain, for colds, and to treat wounds. The inner bark, outer bark, and leaves were used to treat scurvy. The boiled inner bark was used for sores and swellings, and the dried inner bark was used as a cough remedy. Steam from the bark decoction was inhaled for colds, and crushed leaves were used as an herbal steam for headache and backache. The powdered wood was used on chafed babies, sores, and improperly healed navels. A shaved-knot decoction is used for poison ivy. It was also taken for consumption and as an appetite stimulant. The shaved-knot decoction has been described as "better than penicillin." The boiled gum was taken for sore throat, colds, and consumption, and pitch was chewed for a cough. The raw bark was taken for rheumatism, stiff limbs, cramps, and stomach problems.

Tsuga canadensis (*Abies canadensis*) (Canada hemlock, eastern hemlock) is a 50- to 100-foot native coniferous tree found in cool, moist, rocky areas of northern New Jersey and other areas to the south. Leaves are flat, bright green above with two whitish lines on the undersides, $1/4$ to 3/4 inches long including a short petiole, and evergreen, on slender, horizontal branches. Cones are 1 inch long with few, rounded scales. Pollen is shed from April to May.

Native Americans used a cold infusion prepared from twigs and bark as a sudorific for colds and fevers and for kidneys. The inner bark was used to treat scurvy and chapped skin, to check diarrhea, and for dysentery. The root was chewed for diarrhea, and a root decoction was used in an herbal steam for rheumatism. A bark poultice was used for "itching armpits," and the powdered inner bark was used as a styptic for wounds.

081 *Plantaginaceae*

The plantain family of annual or perennial herbs, with leaves alternate or opposite. Most of the species belong to the genus *Plantago* and are distributed globally.

Plantago aristata (bracted plantain, buckthorn) is a 1- to 6-inch native perennial weed found in lawns, dry waste areas, and pastures statewide. Leaves are basal, narrow, dark green, and flat (not fleshy). The flower spike is 1 to 6 inches, with stiff bracts protruding from the flower clusters. Flowers are greenish white and appear in June.

Native Americans used poulticed leaves for headache, burns, blisters, ulcers, and insect stings. Leaf juice was used for sore eyes. An infusion was taken for bowel complaints, "bloody urine," and used as a douche. The root infusion was taken for dysentery and diarrhea in babies.

Plantago lanceolata (English plantain) is a 10-inch to 2-foot natural-

Plantaginaceae

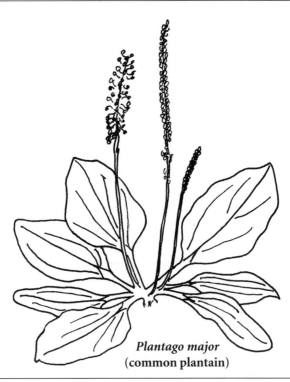

Plantago major
(common plantain)

ized perennial weed found in lawns, waste places, and pastures state-wide. Leaves are basal and lance-shaped, with three to five ribs. The flower spike is dense, short, and cylindrical, on a grooved stalk. Flowers are greenish white and appear in April.

Native Americans used English plantain as they did *P. aristata*. In addition, the leaf infusion was dropped into the ear for earache.

Plantago major (common plantain, white man's foot) is a 6- to 18-inch naturalized perennial weed found in lawns, pastures, salt marshes and along roadsides statewide. Leaves are basal, broadly oval, and ribbed. Leaf margins may be toothed. The flower spike is slender, elongated, and blunt-tipped. Flowers are greenish white and appear in June.

Native Americans used common plantain as they did bracted and English plantain. In addition, a poultice of fresh, chopped leaves was applied for rheumatism, inflammation, snakebite (roots and leaves), and bruises, and to draw thorns and splinters. The leaf was rubbed on the body as a sudorific, and a leaf infusion was taken for urinary problems. The root decoction was taken as a febrifuge and for constipation, colds, pneumonia, and stomach trouble.

In Chinese medicine, the whole plant or the seeds alone are prepared as a decoction for treatment of urinary tract problems, prostatitis, and conjunctivitis.

082 *Platanaceae*

The sycamore or plane tree family of large trees, with dark outer bark and white or greenish inner bark. Leaves are palmately lobed to cleft, and simple. The family is composed of a single genus, *Platanus*, occurring in the Northern Hemisphere. The sycamore of ancient history was probably *Ficus sycomorus* or *Sycomorus antiquorum*, also known as pharaoh's fig.

Platanus occidentalis (buttonwood, sycamore) is a 130- to 170-foot native tree found in swamps, along streams, and in other rich-soiled, moist areas of northern New Jersey. Those found in the inner-coastal plain of southern New Jersey are escapes. The trunk may be 10 feet in diameter, with the bark creamy white, mottled, and peeling. Leaves are toothed and broadly oval, with three to five lobes. Flowers appear in May, producing 2-inch globular, persisting fruit in October.

Native Americans used an inner-bark infusion for dysentery, milky or yellow urine, measles, and cough. The bark infusion was used for pulmonary tuberculosis, colds, and hemorrhage, as a wash for dry small-pox pustules (to prevent scars), and as a blood purifier. The expressed

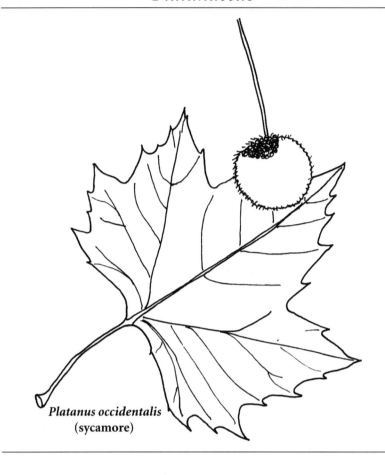

Platanus occidentalis
(**sycamore**)

Polemoniaceae

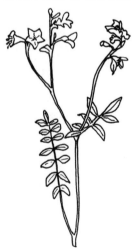

Polemonium reptans
(**Jacob's ladder**)

bark juice was used as a wash for infected sores and for infant rash. The root decoction was taken as an emetic and purgative. The plant was also used to remedy catarrh and to treat internal ulcers.

083 *Polemoniaceae*

The phlox family of herbs, shrubs, and, rarely, small trees. Leaves are entire, lobed, dissected, or compound. The family occurs in the Western Hemisphere and, with the exception of a few species in northern Eurasia, is centered in California and neighboring states. A number of species of *Polemonium* (Jacob's ladder) occur from the mountainous west through northeastern North America.

Polemonium reptans (abscess plant, Greek valerian, Jacob's ladder) is a 6-inch to 2-foot native and escaped perennial found in rich-soiled, moist areas of northern New Jersey and along the inner-coastal plain as an escape. Leaves are alternate and divided, with 11 to 17 lance-shaped or oval, paired leaflets. Stems are weak and bending. Flowers are blue and appear in May.

Native Americans used the root of Greek valerian in a compound diuretic and cathartic preparation. A decoction prepared from this species of valerian was used as a hair and scalp wash.

084 *Polygalaceae*

The milkwort family of herbs, shrubs, small trees, and saprophytic vines. Leaves are usually alternate and without stipules. The family occurs in both tropical and temperate regions, with many species in the southern and eastern portions of North America.

Polygala leutea (orange milkwort, yellow bachelor's buttons) is a 6-inch to 1-foot native perennial found in sandy swamps of southern New Jersey, especially in the pinelands. Leaves are small, narrow, lance-shaped, and alternate. Flowers are small and orange-yellow, in dense, cloverlike heads, appearing in mid-June.

Native Americans used a wetted poultice of dried milkwort flowers for swelling.

Polygala paucifolia (flowering wintergreen, fringed polygala, gay wings) is a 3- to 6-inch native perennial found in light, moist, rich soils of northern New Jersey. Leaves are alternate, egg-shaped, and clustered at the top of the stem. Flowers are few, arising from leaf axils. They are rose-purple, less than 1 inch long, and fringed at the tip. Flowers appear in late April and produce fruit in July.

Native Americans used a plant decoction as a wash for boils and for babies with syphilitic sores. A plant infusion was taken for and a leaf poultice applied to abscesses.

Polygala polygama (racemed milkwort) is a 4-inch to 1-foot rare native perennial found in dry woods and clearings statewide. Leaves are about 1 inch long, alternate, lance-shaped, and numerous. Flowers are usually rose-purple but occasionally white in a 1- to 4-inch raceme, appearing in June and producing fruit in July.

Native Americans used a plant decoction of milkwort as a cough medicine.

Polygala senega (Seneca snakeroot, senegaroot) is a 6- to 18-inch rare native perennial found in dry or moist, rocky, wooded areas of northern New Jersey. Leaves are small, alternate, and lance-shaped. Flowers are white and legumelike, appearing in May in a terminal spike.

Native Americans used Seneca snakeroot for colds, croup, pleurisy, rheumatism, dropsy, and inflammation, and also as a sudorific, diuretic,

Polygalaceae

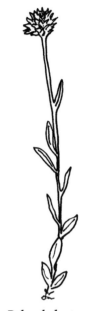

Polygala leutea
(orange milkwort)

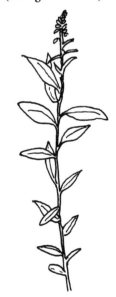

Polygala senega
(Seneca snakeroot)

cathartic, and abortifacient. For snakebite, the root was chewed, some was swallowed, and the remainder applied as a poultice.

Bigelow described senegaroot as sudorific and expectorant in small doses, and emetic and cathartic in large doses. Senegaroot was used by physicians in advanced pulmonary disease, asthma, croup, dropsy, rheumatism, and amenorrhea.

Polygala verticillata (whorled milkwort) is a 4- to 20-inch native, branched perennial found in dry or moist areas statewide. Upper leaves are in whorls of three to five, while lower leaves may be alternate or opposite. Flowers may be purplish or greenish white, in terminal, tapering clusters. Flowers appear in late June.

Native Americans used an infusion of milkwort internally for "summer complaint" in adults and babies.

085 *Polygonaceae*

The buckwheat family of primarily herbs, but occasionally shrubs, trees, and vines. The name is from the Greek term for "many-jointed," and the common names include jointweed and knotweed. Leaves are simple and alternate, with stipules usually present. The family is essentially limited to the temperate regions of the Northern Hemisphere. Buckwheat and rhubarb are the major food plants in the family. A sour or pungent taste is characteristic. Rhubarb (*Rheum rhaponticum*) leaf petioles are edible and widely cultivated for use as a vegetable and pie filling. The leaf blades contain high concentrations of soluble oxalates and anthraquinone glycosides that, if consumed, can cause severe diarrhea and vomiting and may inhibit blood clotting.

Roots of the Chinese herb *P. multiflorum* (fo-ti, ho shou-wu) have been credited with truly magical powers in maintaining the youthful state of appearance and energy. Consuming a preparation from a 300-year old root is said to make one immortal. The 50-year old root is said to restore and retain natural hair color. I do not know what to expect from the 1-year-old plants in my garden.

Polygonum aviculare (common knotgrass, doorweed, prostrate knapweed) is an 8-inch to 2-foot native and naturalized common weed found in waste places statewide. It is usually prostrate but may be half or fully erect. Leaves are blue-green, alternate, entire, and $1/2$ to 1 inch in length. Flowers are green with white or pink margins and appear in July.

Native Americans used knotgrass for gravel and bloody urine, as an astringent for children's diarrhea, for stomachache, and to prevent abortion. The plant was poulticed for application to swellings, inflammations, and pain. The plant was also used as a fish poison.

Polygonaceae

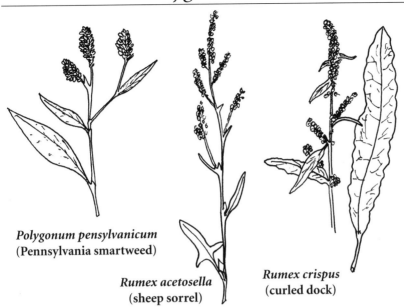

Polygonum pensylvanicum
(Pennsylvania smartweed)

Rumex acetosella
(sheep sorrel)

Rumex crispus
(curled dock)

Polygonum hydropiper (common smartweed, water pepper) is an 8-inch to 2-foot naturalized annual weed found in moist areas statewide. Stems are pinkish red with alternate, entire, lance-shaped leaves. Flowers are green, in 1- to 3-inch slender spikes, appearing in July.

Native Americans used smartweed as they did knotgrass. In addition, a plant decoction was taken for fever, chills, and "when cold." In small amounts it was taken for indigestion.

In Chinese medicine, a decoction of the whole plant is taken for bacterial dysentery, heat stroke, and rheumatoid arthritis.

Polygonum pensylvanicum (heart seed, Pennsylvania persicaria, Pennsylvania smartweed, pink knotweed, pinkweed) is a 1- to 5-foot prostrate or erect native annual weed found in well-drained, rich-soiled, moist areas statewide. Leaves are alternate, entire, lance-shaped, and long-pointed. Upper portions of the stems are covered with glandular hairs. Flowers are pink, in dense clusters, appearing in June.

Native Americans used an infusion prepared from plant tops for epilepsy and a leaf infusion to stop "hemorrhage of blood from the mouth." The plant was also used as an anal wipe for piles and bloody diarrhea.

Polygonum persicaria (heart's ease, lady's thumb, smartweed) is a 6-inch to 2-foot prostrate, naturalized perennial weed found in moist areas statewide. Stems are reddish, with alternate lance-shaped leaves showing a dark blotch in the center. Flowers are pink or purple, in elongated clusters, appearing in July.

Native Americans used a leaf infusion for gravel and a leaf-and-flower decoction for stomach pain. Crushed leaves were rubbed on poison ivy rashes, and a plant decoction was used as a foot and leg soak for rheumatism. The plant decoction was also mixed with meal to make a poultice for pain. Smartweed was also used for heart trouble and was rubbed on horses to repel flies.

Rumex acetosa (Belleville dock, French sorrel, green sorrel, sour dock) is a 3- to 5-foot erect, naturalized perennial weed found in open areas of northern New Jersey. Leaves are alternate, entire, arrow-shaped, relatively thin, and light green. The inflorescence is large and may be partially or totally sterile; it appears in May.

Native Americans used a sour dock leaf-and-stem decoction as a treatment for diarrhea.

Rumex acetosella (red sorrel, sheep sorrel, sourgrass) is a 4- to 15-inch naturalized perennial weed found in open, dry waste areas statewide. Leaves are alternate, entire, and arrow-shaped, with a distinct sour taste. Flowers are reddish or greenish, in branching, leafless racemes, appearing in April.

Native Americans chewed fresh leaves as a digestive aid and for tuberculosis. Bruised leaves and blossoms were applied as a poultice for old sores. A poultice of steamed leaves was applied to warts and bruises.

Rumex crispus (curled dock, sour dock, yellow dock) is a 1- to 6-foot naturalized perennial weed found in open areas statewide. Leaves are large, alternate, lance-shaped, and entire, with curled margins. Flowers are small and green, on branched racemes, appearing in May.

Native Americans used curled dock infusion for dysentery and kidney problems, and as an emetic. The root infusion or decoction was taken for hemorrhage of the lungs, venereal disease, and liver complaints; to heal cuts; as an appetite stimulant, a cathartic, and a general tonic. A cold leaf infusion was used for mouth sores, and a leaf-and-seed decoction was applied to sores. A seed infusion was given to babies for dysentery. The root poultice was applied to sores, ulcers, swellings, rheumatic pains, burns, and bruises. A leaf poultice was applied to boils to draw pus.

Polypodiaceae

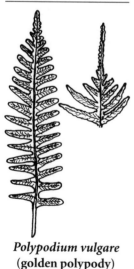

**Polypodium vulgare
(golden polypody)**

086 *Polypodiaceae*

A fern family of low-growing plants characterized by the appearance of their fronds and the morphology and distribution of reproductive structures. They are easily identified as ferns, but nearly impossible for the amateur botanist to separate into families. Individual species are much simpler to identify.

Polypodium vulgare (*P. virginianum*) (golden polypody, rock polypody) is a 1-foot, spreading, evergreen native fern found statewide, with the exception of the central pinelands. Leaves are oblong, dark green, leathery, and divided nearly to the midrib into 10 to 20 blunt, alternating leaflets.

Native Americans used a polypody decoction for stomach pains, and the root was chewed for swollen sore throat.

087 *Portulacaceae*

The portulaca family of herbs and, occasionally, shrubby plants. The leaves are more or less succulent, simple, and alternate or opposite. Stipules may or may not be present. The family includes both weeds and cultivated species and is distributed widely.

Portulaca oleracea (pig pursley, purslane) is a prostrate, smooth, herbaceous native weed found in gardens and waste areas statewide. Stems are reddish, with leaves alternate, entire, spatula-shaped, and scattered along the stem with clusters at the ends of branches. Flowers are in the leaf cluster. They are small and yellow and appear only for a few hours in the morning sun, beginning in June.

Native Americans used the entire plant to poultice bruises and burns.

In Chinese medicine, the fresh whole-plant poultice is applied for hemorrhoids, erysipelas, boils, and ulcers, and snake and insect bites. A decoction is taken internally for dysentery and urinary tract infections.

088 *Primulaceae*

The primrose family of herbs and slightly woody plants. The leaves are usually simple, and opposite or whorled. The family is distributed globally.

Anagallis arvensis (cure-all, scarlet pimpernel, shepherd's weather glass) is a small, prostrate, native(?) annual weed found in waste areas statewide. Leaves are small, opposite, entire, and egg-shaped. Flowers are red or sometimes blue and starlike, $1/4$ inch, in leaf axils. Flowers appear in June, opening only in sunlight.

Native Americans apparently did not use scarlet pimpernel as a medicinal plant. In England, the plant juice is used as a gargle. In India, it has been used to treat gout, cerebral affections, hydrophobia, leprosy, dropsy, epilepsy, and "mania." The poultice is used to treat snakebite and is also used as a fish poison. When taken in large doses, toxicity to livestock and humans has been noted in both England, India, and the United States.

Glaux maritima (sea milkwort) is a 2-inch to 1-foot endangered

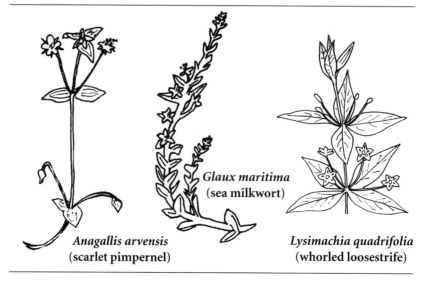

Glaux maritima
(sea milkwort)

Anagallis arvensis
(scarlet pimpernel)

Lysimachia quadrifolia
(whorled loosestrife)

native perennial found in salt marshes and on sea beaches of eastern New Jersey. The plant is light-colored, with leaves opposite, entire, oblong or narrow, about $1/2$ inch long, and fleshy. Flowers are stalkless, white, pink, or purple, without petals, and appearing in June and July only.

Native Americans ate the boiled root as a sedative.

Lysimachia quadrifolia (whorled loosestrife) is a 1- to 3-foot native perennial found in moist or dry, wooded areas statewide. Leaves are in whorls of four or five. Flowers are yellow with red dots or streaks, on long stalks arising from the leaf axils, and appearing in June.

Native Americans used the root infusion or decoction as an emetic and for kidney and urinary problems, "female trouble," and "bowel trouble."

089 *Ranunculaceae*

The buttercup family of mainly herbs but sometimes bushes and woody vines such as *Clematis*. They may be annuals or perennials with variable leaves. The family is distributed globally but mainly located in the Northern Hemisphere. Monkshood (*Aconitum napellus*) is native to Europe and cultivated here as a showy perennial. The plant contains the toxic polycyclic diterpene alkaloid aconitine. Poisoning with aconitine causes blindness, numbness, respiratory failure, and death within 2 hours. The root is the most toxic, but the leaves are also quite dangerous, especially just before flowering.

Actaea alba (*A. pachypoda*) (doll's eyes, white baneberry, white cohosh) is a herbaceous 1- to 2-foot native perennial found mostly in northern New Jersey and less frequently in the south, in rich-soiled, forested areas, especially at the forest edge. Leaves are large and compound, twice-divided pinnately. The leaflets are oblong and sharp-toothed. Flowers appear from mid-May to June in oblong clusters on thick, red stalks. Fruit appears in late July to September as white, fleshy berries with a dark spot at the blossom end, hence the common name "doll's eyes."

Native Americans used the root infusion as a gargle and to cure "itch." It was given to children and adults for convulsions. The root decoction was taken "when a man urinates blood," to relieve the pains of childbirth, and as a stimulant "to relieve and rally a patient at the point of death." As a toothache remedy, it "will kill the teeth of young people if not careful with it." Only the roots and stems were used medicinally, but all parts of the plant should be considered poisonous due to an essential oil that can cause skin blisters on contact. As few as six berries can accelerate the heartbeat and cause severe gastroenteritis. Cases of poisoning are rarely if ever fatal and are best left untreated. Symptoms are said to disappear in 3 to 4 hours.

Actaea rubra (red baneberry, snakeberry) is native and similar to *A. alba* in all respects including distribution in New Jersey, namely, primarily in the northern regions but occasionally in the south, but is encountered less frequently. The berries are red.

Native Americans used the root decoction for colds and coughs, to treat sores; stimulate the appetite, reduce excessive menstrual flow; as a wash for rheumatism, a gynecological aid after childbirth to "purge the patient of afterbirth," a remedy for syphilis, and a cure for emaciation. The root was eaten for stomach troubles. The plant was used as a purgative, and a stem infusion was taken by pregnant and nursing mothers to increase milk flow. The root was recognized as poisonous in large quantities. Toxicity is similar to that described above for *A. alba*.

Anemone canadensis (Canada anemone) is a 1- to 2-foot native perennial rarely seen in New Jersey. It is essentially limited to the northern portion of the state and mostly along the Delaware River. Basal leaves are long-stalked, with five to seven lobes. The lower-stem leaves are in a whorl of three. They are deeply lobed, wedge-shaped, and stalkless, while the upper leaves are paired. The flowers are showy white with five "petals" (actually sepals) appearing in late May.

Native Americans used a root decoction for worms. An infusion was used as a wash for sores, for "cross eyes," eye twitch, and eye "poisoning." The root poultice was applied to wounds, and the leaves were used as a hemostat for nosebleed and bleeding sores and wounds. Many members of the buttercup family are poisonous, and all poisonous members of the genus *Anemone* contain toxic alkaloids.

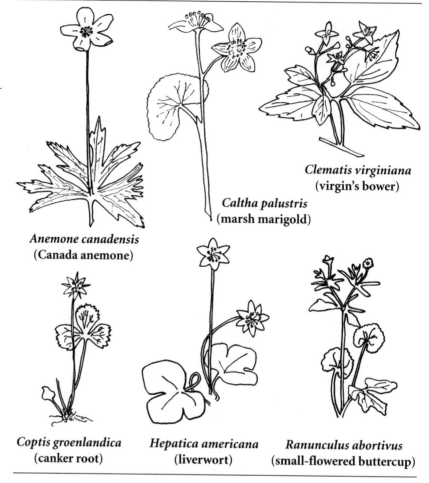

Anemone canadensis
(Canada anemone)

Caltha palustris
(marsh marigold)

Clematis virginiana
(virgin's bower)

Coptis groenlandica
(canker root)

Hepatica americana
(liverwort)

Ranunculus abortivus
(small-flowered buttercup)

Anemone cylindrica (long-fruited anemone, long-headed anemone, thimbleweed) is a 1- to 3-foot native perennial also rare in New Jersey and limited to the north. It is found in dry, open-wooded areas. Lower-stem leaves are in a whorl of five to nine, with three leaves larger than the others. The flowers are greenish white, appearing from June through September, and giving rise to $^3/_4$- to $1^1/_2$-inch-long cylindrical fruit.

Native Americans used a root infusion for lung congestion in tuberculosis and for headache and dizzy spells. A stem-and-fruit decoction was used as an eyewash, and a leaf poultice was applied to burns. As with other members of the genus *Anemone*, thimbleweed should be regarded as poisonous.

Anemone virginiana (*A. riparia*) (tall anemone, thimbleweed, wood anemone) is a 2- to 4-foot native perennial found in dry, rich-soiled, open areas statewide. Leaves are opposite or in whorls of three. The leaves are strongly veined, divided, and toothed. Flowers with petallike sepals are greenish or white, appearing in June, and giving rise to thimble-shaped fruit in late July.

Native Americans used tall anemone root infusion for whooping cough, diarrhea, tuberculosis, and as an emetic. The root poultice was applied to boils. Smoke from the seeds was inhaled for catarrh.

Anemonella thalictroides (rue anemone, windflower) is a 4- to 9-inch native perennial found in rich-soiled, dry or moist, open areas of northern and southwestern New Jersey. Leaves are in a whorl of three below the flower cluster and basally in three groups of three long-stalked leaves on the stem. Flowers with petallike sepals are white or pink, appearing in April.

Native Americans used the root as an antiemetic and for diarrhea.

Aquilegia canadensis (meeting houses, wild columbine) is a 1- to 3-foot native perennial found in dry or moist, rich-soiled, wooded areas statewide, with the exception of the central pinelands. Leaves are alternate and divided into three toothed leaflets. Flowers are showy and nodding. Each petal has a long, narrow spur at the back. The flowers are scarlet with yellow centers and protruding stamens, and appear in April.

Native Americans used an infusion for heart trouble and a cold infusion for bloody diarrhea. The root decoction was taken for diarrhea, and the infusion for kidney trouble. The root was chewed for stomach and bowel troubles. A crushed-seed infusion was taken for headache and fever.

Species of *Aquilegia* should be regarded as poisonous as they contain aconitine (as discussed in the description of the family).

Aquilegia vulgaris (blue columbine, European columbine) is a 1- to 2-foot escaped perennial found along roadsides and in shaded areas statewide. Leaves are alternate and divided into three toothed leaflets. Flowers are showy and similar to those of *A. canadensis* with the exception that they are blue, purple, or white and that the stamens do not protrude. Flowers appear in May.

Native Americans apparently did not use blue columbine as a medicinal plant possibly because they recognized this as a poisonous plant. Blue columbine poisoning is similar to that observed for the alkaloid acotine. Seeds have caused deaths in children.

Caltha palustris (cowslip, king cup, marsh marigold) is a 1- to 2-foot native aquatic perennial found in wet soils, bogs, and swamps statewide, except for the central pinelands. Leaves are glossy, heart-shaped, and toothed on long, succulent, hollow stems. Flowers are buttercuplike, showy, 1 to 1^1/$_2$ inches, with five to nine deep yellow, petallike sepals, appearing from April to May.

Native Americans used the root decoction as a diaphoretic, expectorant, and emetic. A boiled and crushed root poultice was applied to sores including those of scrofula. The leaf infusion was taken for constipation.

Marsh marigold poisoning is similar to that associated with other buttercups, but only the raw plant is poisonous. Boiled stems and leaves are edible, and the flower buds make "capers."

Cimicifuga racemosa (black cohosh, black snakeroot) is a 3- to 8-foot native perennial found in rich-soiled, moist, wooded areas of northern and inner-coastal southern New Jersey. Leaves are alternate and divided into leaflets, which are further divided into pointed-oval, toothed subleaflets. Flowers are malodorous and white, on long, showy spikes, and appear in June.

Native Americans used black cohosh as an abortifacient, tonic, anodyne, and diuretic. They also used it for colds, coughs, and constipation, and as a soak and steam bath for rheumatism. The root infusion was taken to promote lactation and to treat kidney problems. A crushed-leaf poultice was applied to the backs of babies for soreness.

Bigelow described black snakeroot tea as a useful astringent gargle for sore throat and a cure for psora (itchy skin). It was used as an aid in childbirth, for rheumatism, and dropsy.

Clematis virginiana (devil's darning needle, virgin's bower) is a 12- to 15-foot native, climbing perennial vine found in low, moist, shaded areas statewide, with the exception of the central pinelands. Leaves are divided into three toothed leaflets. Leaf or leaflet stalks may be twisted around supporting vegetation. Flowers are white, with four petallike sepals, appearing in late July.

Native Americans used virgin's bower as an ingredient in green corn medicine. The root infusion was taken for kidneys "when it burns," stomach trouble, nerves, and with root powder for the treatment of venereal disease sores. A stem decoction was used as a hallucinogenic wash.

All species of *Clematis* contain toxins similar to those found in the anemones. The juice is violently purgative and may cause death. The leaves of virgin's bower may cause contact dermatitis.

Coptis trifolia (*C. groendlandica*) (canker root, coptis, golden thread) is a 3-inch, running, mat-forming native perennial found in moist, well-shaded woods of northern New Jersey. The root is bright yellow and threadlike. Leaves are basal and divided into three shiny, evergreen, strawberrylike, toothed leaflets. Flowers are white, with five to seven petallike sepals, and appear in late April.

Native Americans used golden thread root infusion or decoction as an antiemetic and antiseptic mouthwash for babies. The root was also used for jaundice and as eye drops. The stem was chewed for mouth sores and irritation due to tobacco smoking.

Bigelow described coptis as a pleasant tonic, promoting appetite and digestion.

Hepatica americana (liverwort, round-lobed hepatica) is a 4- to 8-

inch native perennial found in rich-soiled, dry, wooded areas of northern and inner-coastal southern New Jersey. Leaves are basal and somewhat thick, with three deep lobes. Flowers are blue, pink, or white, with 6 to 12 petallike sepals and 3 green sepallike bracts. Flowers appear in late March.

Native Americans used liverwort root decoction for liver ailments, convulsions (especially in children), and menstrual complaints. An infusion was used to relieve vertigo. Plants were poulticed for inflammations and bruises, and the petals were chewed "to prevent fever in summer."

Hydrastis canadensis (goldenseal, turmeric) is a 6- to 15-inch native perennial found in rich-soiled, wooded areas of northern New Jersey. The root is bright orange-yellow. The leaves are large, alternate, deeply lobed, and toothed. The single greenish white flower, a globe-shaped cluster of stamens, arises from the uppermost leaf in April and gives rise to scarlet fruit in August.

Native Americans used goldenseal for cancer, diarrhea, whooping cough, fevers, pneumonia, tuberculosis (especially scrofula), liver trouble, and biliousness, and as a general tonic for debility and dyspepsia. The root was also used to treat chapped or cut lips.

Ranunculus abortivus (crowfoot, kidney-leaved buttercup, small-flowered buttercup) is a 6-inch to 2-foot native perennial found in moist, open-wooded areas of northern and southwestern New Jersey. Leaves are alternate and divided, with some of the basal leaves heart-shaped and toothed. Flowers are small (less than $^1/_2$ inch) and yellow, and appear in May.

Native Americans used crowfoot root decoction for stomach trouble and as an emetic remedy for poisonings. It was also used as a gargle for sore throat ("thrash"), a sedative, an eyewash, a wash for snakebite, and to dry up smallpox. It was used as a poultice for abscesses and as a styptic for nosebleed.

Bigelow described crowfoot as any one of several species of *Ranunculus* characterized by "violent acrimony" no longer used as rubifacients because they sometimes caused "deep running sores" that were difficult to heal.

Ranunculus acris (crowfoot, tall buttercup) is a 2- to 3-foot naturalized annual or perennial weed found in open areas of northern and southwestern New Jersey. Leaves are alternate and divided into five to seven long-toothed lobes. Flowers are showy and golden-yellow, appearing in May.

Native Americans used crowfoot infusion as a gargle for sore throat ("thrash") and for diarrhea. The juice was used as a sedative. The root poultice was applied to boils and abscesses and was also applied for chest pains and colds. The crushed leaves were inhaled for headache.

The coffeeberry, or buckthorn, family of shrubs, trees, climbing vines, and herbs, with simple, usually alternate leaves. The family is composed primarily of shrubs and is global in distribution.

Ceanothus americanus (New Jersey tea, redroot) is a 1- to 4-foot native perennial shrub found in open, dry areas of northern and inner-coastal southern New Jersey. Leaves are alternate, toothed, and pointed-oval, with three distinct parallel veins. Flowers are white, in clusters on new wood, appearing in June.

Native Americans used New Jersey tea root decoction as a wash for leg or foot injuries. The root was also used as a powerful astringent for bloody diarrhea, pulmonary troubles, toothache, suppressed menses, and to abort a fetus before the third month. It was also used for snakebite and venereal disease, as a cure-all for stomach problems, and was taken by women with urinary problems caused by colds. A bark decoction was applied to open sores caused by venereal disease and was also used as a wash for "sore roof of the mouth." Although the leaves do not produce a pleasant beverage, they were used as a tea substitute prior to the Revolutionary War.

Millspaugh considered the twigs of New Jersey tea to be very useful because of their mild astringency, as an injection in gonorrhea, for gleet (a persistent transparent urethral mucous discharge) and for leucorrhea. The plant was being "proven for a place in our Materia Medica."

Rhamnaceae

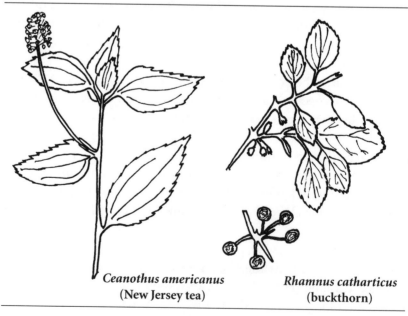

Ceanothus americanus
(New Jersey tea)

Rhamnus catharticus
(buckthorn)

Rhamnus catharticus (*R. cathartica*) (buckthorn) is a 6- to 20-foot naturalized perennial shrub originally cultivated as a hedge and now found in open, dry areas of northern New Jersey. Leaves are oval and toothed. Stems may have spiny tips. Flowers are small and greenish, in axillary clusters appearing in May, and giving rise to black fruit in late August.

Native Americans used a buckthorn bark decoction as an eyewash and as a treatment for "itch." The bark, fruit, and root were used as a cathartic.

Bigelow described buckthorn as a European shrub, not found in the United States. The berries were described as highly cathartic and unpleasant.

Buckthorn berries contain anthraquinone glycosides, and the purging and dehydration associated with ingestion may be followed by loss of consciousness.

091 *Rosaceae*

The rose family of herbs, shrubs, trees, and vines. Leaves are simple, pinnate, and alternate. This is a large, global family, well represented in the northern temperate regions. The genus *Rubus* is probably the most easily identified; however, division into species, although attempted here, should be regarded as a willingness to accept the species differences reported by others. The genus *Prunus* (cherry) contains a number of medicinal species. The leaves, bark, and stones contain cyanogenic glycosides (amygdalin) that release cyanide when ingested. Consuming large quantities should be avoided.

Agrimonia gryposepala (agrimony, tall hairy agrimony) is a 2- to 6-foot native perennial found in moist and dry, open areas of northern New Jersey. This is the most common species of agrimony, with alternate leaves divided into five to nine toothed leaflets. Flowers are small, $1/2$ inch or less, and yellow, in slender, hairy racemes, appearing in late July.

Native Americans used agrimony root infusion as a children's appetite suppressant and as a "blood builder," and the infusion or decoction was used to check diarrhea. The root was also used as a styptic for nosebleed. A fruit infusion was taken for fevers and as an antidiarrheal.

Agrimonia parviflora (many-flowered agrimony; small-flowered agrimony) is a 3- to 6-foot native perennial found in shaded, moist, wooded areas statewide, with the exception of the central pinelands. The stem is densely hairy, with leaves alternate and divided into 11 to 15 relatively large, lance-shaped, toothed leaflets. Flowers are small and yellow, in slender, branched racemes, appearing in July.

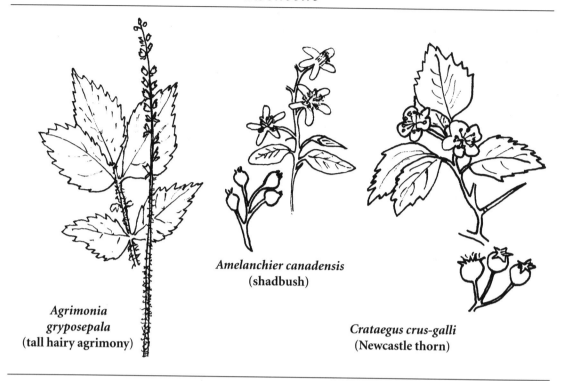

Amelanchier canadensis
(shadbush)

**Agrimonia
gryposepala**
(tall hairy agrimony)

Crataegus crus-galli
(Newcastle thorn)

Native Americans used many-flowered agrimony as they used *A. gryposepala* with the possible exception of the use of the root as a styptic.

Agrimonia pubescens (*A. eupatoria*) (common agrimony, soft agrimony) is a 2- to 3-foot naturalized (also described as native) perennial found in dry, rich-soiled, open areas of northern and southern New Jersey. Leaves are alternate, divided, and aromatic. Flowers are small (not showy) in racemes, and appear in mid-July.

Native Americans apparently did not use common agrimony as a medicinal plant. In India, the root is described as astringent, tonic, and diuretic. The leaves are reported to be anthelmintic. In Europe, the aromatic, astringent tea is taken for diarrhea and fevers and also used as a beverage drink.

Amelanchier arborea (common shadbush, Juneberry, serviceberry) is a 6- to 40-foot native shrub found in rich-soiled, dry areas of primarily northern and decreasingly southern New Jersey. Leaves are alternate and toothed, with white-woolly undersides at flowering time. Flowers are white, 1 to 1^1/$_2$ inches with five petals and in small clusters appearing in mid-April (shad-fishing time). The fruit is dry and tasteless.

Native Americans used a bark infusion for gonorrhea.

Amelanchier canadensis (sand cherry, serviceberry, shadbush, swamp shadbush) is a 4- to 20-foot native shrub found in swamps and wet, wooded areas statewide. Leaves are oblong, fine toothed, and white-woolly on the undersides at flowering time. Flowers are white, $1/2$ to $3/4$ inches, with five petals, in clusters of five or more, and appear in late April. The fruit is juicy.

Native Americans used serviceberry bark infusion as a bath. The infusion was given to children for worms and was taken to prevent abortion after injury.

Amelanchier laevis (Juneberry, smooth shadbush) is a 6- to 40-foot native shrub found near swamps and in rocky, wooded areas of northern and southwestern New Jersey. Leaves are smooth at flowering time. Flowers are white, 1 to $1^1/2$ inches with five petals, in clusters of five or more, and appear in mid-April, producing sweet, juicy fruit from June through August.

Native Americans used a bark infusion as a gynecological aid during pregnancy.

Crataegus crus-galli (cockspur, Newcastle thorn) is typical of this complex genus. There are at least 1,000 species of *Crataegus* (hawthorns), with perhaps 10 in New Jersey. The species *crus-galli* is a native shrub or tree of up to 40 feet in height found along streamsides and in dry to moist, open-wooded areas statewide. Spines are numerous and slender. Leaves are sharply toothed and elongated, with rounded ends. Flowers are pinkish, with rose or purple anthers, and appear in mid-May, producing globose, red fruit, with thin, dry flesh and two stones. Fruits appear in October through November and may persist.

Native Americans used species of hawthorn for "pain in the side," bladder ailments, general debility, and as a stomach medicine. Spines are used to probe boils and ulcers. In Asia and Europe, the fruit and flowers are used as a cardioregulating tonic and remedy for several heart diseases. The bark has been shown to be a febrifuge in cases of malaria.

Duchesnea indica (Indian strawberry, mock strawberry) is a 4- to 6-inch naturalized trailing perennial found in moist, open ground and waste places of northern and inner-coastal southern New Jersey. Leaves are alternate and divided strawberrylike into three toothed leaflets. Flowers are yellow, appearing in late April. Red, tasteless, strawberrylike fruits develop in late August.

Native Americans apparently did not use mock strawberry as a medicinal plant. In Asia, the plant tea is taken for pulmonary complaints and is poulticed or used to prepare an astringent wash for abscesses, boils, rheumatism, and bruises.

Filipendula rubra (queen-of-the-prairie) is a 2- to 8-foot native perennial found in moist meadows and wooded areas of northern New Jersey. Leaves are alternate and divided into three to seven broad, deeply lobed, toothed leaflets. Lower leaves are very large. Flowers are small and deep pink, in large, branching clusters, appearing in late June.

Native Americans regarded queen-of-the-prairie root as a "very important medicine for treating various heart diseases."

Filipendula ulmaria (*Spiraea ulmaria*)(Eurasian queen-of-the-meadow) is a 2- to 6-foot naturalized perennial found in shaded areas and roadsides of inner-coastal central New Jersey. Leaves are smooth above, white-woolly on the underside, and divided, with the terminal leaflet three- to five-lobed and 2 to 4 inches long. Lateral leaflets are smaller, ovate, and toothed. Flowers are white, in dense, branching, flat-topped clusters, appearing in June.

Native Americans apparently did not use the Eurasian queen-of-the-meadow for medicinal purposes. The leaves are aromatic and were used in Europe for flavoring. The roots are astringent and were used to control for diarrhea and kidney and lung problems. Flowers were used for rheumatism and to produce a diuretic tea. Salicylic acid was originally isolated from *Spiraea* in 1839, beginning a series of investigations that led to the discovery of aspirin.

Fragaria vesca (sow-teat strawberry, woodland strawberry) is a 3- to 6-inch naturalized perennial found in rich-soiled, moist, open areas of northern New Jersey. Leaves are basal and divided into three toothed leaflets. Flowers are white, in clusters above the leaves, and appear in May, and producing edible red (strawberry) fruit.

Native Americans used European woodland strawberry root to treat stomach complaints.

Fragaria virginiana (scarlet strawberry, Virginia strawberry) is native and similar to *F. vesca* but occurs statewide and has larger leaves and flowers. The fruit is somewhat more rounded, with deeply embedded seeds.

Native Americans used a scarlet strawberry infusion as a nerve medicine. It was also taken for dysentery, kidney problems, bladder and liver problems, scurvy, stomachache, and irregular menses. The root infusion was given for infant cholera, and the fruit was held in the mouth to remove tartar from teeth.

Geum canadense (white avens) is a 1- to 3-foot native perennial found in rich-soiled, moist, shaded areas statewide. The stem is smooth or only slightly hairy. Leaves are alternate, divided, and toothed, with the basal leaves more divided than those of the stem. Flowers are white, appearing in May.

Native Americans used avens root for "female weakness."

Geum rivale (*G. nivale*) (chocolate root, purple avens, water avens) is a 1- to 3-foot native perennial found in wet areas of far northern New Jersey. Leaves are alternate, divided, and toothed, with the basal leaves

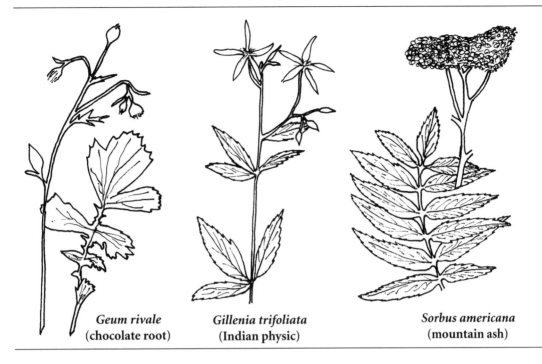

Geum rivale
(**chocolate root**)

Gillenia trifoliata
(**Indian physic**)

Sorbus americana
(**mountain ash**)

more divided than those of the stem. Flowers are purplish and nodding, appearing in late May.

Native Americans used chocolate root infusion or decoction for fevers, diarrhea, dysentery, coughs, and colds, especially in children.

Bigelow described chocolate root as one of the strongest astringents, useful in uterine hemorrhage, leucorrhea, and diarrhea. It was used in New York and in Europe for intermittent fevers.

Gillenia trifoliata (bowman's root, false ipecac, gillenia, Indian physic) is a 2- to 4-foot rare native perennial found in rich-soiled, wooded areas of northern New Jersey. Leaves are alternate and divided into three lance-shaped, toothed leaflets. Flowers are pinkish, with long, narrow petals, appearing in late May.

Native Americans used the root infusion or decoction for grippe, colds, chills and fever, and sore throat, and as a diaphoretic. The root was also used for kidneys and toothache, and as an emetic and a wash for leg scratches. A poultice was applied for "leg swelling" and rheumatism.

Bigelow described gillenia root bark as emetic if recently dried and powdered, and tonic in small doses.

Physocarpus opulifolius (ninebark) is a 3- to 10-foot native shrub found in moist areas of northern and inner-coastal New Jersey. The branches are spineless, with bark that peels with age. Leaves are alternate, oval, lobed, and toothed. Flowers are white and numerous, in rounded clusters appearing in May.

Native Americans used the inner-bark decoction as an emetic, a laxative, and a wash for gonorrhea. It was taken and used as a wash for scrofulous glands in the neck and as a cleansing drink for female maladies. The root infusion was taken as an emetic, and the bark decoction was taken as an emetic and purgative with the knowledge that a large dose could be fatal.

Potentilla arguta (five fingers, tall cinquefoil) is a 1- to 3-foot native perennial found in dry, rocky areas statewide. The stem is erect and hairy. Leaves are alternate and divided into 7 to 11 ovoid, toothed leaflets. Flowers are white in a cluster, appearing in late May.

Native Americans used a five fingers root decoction for dysentery. A poultice of moistened, dried, powdered root was applied to cuts. The dry, powdered root was also pricked into temples and stuffed into nostrils for headache.

Potentilla canadensis (Canadian cinquefoil, dwarf cinquefoil, five fingers) is a prostrate native perennial found in dry, open areas statewide. Leaves are basal and divided strawberrylike into five toothed leaflets. Flowers are yellow, appearing in late April.

Native Americans used a crushed dwarf cinquefoil root infusion for diarrhea.

Potentilla simplex (common cinquefoil) leaves are less strawberrylike than dwarf cinquefoil and have teeth around three-quarters of the leaflet border, while dwarf cinquefoil teeth do not extend beyond the middle. Flowers are yellow, appearing in mid-April.

Native Americans used a common cinquefoil root infusion for dysentery and as a mouthwash for "thrash."

Prunus americana (wild plum) is a 15- to 20-foot native shrub found in moist, shaded areas statewide, with the exception of the central pinelands. Branches are gray or gray-brown and thorny, with pointed-oval, toothed leaves in clusters. Flowers, large and white in clusters, appear in late April before the leaves, giving rise to small, hard, red to yellow fruit in late August.

Native Americans used wild plum bark to make cough syrup. The bark infusion was taken for kidney and bladder problems, and the decoction was used as a disinfecting wash. The root bark infusion was used as an astringent for mouth cankers, and a twig infusion was taken for asthma. A poultice of boiled root bark was applied to abrasions, and crushed fruit was used for mouth disease.

Bigelow described the dried fruit of the plum tree (prunes) as nutritious and laxative, to be taken habitually to obviate costiveness.

Prunus cerasus (egriot, pie cherry, sour cherry) is a 10- to 15-foot escaped tree forming thickets in well-drained areas statewide. These are rather low, round-headed trees with gray bark and no central lead stem. New shoots sprout from the roots, leading to the formation of dense thickets. Leaves are alternate, pointed-oval, and toothed. Flowers appear in May slightly before the leaves, with red, soft-fleshed, acidic fruit forming in late June.

Native Americans used a sour cherry bark infusion at the beginning of labor pains. It was also taken for coughs and colds, for "thrash," fevers, and "the great chill." The inner-bark infusion or decoction was taken for laryngitis, and the root bark was used to prepare a wash for old sores and ulcers. The boiled fruit was used for "blood discharged from the bowels" and in steam for digestive complaints.

Prunus serotina (rum cherry, wild black cherry) is a 40- to 90-foot native tree found in open areas statewide. The bark is rough and dark with a somewhat red undersurface. Leaves are lance-shaped and blunt-toothed. Flowers are white, in long, dense racemes, and appear in May, producing purplish black, sweet, fleshy fruit in late August.

Native Americans used a wild black cherry bark infusion for coughs and colds, fevers, including "the great chill," childbirth, "thrash," infant cholera; as a steam bath for babies with bronchitis; and to treat smallpox. The inner-bark infusion or decoction was taken for laryngitis, chest pain, and soreness. The astringent root bark was used as a wash for old sores and ulcers, and a poultice of fresh roots or the root decoction was used as a wash for a "scrofulous neck." The powdered root was applied to burns and ulcers. A bud, leaf, or bark infusion was taken with sugar for colds. The bark or berry infusion, sweetened with honey, was taken for cough with the caution that it would be poisonous if "stale." The fruit was used as a tonic and to produce a wine used as a remedy for dysentery.

Prunus virginiana (chokecherry) is a 2- to 20-foot native tree found in thickets of northern New Jersey. Leaves are pointed-oval and sharply toothed. Flowers are white and in racemes similar to those of the black cherry. Flowers appear in late April and produce reddish fruit in August.

Native Americans used chokecherry for the same medicinal purposes as they did wild black cherry. In addition, the bark decoction was used as a strengthening and growth-stimulating hair wash and an eyewash. The dried, powdered bark was smoked for headache or head colds, and steam from the boiling bark was used to treat snow blindness. The inner bark was tonic and taken for nervousness and cramps, and was sweetened to treat children's diarrhea. A pounded inner-bark poultice was applied to wounds or "galls." The root bark infusion was taken for stomach troubles and as a sedative, and was applied as a rectal douche for piles. An infusion prepared from wood scrapings was used to treat bowel troubles of children and adults. The unripe berries were eaten by children for diarrhea. Crushed ripe berries were given to children as an appetite stimulant and laxative. A preparation from the leaves was taken as an emetic, and a leaf, bark, or root decoction was taken for tuberculosis.

Bigelow listed only *P. virginiana* with the common name "wild cherry tree." The bark was described as bitter and aromatic, with a taste strong and penetrating but not disagreeable. It was a useful tonic with narcotic and, in fresh bark, antispasmodic properties.

Rosa blanda (meadow rose; smooth wild rose) is a 2- to 5-foot native shrub found on rocky slopes and the shores areas of inner-coastal New Jersey. Upper stems are smooth and nearly without thorns. Leaves are divided into five to seven dull green leaflets. Flowers are pink, 2 to $2^1/_2$ inches, appearing in June, with red fruit in August.

Native Americans used a fruit decoction to treat "itch," including itching piles. The fruit skin was used to treat stomach troubles. A root infusion was used as an eyewash and was taken for headache or lumbago. The dried, powdered flowers were used to relieve heartburn.

Rosa eglanteria (sweet briar, eglantine rose) is a 4- to 8-foot naturalized shrub found in open areas and along roadsides in northern New Jersey. It is a dense shrub with hooked thorns. Leaves are divided into five to seven dark green, fragrant leaflets. Flowers are bright pink, $1^1/_2$ to 2 inches, appearing in May, with fruit in September.

Native Americans used sweet briar as an ingredient in a urinary aid.

Rosa palustris (swamp rose; wild rose) is a 2- to 8-foot native shrub found in wet areas statewide with the exception of the central pinelands. Leaves are divided into seven dull green, fine-toothed leaflets. Flowers are pink, 2 inches, and appear in June with fruit in September.

Native Americans used a bark-and-root infusion for worms, and the root decoction was taken for dysentery.

Rosa rugosa (rugose rose, wrinkled rose) is a 2- to 8-foot naturalized shrub found in seashore thickets, on sand dunes, and along roadsides of coastal New Jersey. Leaves are divided into five to nine shiny, dark green, deeply veined leaflets. Flowers are purple or white, 3 to 4 inches, and appear in May, with fruit in September.

Native Americans apparently did not use the wrinkled rose for medicinal purposes. They used various available species of *Rosa* as purgatives for stomach pain, as antidiarrheals and eyewashes, and as ingredients in compound medicines.

Rosa virginiana (*R. lucida*) (glossy rose, low rose, pasture rose) is a 2- to 8-foot native shrub found in moist or dry thickets and borders of wet areas statewide. Leaves are divided into seven to nine dark green, shiny, coarsely toothed leaflets. Flowers are pink or white, 2 inches, and appear in May, with fruit in September.

Native Americans used a pasture rose root decoction as a bath and gave it to children for worms. The wash was also used for sore eyes and bleeding cuts.

Rubus allegheniensis (common blackberry, mountain blackberry, sow-teat blackberry) is a 2- to 8-foot native perennial found in open, dry areas of northern New Jersey. Stems are prickly and erect or arched. Leaves are alternate and divided into three to five leaflets. Flowers are white and appear in May, with fruit in August.

Native Americans used an infusion for urinary troubles, and the root or leaf infusion for diarrhea. The root infusion was taken by women threatened with miscarriage, and the decoction was taken as an antidote for poison. The root extract was used for stomach trouble and to treat sore eyes. A poultice of crushed roots was applied to the sore navel after birth, and the washed root was chewed for a coated tongue. Blackberry infusion was taken for rheumatism, for venereal disease, as a tonic and stimulant, and with honey as a wash for sore throat.

Rubus argutus (tall blackberry, thimbleberry) is similar to the common blackberry, but stems are more erect, stout, and prickly. Leaves are relatively small.

Native Americans used tall blackberry essentially as they did *R. allegheniensis*. The root was not poulticed.

Bigelow uses the common name "high" or "tall blackberry" to refer to *R. villosus* instead and gives uses as described for *R. flagellaris*.

Rubus canadensis (smooth blackberry, Millspaugh's blackberry) is similar to the common blackberry, but stems are thornless and weak.

Native Americans used thornless blackberry vines and berries to treat dysentery.

Rubus flagellaris (*R. baileyanus*) (dewberry, northern running dewberry) is a 3- to 4-inch trailing perennial found in dry, open areas statewide. Leaves are divided into three or five toothed leaflets. Flowers are white, appearing in May, with fruit in July.

Native Americans used dewberry as they did *R. allegheniensis* described above. The root was not poulticed.

Bigelow used the name *R. trivialis* for dewberry and described the root bark as highly astringent and rich in tannin and gallic acid. The root bark tea was used in infant cholera, dysentery, and diarrhea.

Rubus occidentalis (black raspberry, thimbleberry) is a strong, erect native bush with stems that arch over and root at the tips. It is found in rich-soiled, dry or moist, open areas statewide. Leaves are alternate and divided into three toothed leaflets. Upper leaf surfaces are dull green, while the lower are white. Flowers are white, in small, dense, prickly clusters, with petals shorter than the sepals. Flowers appear in May, with fruit in June.

Native Americans used a strong black raspberry leaf infusion for pains at childbirth, as an astringent for bowel complaints, and a wash for old sores. The root infusion was taken as an emetic and cathartic, as a tonic for boils and, in decoction, as a wash for eyes. A root, stalk, and leaf decoction was given to children for whooping cough, and a scraped-root decoction was given to children as a remedy for bowel complaints. The crushed-root decoction was taken for stomach pain, and the root was chewed for toothache and cough. A thorny branch was used as a scratch for rheumatism.

Rubus odoratus (purple flowering raspberry; thimbleberry) is a 3- to 6-foot native shrub found in moist, shaded, rocky woods of northern New Jersey. Leaves are alternate and large, with three to five lobes and heart-shaped at the base. Flowers are rose-purple, 1 to 2 inches, in clusters appearing in June, with red, dry, tasteless fruit in July.

Native Americans use purple flowering raspberry as they did *R. occidentalis*. A decoction is taken as a blood medicine and given to newborn babies for bowel problems.

Rubus pensilvanicus (*R. frondosus*) (bush blackberry, leafy-flowered blackberry) is a native cultivated blackberry similar to *R. allegheniensis* but less common and not recognized as a separate species by most botanists.

Native Americans used the root decoction as an abortifacient.

Rubus pubescens (dwarf raspberry, dwarf red blackberry, running raspberry) is a trailing, 1- to 2-foot, native, herbaceous perennial found in moist, rocky areas of northern New Jersey. The stem is without thorns, and the branches are erect and leafy. Leaves are thin, soft, light green, and divided into three or five ovate, coarsely toothed leaflets. Flowers are small and white, appear in May, and produce small, red fruit in June.

Native Americans used dwarf raspberry leaf decoction as an antihemorrhagic for internal bleeding, as a stomach tonic, and as an abortifacient for irregular menses. The root decoction was also taken as a stomach tonic.

Rubus strigosus (*R. idaeus*) (red raspberry) is a 2- to 6-foot upright native shrub found in dry or moist, rocky, open areas of northern New Jersey. It is similar to *R. occidentalis* except that the stems are not so whitened, are hairy rather than thorny, and do not root at the tips. Flowers are white, appearing in May, with red fruit in July.

Native Americans used red raspberry for the treatment of more complaints than any other member of this genus. Red raspberry was used as described for *R. occidentalis*. In addition, the root bark infusion was used as a wash to heal cataracts and sore eyes. The root or stem decoction was taken for measles, for high or low blood pressure, and was used as a blood purifier. The root and berries were used as seasoners in medicines. The leaf decoction was taken for kidneys and for "burning pain when passing water."

Sorbus americana (*Pyrus americana*) (dogberry, mountain ash) is a 5- to 30-foot native shrub or tree found in moist woods and mountain slopes of northern New Jersey. The bark is smooth, and buds are red and gummy. Leaves are alternate and divided into 11 to 17 toothed leaflets. Flowers are white, in flat, broad clusters appearing in May and producing fruit in September.

Native Americans used a bark decoction to "purify the blood" and to stimulate the appetite. The bark was also used to treat boils and to treat "mother pains." A root bark infusion was used to treat gonorrhea. The plant was also used as an emetic.

Spiraea tomentosa (hardhack, steeplebush) is a 1- to 4-foot native shrub found in moist or wet areas statewide. Stems and leaf undersides are white-woolly. Leaves are alternate, oblong, and toothed. Flowers are pink or white, in a steeplelike cluster composed of smaller steeplelike clusters, appearing in early July.

Native Americans used the leaf infusion for dysentery. A leaf-and-flower infusion was taken for sickness during pregnancy and to ease childbirth.

Bigelow described hardhack roots and leaves as highly astringent and useful in "various discharges from debility, and particularly in hemorrhage from the bowels."

092 *Rubiaceae*

The madder family of herbs, shrubs, trees, and tropical woody vines. Stipules are present and sometimes as large as leaves. The leaves are simple, toothed, and usually entire. The leaves are opposite, but with their four stipules may appear to be a whorl of six leaves. It is the largest of the plant families occurring in the tropics and subtropics. The most abundant North American genus is *Galium*. Economically, the family is important as the source of quinine and coffee.

Cephalanthus occidentalis (buttonbush, honey balls) is a 3- to 20-foot native shrub found in wet areas statewide. Leaves are opposite, pointed-oval, and entire. Flowers are white, in round, balllike heads, with strongly protruding stamens; they appear in early July.

Native Americans chewed the bark of buttonbush for toothache and used a strong bark decoction as a favorite medicine for dysentery and an astringent wash for sore eyes. The inner bark was a very important emetic. Tree and root barks were used as a tonic and febrifuge. The root bark was also taken for hemorrhages and "enlarged muscles." A poultice

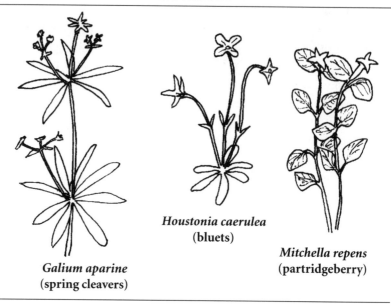

Houstonia caerulea
(bluets)

Galium aparine
(spring cleavers)

Mitchella repens
(partridgeberry)

of warmed root was applied to the head for eye problems, and a leaf decoction was taken for rheumatism.

Galium aparine (goosegrass, spring cleavers) is a 1- to 2-foot native annual found in rich-soiled, moist areas of northern and inner-coastal New Jersey. The stem is prickly, weak, and drooping, with 1- to 3-inch lance-shaped leaves in whorls of eight. Flowers are white and inconspicuous, arising from the leaf axils in late April, with bristly fruit forming in late May.

Native Americans used goosegrass infusion as a laxative and diuretic, for kidney trouble and gonorrhea, and in a decoction as an emetic. It was used as a rub for skin trouble and was regarded as poisonous.

Galium triflorum (fragrant bedstraw, sweet-scented bedstraw) is a 1- to 3-foot native perennial found in shaded, dry areas of northern and southwestern New Jersey. Leaves are lance-shaped and entire, in whorls of six. Flowers are greenish white, arising from leaf axils in early June.

Native Americans used a fragrant bedstraw infusion for gallstones and kidney troubles. The plant was rubbed on the skin for chest pains, and the whole-plant poultice was applied for backache in babies and to the hair as a growth stimulant.

Houstonia caerulea (bluets, innocence, Quaker ladies) is a 2- to 8-inch native perennial found in northern and inner-coastal New Jersey. The stem is not creeping at the base. Stem leaves are few, opposite, and entire. Flowers are small, pale-blue or white, with a yellow center; they appear in late April.

Native Americans used a bluets infusion as a urinary aid to stop bedwetting.

Mitchella repens (partridgeberry, two-eyed berry) is a native trailing perennial found in rich-soiled, dry or moist areas, often forming mats under evergreen trees statewide. Leaves are opposite and entire, oval, shining, and evergreen. Flowers are white or pinkish, in pairs at the ends of branches, and appearing in late May, with persisting, scarlet, tasteless, edible fruit in June.

Native Americans used partridgeberry for menstrual cramps, suppressed menses, and to facilitate childbirth. It was used for sore nipples and was given to babies to promote suckling. Pregnant mothers took the plant decoction to prevent rickets in the baby. The decoction was taken for hives, as a diaphoretic and diuretic, and was given to babies as a laxative for stomach gas. It was also given to babies with rashes. A preparation was taken for bladder stricture and to treat insomnia. The root and bark infusion or decoction was taken for kidney troubles and was used as an herbal steam for rheumatism. A decoction prepared with milk was taken for dysentery and piles, and berries were cooked into a jelly for the treatment of fever. A crushed-plant poultice was applied to cuts as a hemostat and was applied to babies with swollen abdomens. The hot poultice was also applied to the chest for fevers. The leaves were smoked as a ceremonial medicine.

093 *Rutaceae*

The citrus family of trees, shrubs, and herbs, with simple, palmate, or pinnate leaves that may be alternate or opposite. This is a large tropical and subtropical family that extends into the warm temperate regions. Members of the family include the orange, lemon, lime, grapefruit, and so on, which are usually cultivated as economic crops.

Ptelea trifoliata (stinking ash, three-leaved hop tree, wafer ash) is a 5- to 20-foot native small tree or shrub found in rich-soiled moist areas of northern New Jersey. Leaves are alternate and divided into three black-dotted leaflets. Flowers are small and greenish white in branching clusters, appearing in late May and producing round, winged fruit in September.

Native Americans regarded the hop tree root as a sacred medicine and panacea. It was added to other medicines as a seasoner to make them more potent.

Xanthoxylum americum (*Zanthoxylum americanum*) (angelica tree, northern prickly-ash, toothache tree) is a native shrub or small tree attaining 25 feet and found in rich-soiled, moist areas of northern New

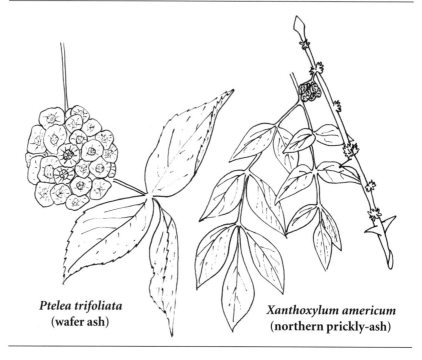

Ptelea trifoliata
(wafer ash)

Xanthoxylum americum
(northern prickly-ash)

Jersey. Branches are prickly, with leaves divided into 5 to 11 toothed leaflets that are lemon-scented when crushed. Flowers are small and greenish in axillary clusters, appearing in April, shortly before the leaves. Greenish red, aromatic fruits appear in July. This was a very important medicine for Native Americans.

Native Americans used the chewed, pounded, or powdered inner bark for toothache. The bark was put into the cavity and packed around the tooth or smoked for toothache or neuralgia. The inner-bark infusion was used sparingly for heart trouble. The bark infusion was used as a wash for itching or swollen joints; for colds, coughs or other pulmonary problems, fever or sore throat, heart trouble, cramps, and worms; and to induce abortion. The bark and berries were used to make an expectorant and cough syrup, and another bark-and-berry preparation was used as a hemostat for hemorrhages. The bark or berries were used to treat sore throat and tonsillitis, and mouth sores. The berry infusion was sprayed on the chest or throat for bronchial disease. The inner-bark poultice was applied for sharp pains and rheumatism. A root infusion was taken as a diuretic, and a root bark poultice was applied for swellings.

Bigelow described prickly-ash as having "acquired much reputation as a remedy in chronic rheumatism, producing a sense of heat in the stomach, a tendency to perspiration, and relief of rheumatic pains."

094 *Salicaceae*

The willow family of shrubs and trees, composed of two genera, *Populus* in the temperate regions and *Salix* in both the temperate and arctic regions. With the exception of the South Pacific, the family is global.

Populus alba (silver-leaved poplar, white poplar) is a naturalized weed tree found in open areas statewide. The tree is highly branched, with whitish bark on the young branches becoming dark and rough when mature. Leaves are roundish and large-toothed, with a white-woolly undersurface. Flowers are in 2-inch catkins, appearing in April. Reproduction is vegetative.

Native Americans used an infusion prepared from the crushed plant as a wash for general illness and rheumatism. An inner-bark infusion was taken as a tonic, and a bark-and-root infusion was taken for blood diseases.

Populus candicans (*P. gileadensis*) (balm of Gilead) is an escaped tree found in moist areas statewide. Spring buds are large, hairy, resinous, and fragrant, with leaves broad, heart-shaped, and hairy. The trees are pistillate, flowering in April, and reproduce vegetatively by spreading.

Native Americans used a bud tincture for chronic rheumatism, chronic venereal complaints, and as a gastrointestinal aid. Buds were also used for toothache, head colds, and in a salve for wounds.

Populus deltoides (eastern cottonwood, necklace poplar) is a large, native tree attaining 150 feet and found in rich-soiled, moist areas along the Delaware River. Leaves are broadly oval to triangular and coarsely toothed with flattened petioles (stalks). Petioles show two or three glands at the top. Flowers are in long, loose catkins, appear in late March, and produce cottony seeds.

Native Americans used the inner bark as an antiscorbutic (to prevent scurvy) food and for "kinnikinnick" (a mixture of dried leaves and bark of certain plants to be smoked).

Populus tremuloides (American aspen, quaking aspen) is a common native tree attaining 60 feet found in dry or moist, open areas statewide, but decreasing southward. The bark is smooth and greenish to whitish. Leaves are small, broadly oval, fine-toothed, and downy when young, smooth when mature. Petioles are long, slender, and flattened, so that the leaves "quake" in the slightest breeze. Flowers are in catkins, with pistillate flowers 3 to 4 inches long appearing in late March, with fruit in late April.

Native Americans used quaking aspen bark as a purgative, for worms, to stimulate appetite, and as a diaphoretic for colds. The inner bark was used as an antiscorbutic food and as an ingredient in "kinnikinnick" (a mixture of dried leaves and bark of certain plants to be smoked). A

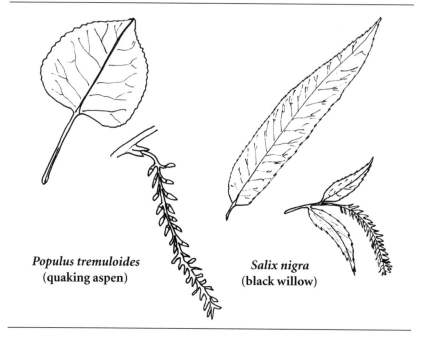

Populus tremuloides
(quaking aspen)

Salix nigra
(black willow)

poultice of bark, chewed bark, or root was applied to cuts and wounds. A root, root bark, or bark decoction was taken for venereal disease. A poultice of wetted bark was applied for pleurisy, and a leaf decoction was taken for urinary trouble. A bud decoction was used as a nasal salve for colds, and the plant was smoked as a ceremonial medicine.

Salix alba (white willow) is a large naturalized tree attaining a 90-foot height and found in wet areas statewide. The trunk is short and thick, and the branches are yellowish brown. The leaves are 2 to 4 inches, lance-shaped, ashy gray, and silky, making the entire tree appear white.

Native Americans used a white willow bark infusion as a tonic, an antidiarrheal, and as a growth-stimulating hair wash. The root was chewed for hoarseness, and an inner-bark decoction was taken for laryngitis.

Bigelow described white willow bark as "extremely bitter" and astringent, used as a tonic and stomachic.

Salix babylonica (weeping willow) is a 30- to 40-foot escaped tree found in moist areas statewide. Branches are olive-green or purplish and slender, producing the weeping habit. Leaves are 2 to 6 inches and lance-shaped.

Native Americans used weeping willow essentially as they did *S. alba.*

Salix candida (hoary willow, sage-leaved willow) is a 2- to 5-foot native shrub found in cold, wet areas of northern New Jersey. Young branches are whitish, becoming smooth and red with age. Leaves are 2 to 4 inches, lance-shaped, dark green, and wrinkled above, white and pubescent beneath. Flowers appear in late April, with fruit in late July.

Native Americans used a hoary willow inner-bark decoction for coughs. The plant was also used as a gastrointestinal aid, a sedative, and a stimulant.

Salix discolor (glaucous swamp willow, large pussy willow) is a 10- to 20-foot native shrub or short-trunked tree found in wet or moist areas of northern and inner-coastal New Jersey. The buds are very large and nearly black. Leaves are smooth and bright green on the upper surface and whitish on the lower. Flowers appear in early April before the leaves, giving rise to fruit in late April.

Native Americans regarded large pussy willow bark as a panacea. The bark infusion was used as a hemorrhoid remedy and hemostat. The plant was also used as a gastrointestinal aid, a sedative, and a stimulant.

Salix fragilis (brittle willow, crack willow) is a 50- to 60-foot naturalized tree found in moist areas statewide. The trunk extends to the top of the tree, with brown branches obliquely ascending. Leaves are lance-shaped, smooth or only slightly hairy, and only slightly paler on the undersurface. Flowers appear with the leaves in April.

Native Americans used crack willow bark and a bark poultice as a styptic and healing aid for sores.

Salix lucida (glossy willow, shining willow, squaw bush) is a 6- to 15-foot native shrub or bushy tree found in moist or wet areas of northern New Jersey. Branches are yellowish brown and shiny. Buds are large, flat, and curved downward. Leaves are large, broadly lance-shaped, toothed, dark-green, and shiny. Flowers appear in late April, with fruit in July.

Native Americans smoked the dried bark of squaw bush for asthma. A bark poultice was used to heal sores and as a hemostat for cuts. A leaf infusion was taken and the bark poultice applied for headache.

Salix nigra (black willow) is a 30- to 40-foot native tree found in low, rich-soiled, moist areas statewide. The bark is flaky, becoming shaggy. Twigs are brittle at the base, and buds are small. Leaves are lance-shaped, fine-toothed, and green on both sides. Catkins are 1 to 2 inches, appearing in early May, with fruit in June.

Native Americans used a black willow bark infusion or decoction as a tonic, febrifuge, and antidiarrheal, and as a growth-stimulating hair wash. An inner-bark infusion was taken for laryngitis, and the root was chewed for hoarseness. A root decoction was taken for fever, headache, and dyspepsia.

Salix sericea (silky willow) is a 4- to 8-foot native shrub found in wet, rocky areas of northern and southwestern New Jersey. Branches, spreading from the base, are often reddish. Leaves are lance-shaped and silky on the undersurface. Catkins are densely flowered, often with orange-red stamens, appearing with the leaves in early April. Fruits appear in mid-May.

Native Americans used silky willow as an oral aid for the treatment of abscesses in the mouth and throat.

Sarraceniaceae

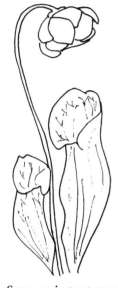

Sarracenia purpurea
(pitcher-plant)

095 *Sarraceniaceae*

The pitcher-plant family of perennial herbs, with simple, tubular, basal leaves, growing in moist soils, peat moss, or marshes. The family occurs only in North and South America, and primarily in eastern North America. The entire leaf forms a pitcher in which insects are trapped.

Sarracenia purpurea (huntsman's cup, Indian cup, pitcher-plant) is an 8-inch to 2-foot native insectivorous perennial found in wet, acidic areas statewide, including the pinelands. Leaves are 4 to 10 inches, basal, red- or purple-veined, hollow and pitcher-shaped. Flowers are large, dark red, and nodding. Flowers appear in late May with fruit in July.

Native Americans used a pitcher-plant leaf infusion as a febrifuge and treatment for smallpox. The root infusion was used as a gynecological aid in childbirth, for sore throat, to treat smallpox, and as an antihemorrhagic for consumption. The plant decoction was taken for whooping cough, consumption, and kidney trouble.

096 *Saururaceae*

Saururaceae

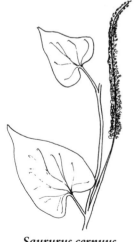

Saururus cernuus
(lizard's-tail)

The lizard's-tail family of perennial herbs, found in moist environments. The leaves are simple and usually ovate. The family, consisting of only three genera, is found in Southeast Asia, Mexico, the United States, and Canada.

Saururus cernuus (Indian pepper, lizard's-tail, swamp lily, water dragon) is a 2- to 5-foot native perennial found in low, wet areas statewide, with the exception of the pinelands. Leaves are alternate, entire, and heart-shaped. Flowers are fragrant, small, and white, with long stamens and no petals or sepals, in dense, nodding spikes, appearing in early June.

Native Americans used a plant infusion for stomach trouble and rheumatism. A poultice prepared from the roasted or boiled root was applied as a dermatological aid for wounds.

The saxifrage family of herbs and shrubs, and, rarely, small trees. The leaves may be simple or compound and alternate or opposite; they are without stipules and usually deciduous. The distribution of the family is essentially global, but about one-third of the genera are concentrated in North America.

Saxifragaceae

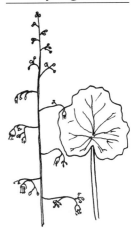

Heuchera americana
(alum root)

Heuchera americana (alum root, rock geranium) is a 1- to 3-foot native perennial found in rich-soiled, dry areas of northern and decreasingly southern New Jersey. Leaves are basal, rounded, and geranium-shaped. Flowers are small and greenish white, in a loose spike, and appear in late May.

Native Americans used the astringent root as a tonic, for "thrash" and "sore mouth," for dysentery, and for piles and hemorrhages, including excess menstrual flow. The leaves and the roots were used on slow-healing sores. The root was chewed to remove coating from the tongue and for a "disordered stomach." The powdered root was used on malignant ulcers.

Bigelow described alum root as one of the strongest plant astringents, applied externally where an astringent was indicated.

Hydrangea arborescens (sevenbark, wild hydrangea) is a 4- to 10-foot native shrub found in rich-soiled, rocky areas of northern New Jersey. Leaves are opposite, 3 to 6 inches long, pointed-oval, and sharply toothed. Flowers are white, in branched clusters, and appear in early June.

Native Americans used sevenbark bark infusion as an antiemetic, purgative, and antiseptic. The bark was chewed for stomach trouble and high blood pressure, and the inner bark and leaves were used as a stimulant. A poultice of scraped bark was used for burns, sore muscles, sprains, and cancerous tumors.

Ribes americanum (wild black currant) is a 1- to 5-foot native shrub found in rich-soiled, moist areas of northern New Jersey. Stems are thornless, with leaves toothed and lobed maplelike. Flowers are whitish to yellowish and bell-shaped, in nodding racemes. They appear in late April and give rise to black fruit in June.

Native Americans used a wild black currant root infusion or decoction as an anthelmintic for intestinal worms and for kidney and uterine problems. The leaf decoction was taken for lifting (internal muscle) injury, and the bark poultice was applied to swellings.

Tiarella cordifolia (coolwort, false miterwort, foamflower) is a 6-inch to 1-foot native perennial found in rich-soiled moist areas of northern New Jersey. Leaves are basal, toothed, and lobed maplelike. Flowers are white, with conspicuous stamens, in upright racemes, and appear in early May.

Native Americans used a foamflower infusion as a mouthwash for coated tongue. The crushed-root infusion was given to babies with sore mouths. The root-and-leaf infusion was given as tonic and as a dietary aid to fatten children. A dried-leaf infusion was used as an eyewash. Roots were used to treat diarrhea, and a crushed-root poultice was applied to wounds.

098 *Scrophulariaceae*

The snapdragon family of herbs, shrubs, and vines. Leaves are simple or pinnate. The family of 2,000 to 3,000 species is distributed globally and is common throughout North America.

Castilleja coccinea (Indian paintbrush, scarlet painted-cup) is an 8-inch to 2-foot native annual found in moist meadows of northern and southwestern New Jersey. Stem leaves are alternate and divided into two to five deep lobes, while the basal leaves are entire and in a rosette. Flowers are yellowish, in a terminal spike surrounded by leafy, three-lobed, red-tipped bracts, and appear in early May.

Native Americans used a painted-cup flower infusion for colds and a decoction to treat paralysis. Indian paintbrush was also used as a poison "to destroy your enemies."

Chelone glabra (snakehead, turtlehead) is a 1- to 3-foot native perennial found in wet areas of northern and southwestern New Jersey. Leaves are opposite, lance-shaped, and toothed. Flowers are white or pink in a terminal cluster, appearing in August.

Native Americans used turtlehead as a contraceptive and to increase appetite. It was also used as a dermatological aid for sores and skin eruptions. The flower infusion was taken as a febrifuge, laxative, and anthelmintic for intestinal worms.

Digitalis purpurea (purple foxglove) is a 3- to 6-foot naturalized and escaped biennial found in open areas such as old fields of northern New Jersey. First-year leaves are lance-shaped and soft-hairy in a rosette. Flowers are red to purple on long spikes, arising in June of the second year.

Native Americans apparently did not use foxglove for medicinal purposes.

Foxglove was introduced from England, and dried leaves were used as a diuretic and for dropsy. Today, it is used to increase the systolic contraction in congestive heart failure. It lowers the venous blood pressure in hypertensive heart conditions and raises the pressure in weak heart conditions. The dramatic effect on the heart also makes foxglove a poisonous plant. Leaves of foxglove in the first year form a rosette, and the

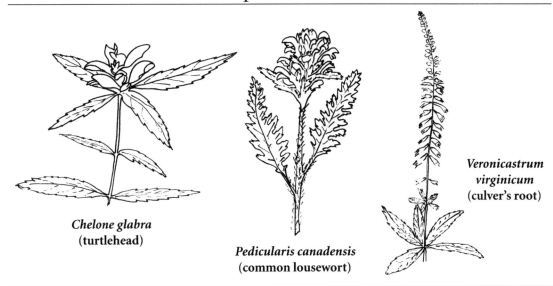

Chelone glabra
(turtlehead)

Pedicularis canadensis
(common lousewort)

Veronicastrum
virginicum
(culver's root)

plant has been mistaken for comfrey. When consumed as a vegetable, the results are usually fatal.

Bigelow described foxglove as a narcotic and circulatory sedative useful in hemorrhages and pulmonary consumptions; inflammations of the brain, lungs, and other viscera; and dropsy.

Linaria vulgaris (butter-and-eggs, yellow toadflax) is a 1- to 3-foot naturalized perennial found in open areas and as a garden weed statewide. Leaves are alternate, entire, narrow, and numerous. Flowers are yellow with orange marks, in a raceme, and appear in early June.

Native Americans used a plant infusion as an emetic, and a cold leaf infusion was taken for diarrhea.

Paulownia tomentosa (empress tree, keri tree, princess tree) is a 30- to 60-foot naturalized tree found in wet areas along the coastal plain, especially along the Delaware River. Leaves are large, 12 or more inches in length or width, heart-shaped, entire, and velvety on the undersurface. Flowers are fragrant, flared thimbles in large clusters, appearing in early April, with upright, hickorylike fruit in September.

Native Americans apparently did not use the princess tree for medicinal purposes. In Asia, an inner-bark tincture was used as a febrifuge, and a bark poultice was applied to bruises. A leaf tea was used as a wash for swollen feet, and a tea prepared from the leaves and fruit was used as a hair wash to prevent graying. The juice from crushed leaves was used to treat warts.

Pedicularis canadensis (common lousewort, wood betony) is a 6- to

15-inch native perennial found in dry, open-wooded areas statewide. The plant is hairy, with leaves alternate, deeply lobed, and fernlike. Flowers are yellow or reddish in a dense terminal cluster, appearing in late April.

Native Americans used common lousewort to repel lice from sheep and dogs. The root infusion or decoction was taken as an analgesic for stomach pain, as an antidiarrheal in flux, and as a rub for sores. A dried-root infusion was taken as a blood medicine for anemia, and a crushed-root infusion was taken for heart troubles. A root poultice was applied to cancerous tumors. The root was also used as a cathartic and added to food as an aphrodisiac. The leaf infusion was used to induce abortion.

Scrophularia lanceolata (hare figwort) is a 3- to 8-foot native perennial found in open, moist areas statewide. Leaves are opposite, pointed-oval, and toothed. Flowers are green or brown and shiny on the outside, with a yellow, undeveloped stamen appearing in May.

Native Americans used a root decoction as a blood medicine and an infusion as a gynecological aid to prevent cramps and colds following childbirth. A poultice was applied to relieve the pain of sunburn, sunstroke, and frostbite.

Scrophularia marilandica (carpenter's square, Maryland figwort) is similar to *S. lanceolata* with less prominently toothed leaves, flowers are dull on the outside, and the undeveloped stamen is purple. Flowers appear in early July.

Native Americans used a root infusion as a gynecological aid in irregular menses.

Verbascum thapsus (common mullein, flannel plant) is a 2- to 8-foot naturalized biennial weed found in dry areas statewide. First-year leaves are soft and white-woolly, in a rosette. Flowers are yellow, in tight, long spikes, appearing in late June of the second year.

Native Americans smoked the dried leaves of mullein for asthma, catarrh, sore throat, consumption, hiccough, or as Indian tobacco. Smudged leaves were inhaled for catarrh. The leaf decoction was taken with sugar or molasses for colds, coughs, and rheumatism, and as a febrifuge, and a leaf infusion was given to babies as a laxative. Poultices of raw, crushed leaves were applied to cuts; to the throat for diphtheria; to sprains, pains, swellings and bruises, abscesses, and sores; and for erysipelas. The heated leaf poultice was applied for earache and rheumatic pain. Leaves were wrapped around the neck for mumps, and scalded leaves were applied to swollen glands. Crushed leaves were rubbed over the body in the sweat bath and rubbed under the armpits for prickly rash. A whole-plant decoction was given to babies with a rash, and a root decoction was given to children with croup. The root decoction was also taken for coughs, "female troubles," and kidneys and was used as a leg bath for dropsy.

Veronica officinalis (common speedwell, gipsyweed) is a creeping, hairy-stemmed, evergreen native perennial found in open and shaded areas statewide. Leaves are opposite, elliptical, and toothed. Flowers are small, lilac- or lavender-colored, and appear in early May.

Native Americans applied a common speedwell poultice to boils and used the warmed juice as drops for earache. A plant decoction was taken for chills, as an emetic, and with sugar for coughs. The root decoction was taken as a gynecological aid to ease childbirth.

Veronicastrum virginicum (bowman's root, culver's root) is a 2- to 5-foot native perennial found in rich-soiled, moist, wooded areas of northern New Jersey. Leaves are lance-shaped and sharply toothed, in whorls of three to seven. Flowers are small and white or purple, in showy spikes, appearing in late June.

Native Americans used culver's root as a purgative, tonic, antiseptic, and diaphoretic. The plant was used to treat rheumatism, and the root was chewed for colic. The root was used as an anticonvulsive and antidiarrheal, as a gynecological aid in labor, and to dissolve gravel in the kidneys. It was taken for a "bad heart" and described by the Iroquois as poisonous.

099 *Simaroubaceae*

The quassia family of shrubs and trees. Leaves are alternate, pinnate, simple, or reduced to scales. The family is primarily tropical but extends into the temperate regions.

Ailanthus altissima (copal tree, tree of heaven) is native to Asia and naturalized statewide in New Jersey. It is found on the edges of wooded waste areas, flowering mid-June to July, with fruit from July through October. Male flowers are malodorous. It is a smooth-barked tree of up to 100 feet, with compound leaves similar to those of the sumacs. Close inspection shows two glandlike pits at the base of each leaflet, and crushing the leaves releases a distinctly peanutlike aroma. It is now considered a weed in many areas, and attempts to remove it may lead to contact dermatitis from flowers and leaves.

Native Americans apparently did not use the copal tree for medicinal purposes. In China and India, bark and root decoctions are used for diarrhea and dysentery as well as for tapeworm and other intestinal parasites.

The nightshade family of herbs, shrubs, trees, and woody vines. Leaves are alternate, simple, or pinnate. The family of about 2,000 species is distributed widely. This is a family of many strong-scented plants and is one of the major sources of foods, drugs, and ornamentals. *Atropa belladonna* (deadly nightshade) is a cultivated perennial in New Jersey. All parts of the plant contain poisonous alkaloids.

Datura stramonium (jimsonweed, thorn apple) is a 1- to 5-foot naturalized annual weed found in dry, open areas statewide. Leaves are alternate and coarsely toothed. Flowers are trumpet-shaped and white to lavender, appearing in late June, with spiny fruit forming in August.

Native Americans smoked jimsonweed for asthma. The leaf decoction was applied to body areas affected with fever and inflammation, and the mash from the decoction was applied as a poultice to the chest for pneumonia. A poultice of crushed leaves was applied to cuts, and a poultice of seeds and leaves was applied to wounds. Crushed seeds in a tallow salve were used to treat piles. A poultice of wilted leaves was applied to boils. The Rappahannock considered jimsonweed to be poisonous.

Bigelow described thorn apple as a powerful narcotic acting as an anodyne and antispasmodic, and in large doses a poison. It was used in epilepsy, tic douloureux, and, when smoked, for asthma.

Jimsonweed seeds and other plant parts contain poisonous alkaloids that can cause death in humans.

Physalis heterophylla (clammy ground cherry) is a 1- to 3-foot native perennial weed found in rich-soiled, dry areas statewide. The stem is covered with sticky hairs. Leaves are alternate, entire to coarsely toothed, and heart-shaped. Flowers are greenish yellow with brown centers, bell-shaped, and nodding. They appear in late June and give rise to fruit enclosed in papery, lanternlike pods in August.

Native Americans used a clammy ground cherry compound leaf-and-root infusion for use as a wash for scalds, burns, and venereal diseases. It was also taken as an emetic for stomach disorders.

Solanum carolinense (ball nettle, horse nettle, sand brier) is a 1- to 4-foot native perennial weed found in dry, open areas statewide. The stem is prickly. Leaves are alternate and coarsely toothed or lobed. Flowers are violet or white and star-shaped, in small clusters, appearing in early June and giving rise to yellow berries in August.

Native Americans used an infusion as an anthelmintic for worms and for "ulcers and proud flesh." Crushed leaves in milk were used as an insecticide for flies. A seed infusion was taken for goiter and gargled for sore throat. The berries were fried in grease and the grease was then used to treat dog mange.

Solanaceae

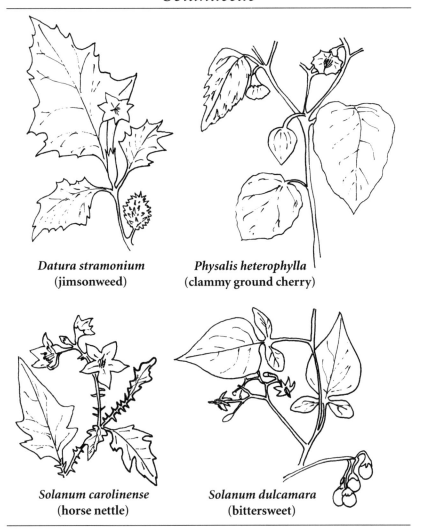

Datura stramonium
(jimsonweed)

Physalis heterophylla
(clammy ground cherry)

Solanum carolinense
(horse nettle)

Solanum dulcamara
(bittersweet)

Solanum dulcamara (bittersweet, blue bindweed, purple nightshade) is a woody, climbing, naturalized vine found in waste areas and moist thickets statewide. Leaves are divided into three leaflets, deeply lobed, or entire. Flowers are violet or purple and star-shaped, and appear in May. Berries are red.

Native Americans used bittersweet to prepare a salve for felons, warts, and tumors. The root was also used as an antiemetic to treat nausea.

Bigelow described bittersweet as a native plant, common also to Europe, efficacious in cutaneous diseases, particularly psoriasis, pityriasis, and especially leprosy.

Bittersweet leaves and green fruit contain the poisonous alkaloid solanine. A few berries can cause vomiting, anorexia, paralysis, and death.

Solanum nigrum (black nightshade, deadly nightshade) is a 1- to 2¹/₂-foot native perennial weed found in open areas and gardens statewide. Leaves are pointed-oval and entire. Flowers are star-shaped and white, with protruding yellow stamens, and appear in late June. Berries are black.

Native Americans considered the plant and berries of nightshade to be poisonous and used a weak infusion prepared from dried leaves as a sedative for sleeplessness. The plant infusion was taken as an emetic, and a decoction was taken for scarlet fever. A poultice of heated leaves was applied to boils, and a poultice of crushed green leaves and grease was applied to sores. The root decoction was given to babies as a treatment for worms. The plant was used as an emetic, and smoke from burning plants was inhaled to relieve the pain of toothache.

In Chinese medicine, a whole-plant decoction is used to treat leucorrhea, cervical cancer, abscesses, and open sores.

Common nightshade contains solanaceous alkaloids and anticholinergics that cause dry mouth and skin, elevated temperature, and delirium.

101 *Taxaceae*

Taxaceae

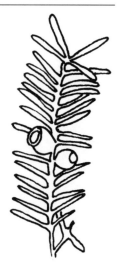

**Taxus canadensis
(Canada yew)**

The yew family of gymnosperms, present on earth from the Jurassic period. There are three living genera, *Taxus*, *Torreya*, and *Austrotaxus*. The wood is very springy, and in the Middle Ages was favored for making bows. These are ornamental woody plants, grown for their dark green foliage and scarlet berrylike fruits. *Taxus brevifolia* and other treelike forms are extremely slow-growing, and the inner bark of *T. brevifolia* was the original source of the anticancer terpenoid taxol.

Taxus canadensis (Canada yew, ground hemlock) is a prostrate, native, evergreen shrub, rarely more than 3 feet tall, found in moist, rocky areas of northern New Jersey. Young branches are smooth and green, while older branches are reddish brown, slender, and spreading. Leaves are ¹/₂ to 1 inch long and yellowish green, becoming reddish in winter. They appear to be opposite, but are not really. Fruit is cuplike, red, and fleshy.

Native Americans used the leaf infusion as a diuretic, and a twig tea was taken for colds. Branches and decoctions were used in herbal steam treatments for chest colds, rheumatism, numbness, and paralysis.

102 *Thymelaeaceae*

The mezereum family of shrubs, small trees, and, rarely, herbs. The leaves are simple, entire, alternate or opposite, and without stipules. Only two species occur in North America. One is found in the San Francisco Bay region of California and the other in the East. These are species of *Dirca*; however, *Daphne mezereon*, used medicinally in Europe, is cultivated widely. *Daphne* contains diterpene alcohols (mezerein) and coumarin glycosides that cause the skin to blister. Ingestion of a few berries causes violent responses leading to death.

Dirca palustris (leatherwood, leaverwood, wicopy) is a 2- to 9-foot native shrub found in rich-soiled, moist areas of northern and south-western New Jersey. Leaves are alternate, pointed-oval, and entire. Flowers are bell-shaped and pale yellow, appearing in mid-April, before the leaves.

Native Americans chewed the green stalk or used a stalk, crushed-root, or bark infusion or decoction as a laxative. The root infusion was also taken for pulmonary problems, typhoid fever, venereal disease, and back pain, as a diuretic, and to heal kidneys. Infusions prepared from the bark or inner bark were taken as diuretics. A branch decoction was applied as a poultice to limb swellings, and a stem decoction was used as an aphrodisiac.

Thymelaeaceae

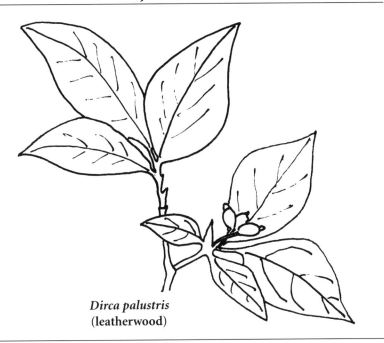

Dirca palustris
(leatherwood)

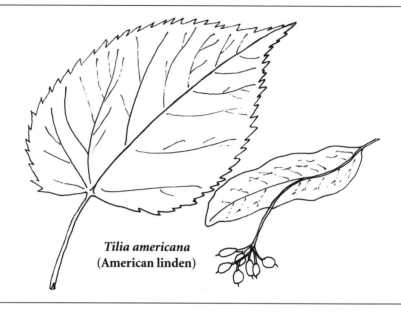

Tilia americana
(American linden)

103 *Tiliaceae*

The linden family of trees, shrubs, and herbs. The leaves are simple, usually alternate, and deciduous. This is a large family, primarily tropical, with a few species native to eastern North America.

Tilia americana (American linden, basswood, whitewood) is a 60- to 120-foot native tree found in moist, rich-soiled areas of northern and southwestern New Jersey. Leaves are broadly oval, pointed, and coarsely toothed, dark green above and light on the undersurface, becoming yellow in autumn. Flowers are yellow, in pendulous clusters, and appear in late June, giving rise to thick-shelled fruit in August.

Native Americans used a basswood inner-bark infusion for dysentery and a bark infusion as a diuretic. The bark decoction was mixed with cornmeal or boiled to prepare a poultice for boils. The inner bark and twigs were used for stomach problems. A twig infusion was taken for lung trouble and as a stimulant. The root was used in a treatment for worms.

104 *Typhaceae*

The cattail family of monocotyledonous perennial herbs. The main stem is a rhizome that gives rise to a leafy flowering stem. The leaves are alternate and basal. The family is composed of a single genus, *Typha*, occurring essentially worldwide with the exception of the coldest regions.

Typha angustifolia (cattail flag, narrow-leaved cattail) is a 4- to 8-foot native perennial found in wet areas statewide. Leaves are alternate, long, and narrow, not over $^1/_2$ inch wide, and green. The mature flower spike is $^1/_2$ inch in diameter.

Native Americans used cattail root to treat gravel.

Typha latifolia (broad-leaved cattail) is similar to *T. angustifolia,* but the leaves are wider, up to 1 inch, and bluish or gray-green. The mature flower spike is 1 inch in diameter.

Native Americans used the basal portion of the leaf and the dried root to prepare an infusion for abdominal cramps. The leaves were used to treat sores, and a stalk decoction was taken for whooping cough. The root infusion was used to dissolve kidney stones, as a wash to stop bleeding from cuts, and to heal the newborn's navel. The root was chewed for gonorrhea, and a crushed-root decoction poultice was applied to sprains, while the crushed-root poultice was applied to inflammations. A poultice of fruit spikes and coyote fat was applied to smallpox pustules and old sores. The down from mature fruit spikes was used as a dressing for burns, scalds, and chafing. The young flowering heads were eaten for diarrhea. The whole plant was used as an emetic. A patient with breast cysts or yellow fever would sleep on a mattress made of the plant.

In Chinese medicine, a pollen decoction is used to control internal bleeding, including hemorrhoids, vaginal bleeding, and menstrual irregularities.

Typhaceae

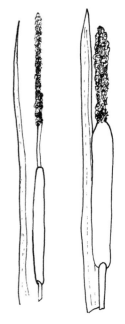

Typha angustifolia **(narrow-leaved cattail)**

Typha latifolia **(broad-leaved cattail)**

105 *Ulmaceae*

The elm family of deciduous shrubs and trees with simple, alternate leaves. The fruit is a samara or drupe. The family is tropical and subtropical, but is also found in much of the Northern Hemisphere.

Ulmus americana (American elm, water elm, white elm) is a native tree attaining a height of 120 feet and is found in rich-soiled, moist areas of northern and inner-coastal New Jersey. The trunk is light gray, with limbs curving outward with pendulous branches. Leaves are alternate, oblong, and sharply toothed. Flowers are in drooping clusters and appear in late March, before the leaves. The fruit is a dry nutlet surrounded by a flat, hairy, membranous wing, appearing in April.

Native Americans used the bark infusion to treat coughs, colds, pulmonary hemorrhage, cramps, and diarrhea. The bark infusion was also used as a wash for gunshot wounds and was taken by pregnant women

Ulmaceae

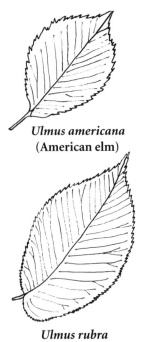

Ulmus americana
(American elm)

Ulmus rubra
(slippery elm)

"to insure stability of children." An inner-bark decoction was taken for menstrual cramps, colds, and coughs. It was also taken and used as a bath for appendicitis. The root bark decoction was used as an eye lotion, and an infusion was taken for excessive menstruation and gonorrhea.

Ulmus rubra (*U. fulva*) (red elm, slippery elm) is a 50- to 70-foot native tree found in rich-soiled, moist areas statewide. Branches are spreading, forming a broad, flat-topped head. Leaves are alternate, oblong, toothed, and very unequal at the base. Flowers are in dense clusters, appearing in late March before the leaves. The fruit is winged and yellowish green, without hairs.

Native Americans used the bark decoction as a gynecological aid in childbirth, a tuberculosis remedy, a gargle for sore throat, and an eyewash, and for kidney problems. The bark or dried root was also chewed for sore throat. The inner bark was used for dysentery, "quinsies," colds, coughs, and catarrh, as a laxative, and as a poultice for sores, burns, and infected wounds.

Bigelow described slippery elm bark as valuable in dysentery and strangury. Externally, the bark was used as an emollient and to promote suppuration.

106 *Umbelliferae*

The parsley family of annual or perennial herbs and shrubs. Leaves are usually pinnate and alternate. The family occurs primarily in the Northern Hemisphere.

Anethum graveolens (dill) is a 2- to 3-foot escaped annual or biennial found along roadsides and waste areas statewide. The stem is smooth, with leaves highly divided and threadlike. Flowers are small and yellowish, appearing in late June.

Native Americans apparently did not use dill as a medicinal plant. Dill seed tea is widely used for flatulent colic in children.

Angelica atropurpurea (alexanders, purple-stemmed angelica) is a 4- to 9-foot native biennial found in rich-soiled, wet areas of northern New Jersey. Stems are purple and smooth, with alternate leaves doubly divided into toothed leaflets. Flowers are greenish white in large heads and appear in early June.

Native Americans used a root tonic for flatulent colic, and as an abortifacient and female medicine. The root or plant infusion or decoction was taken for ague (malaria), fever, colds, and influenza. It was used as a gargle for sore throat and mouth and in a steam bath for rheumatism, headache, exposure, and frostbite. The root poultice was applied

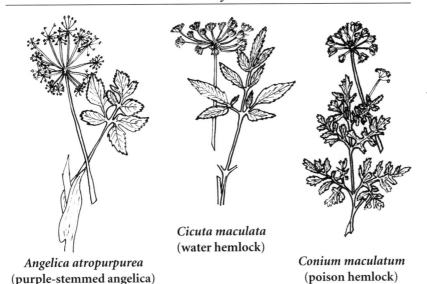

Cicuta maculata
(water hemlock)

Angelica atropurpurea
(purple-stemmed angelica)

Conium maculatum
(poison hemlock)

to broken bones, and a poultice of the cooked, crushed root was applied to swelling and painful areas. The seeds were mixed with tobacco and smoked. The plant was also used as a poison.

Bigelow described angelica as having no poisonous properties and producing roots, stalks, and seeds useful as tonics and carminatives.

Angelica venosa (hairy angelica, pubescent angelica) is a 2- to 6-foot native perennial found in dry, wooded areas statewide. Leaves are alternate and divided into finely toothed leaflets. Flowers are white, in 2- to 4-inch heads, and appear in early July.

Native Americans applied a hairy angelica plant poultice to sprained muscles and twisted joints. The Iroquois used hairy angelica as a poison. The root was eaten to commit suicide.

Cicuta maculata (beaver poison, musquash root, spotted cowbane, water hemlock) is a 1- to 7-foot native biennial found in wet areas statewide, with the exception of the central pinelands. The stem is branched and usually mottled with purple. Leaves are alternate and divided into lance-shaped, toothed leaflets. Flowers are white, in 2- to 4-inch flat heads, and appear in early June.

Native Americans used spotted cowbane as a contraceptive. Women chewed and swallowed the root to become sterile. The root was also chewed to commit suicide. A plant decoction was used on bruises, sprains, sore joints, and broken bones, and a root infusion was used as an insect repellent in which corn was soaked before planting. A poultice of the crushed root was applied for lameness and to cuts and sores.

Water hemlock plants are poisonous, but the roots are most toxic and can be mistaken for parsnips or potatoes. The poison is known as cicutoxin, and the amount found in a single mouthful is a fatal dose.

Conium maculatum (poison hemlock, snakeweed) is a 2- to 6-foot naturalized perennial weed found in moist waste areas statewide. The stem is branched, hollow, grooved, and purple-spotted. The leaves are alternate and highly divided (carrotlike). Flowers are white, in heads appearing in early June.

Native Americans used poison hemlock root as a poison.

Bigelow described hemlock as a powerful narcotic and a cure for jaundice when the dose is high enough to produce dizziness. It was also described as a cure for tic douloureux and to give unequivocal relief in hemicrania, when the pain was not regularly intermittent.

All parts of the plant and especially the young leaves contain the poisonous alkaloid coniine and several other alkaloids. When the young leaves are mistaken for parsley or the seeds mistaken for anise seed, the results are often fatal. The toxins are inactivated on drying. As detailed in the case of Socrates, poison hemlock has been used in judicial procedures.

Daucus carota (Queen Anne's lace, wild carrot) is a 1- to 4-foot naturalized biennial weed found in dry fields and waste areas statewide. The stem is hairy. Leaves are alternate and highly divided. Flowers are white, in 2- to 4-inch heads with a purple floret in the center, and appear in late June.

Native Americans used the flowering head in full bloom to prepare an infusion for the treatment of diabetes. The plant infusion was used as a wash for swelling, and the leaves were taken as a purgative. The root decoction was taken as a diuretic, a blood medicine, an appetite stimulant for men, and for pimples and paleness.

Bigelow described wild carrot seeds as diuretic and the boiled, crushed-root poultice to be mildly stimulating and useful for application to indolent ulcers.

Eryngium aquaticum (button snakeroot, rattlesnake master) is a 2- to 5-foot native perennial found in salt to brackish water and other wet coastal areas. Leaves are alternate and toothed. Flowers are bluish, at the end of branches, and appear in late July.

Native Americans used the root or plant infusion as an emetic and as a venereal aid in the treatment of gonorrhea. The root was used as an anthelmintic for tapeworms and pinworms, an antipoison for snakebite, a diuretic, a stimulant, and an expectorant.

Bigelow described button snakeroot as a substitute for Seneca snakeroot (*Polygala senega*), a diaphoretic, expectorant, and sometimes emetic tea.

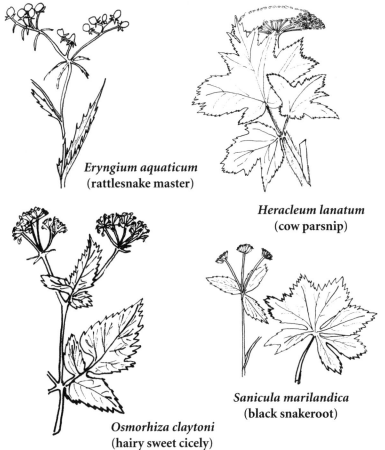

Eryngium aquaticum
(rattlesnake master)

Heracleum lanatum
(cow parsnip)

Sanicula marilandica
(black snakeroot)

Osmorhiza claytoni
(hairy sweet cicely)

Foeniculum vulgare (fennel) is a 4- to 7-foot naturalized annual, biennial, or perennial found in dry waste areas of southern and occasionally northern New Jersey. Leaves are finely divided (threadlike) and strongly anise-scented. Flowers are yellow, in flat heads, and appear in June.

Native Americans used fennel as a tonic. It was also given to women in labor, and taken for colds, colic, and flatulence in children.

In Chinese medicine, a fruit decoction is used for gastrointestinal distress.

Bigelow described fennel as a cultivated biennial with seeds that are carminative and stomachic.

Heracleum lanatum (*H. maximum*) (cow parsnip, masterwort) is a 4- to 10-foot native biennial or perennial found in rich-soiled, moist (including saltwater) areas of northern and southwestern New Jersey. The plant is woolly and strong-smelling with alternate leaves divided into three large, maplelike leaflets. Flowers are white, with notched petals, in 4- to 8-inch heads. Flowers appear in June.

Native Americans used a cow parsnip leaf or root decoction for colds, and a poultice of heated leaves was applied to cuts and sore muscles. Raw- or cooked-root poultices were applied to boils, and dried, crushed roots were mixed with oil as a hair ointment or with water as a hair wash for dandruff. The raw root was placed in tooth cavities for toothache. The root decoction was used to treat rheumatism and as a gargle for ulcerated throat, a cure for erysipelas, a treatment for smallpox and cholera, a purgative, an antidiarrheal, and a remedy for tuberculosis and syphilis. A stem poultice was used for healing wounds, and the plant decoction was used in a steam bath for rheumatism and headaches. The flower infusion was used as a rub to repel mosquitos and flies, and the seeds were used to treat severe headache. The plant tops were used in a smoke treatment for fainting and convulsions.

Bigelow described masterwort root or leaves as externally rubefacient and used internally for epilepsy. Bigelow suggested use with caution.

Cow parsnip foliage is said to be poisonous to livestock, and the roots are known to contain photosensitive compounds such as psoralin.

Osmorhiza claytoni (hairy sweet cicely, sweet javril) is a 1- to 3-foot native perennial found in moist, rich-soiled areas statewide. The plant is soft-hairy with alternate fernlike leaves divided into deeply lobed and toothed leaflets. Flower heads are white and small, with styles shorter than petals, and appear in May. The fruit, formed in June, is club-shaped and blackish, and clings to clothing.

Native Americans used the root decoction for sore throat, as an eyewash, and as a gynecological aid to ease childbirth. The moistened, crushed-root poultice was applied to ulcers, and the root was chewed for sore throat. The root was also eaten as a dietary aid for weight gain.

Osmorhiza longistylis (anise root, smooth sweet cicely) is similar to *O. claytoni*, but stouter and much less hairy. The flower styles are longer than the petals.

Native Americans used a leaf, stem, and root infusion for stomach and kidney disorders. The root infusion was taken for sore throat, and used as an eye lotion and as a gynecological aid to ease childbirth, and to treat amenorrhea. A crushed-root poultice was applied to boils.

Pastinaca sativa (wild parsnip) is a 2- to 5-foot naturalized biennial weed found in moist areas statewide. The stem is stout and deeply grooved. Leaves are alternate and divided into 5 to 15 paired, lobed, and toothed leaflets. Flowers are yellow in heads appearing in early June.

Native Americans used wild parsnip root in small amounts for "sharp pains" and found larger amounts to be poisonous. A root poultice was applied to inflammations and sores.

Sanicula canadensis (short-styled snakeroot) is a 1- to 4-foot native biennial found in dry, open areas statewide, with the exception of the central pinelands. Leaves are alternate and divided palmately into three to seven toothed leaflets. Flowers are greenish white, in small heads appearing in late May and giving rise to rounded burs in June.

Native Americans used a hot decoction prepared from the root for heart trouble. A decoction prepared from the powdered root was used as an abortifacient for "stoppage of periods."

Sanicula marilandica (black snakeroot, Maryland snakeroot, sanicle) is a 1- to 4-foot perennial found in open, rich-soiled areas of northern and southwestern New Jersey. This is the most common species of *Sanicula*, with leaves alternate and divided into five toothed leaflets. Flowers are greenish white, appearing in late May, with fruit in early August.

Native Americans used a plant decoction as a kidney aid for dropsy. The root decoction was taken for kidney trouble and painful or irregular menses, as an aid in slow childbirth, and as a febrifuge, and it was taken and used as a wash for children with sore navels. The root was used to treat rheumatism and snakebite.

Zizia aurea (early meadow-parsnip, golden alexanders) is a 1- to 3-foot native perennial found in rich-soiled, moist or wet, open areas of northern New Jersey. The stem is smooth and branching, with alternate leaves divided threefold into finely toothed leaflets. Flowers are yellow, in heads appearing in late April.

Native Americans used golden alexanders root as a febrifuge.

107 *Urticaceae*

The nettle family of herbs and, rarely, trees, shrubs, and vines, known for their stinging hairs. Most of the family is tropical.

Boehmeria cylindrica (bog hemp; false nettle) is a 1- to 3-foot native perennial found in moist, swampy areas statewide, with the exception of the pinelands. Leaves are opposite, pointed-oval, and toothed. Flowers are greenish, in unbranched spikes, and appear in early July.

Native Americans apparently did not use false nettle as a medicinal plant. It is today one of many plants under investigation as a source for cancer chemotherapeutic agents such as cryptopleurine.

Urtica dioica (*U. gracilis*) (great nettle, stinging nettle) is a 1- to 3-foot naturalized and native perennial found in very rich-soiled, open areas statewide, with the exception of the pinelands. The stem is covered with stinging hairs. Leaves are opposite, pointed-oval, and toothed. Flowers are greenish, in axillary racemes, and appear in mid-June.

Urticaceae

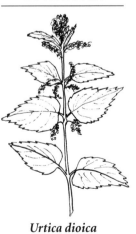

**Urtica dioica
(stinging nettle)**

Native Americans used the stalk as a whip on patients for rheumatism or paralysis. The plant was rubbed on the skin for chest pains, and a moxa of plant fiber was used to cauterize the skin for various ailments. The plant juice was rubbed into the scalp to prevent falling hair and was taken by pregnant women who were overdue. Tips of the plant were chewed by women during labor. A poultice prepared from the sprouts was applied for paralysis, and a poultice of soaked leaves was applied to heat rash. A stalk decoction was used as a body rub for soreness and stiffness, and a stem-and-root decoction was used in a sweatbath for rheumatism, grippe, and pneumonia. A peeled-bark decoction was taken for headache and nosebleed, and a plant decoction was taken for colds. The root infusion or decoction was used as a diuretic, a hair wash, and a wash for rheumatism and taken for dysentery, malaria, and upset stomach. The crushed-root infusion was taken for rheumatism, and a nettle infusion was taken by women shortly before childbirth.

108 *Valerianaceae*

The valerian family of herbs, woody plants, and shrubs, with leaves simple or pinnate. The family occurs in the northern temperate zone and in the Andes of South America.

Valeriana officinalis (garden heliotrope) is a 2- to 5-foot naturalized perennial found in open areas statewide. Leaves are opposite and divided into 5 to 25 lance-shaped leaflets. Flowers are pink, in branched clusters, and appear in late May.

Native Americans apparently did not use the garden heliotrope as a medicinal plant. Other native species of *Valeriana* such as *acutiloba*, *capita, ciliata, edulis, septentrionalis, sitchensis*, and *uliginosa* were used.

In Chinese medicine, the crushed root mixed with hot water (an infusion) or a decoction is taken orally for the treatment of influenza, rheumatism, nervous disorders, and traumatic injuries.

Bigelow described valerian as a valuable antispasmodic and soporific, useful in hysteria and nervous agitation. As a soporific, it was described as exceeding all other medications and "is followed by no unpleasant consequence." It was used as an anodyne in nervous headache, hemicrania, tic douloureux, and epilepsy.

In Europe, the garden heliotrope root is a well-known herbal medicine, used for many disorders of the nervous system. It is a major over-the-counter calmative and tranquilizer.

109 *Verbenaceae*

The verbena family of herbs, shrubs, and trees. The leaves may be simple, pinnate, or palmate. The family is primarily tropical and subtropical, but the large genus *Verbena* occurs in the temperate regions of the Western Hemisphere.

Verbena hastata (blue vervain, false vervain, simpler's joy) is a 2- to 6-foot native perennial found in low, moist, open areas statewide. The stem is square and grooved. Leaves are opposite, lance-shaped, and toothed. Flowers are blue-violet in numerous branched spikes.

Native Americans used vervain as an abortifacient for "female obstructions and afterpains," and as a tonic for breast complaints. It was taken for coughs and colds and used as a sudorific. The root is astringent and used for diarrhea and as a urinary aid to "clear up cloudy urine." The leaves, seeds, and root were used as an emetic, and a snuff of dried flowers was used for nosebleed.

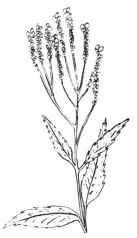

Verbenaceae

Verbena hastata
(blue vervain)

110 *Violaceae*

The violet family of herbs, shrubs, and vines. The leaves are simple and alternate. This is primarily a tropical family but distributed globally.

Viola canadensis (Canadian violet, tall white violet) is a 1-foot endangered native perennial found in rich-soiled, rocky areas of northern New Jersey. The stem is slightly hairy, with leaves alternate, heart-shaped, and toothed. Flowers are white with a yellow throat and a purple tinge on the backs of the petals. Flowers appear in late April.

Native Americans used a root decoction for the treatment of pains "near" the bladder.

Viola conspersa (dog violet, early blue violet) is a 6-inch native violet found in wet, shaded areas of northern and inner-coastal New Jersey. Leaves are alternate, heart-shaped, and blunt. Flowers are pale violet, appearing in late April.

Native Americans used a whole-plant infusion for heart trouble.

Viola cucullata (blue marsh violet, bog violet) is a small native violet found in moist or wet, open areas statewide, with the exception of the pinelands. Leaves are basal, arrow- to heart-shaped, and toothed. Flowers are blue and long-stalked above the leaves, appearing in late April.

Native Americans used a violet infusion as a spring tonic. The infusion was also taken "for the blood," dysentery, colds, and with sugar, for coughs. The infusion was sprayed into the nose for catarrh, and the leaves were applied as a poultice to the head for headache. The crushed-root poultice was applied to boils, and a root infusion was used as an insect repellent in which corn was soaked before planting.

Viola eriocarpa (*V. pensylvanica*) (smooth yellow violet) is a 4- to 8-inch native violet found in moist, wooded areas of northern and southwestern New Jersey. Leaves are heart-shaped and toothed, with one or more basal. Stems and leaves are not hairy or as heavily veined as in *V. pubescens*. Flowers are yellow, appearing in mid-April.

Native Americans used smooth yellow violet as an ingredient in a compound decoction taken for indigestion.

Violaceae

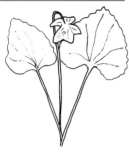

Viola papilionacea (blue meadow violet)

Viola papilionacea (blue meadow violet, common blue violet), the New Jersey state flower, is a 4- to 8-inch native violet found in moist woods of northern New Jersey. Leaves are basal, broad, and heart-shaped. Flowers are blue, appearing in mid-April.

Native Americans used the blue violet as they used *V. cucullata*.

Viola pedata (bird's-foot violet, pansy violet) is a 4- to 8-inch native violet found in dry, open areas statewide. Leaves are basal and divided into narrow, lobed segments. Flowers are dark violet with orange stamens visible in the throat and appear in late April.

Native Americans use the pansy violet as they use *V. cucullata*.

Bigelow described the violets as demulcent in catarrh and strangury and allied to ipecacuanha. *V. pedata* was considered a useful expectorant and lubricating medicine in pulmonary complaints when given as a tea or syrup.

Viola pubescens (downy yellow violet) is a 4-inch to 1-foot native violet found in rich-soiled, dry areas of northern and southwestern New Jersey. Leaves are alternate, very broad, heart-shaped, toothed, prominently veined, and hairy beneath. There may be one basal leaf. Flowers are yellow, appearing in late April.

Native Americans used the downy yellow violet as they used *V. cucullata*. In addition, a plant decoction was used as a wash for facial eruptions. The root decoction was used as a heart medicine and was taken for sore throat.

Viola rafinesquii (*V. kitaibeliana*) (field pansy) is a 4- to 8-inch native(?) annual violet found in dry, open areas, especially along roadsides, statewide, but is more common in southern New Jersey. Leaves are alternate, small, and roundish, with deeply lobed, leaflike stipules. Flowers are bluish white and small, appearing in mid-April.

Native Americans used the field pansy as they use *V. cucullata*.

Viola rotundifolia (round-leaved violet) is a 4- to 6-inch native violet found in rich-soiled, moist, wooded areas of northern New Jersey. Leaves are basal, heart-shaped, and blunt-toothed, expanding from 1 inch long at flowering to 2 to 4 inches in the summer. Flowers are yellow, appearing with the leaves in early April.

Native Americans used the round-leaved violet as they use *V. cucullata.*

Viola sagittata (arrow-leaved violet) is a 2- to 3-inch native violet found in open, moist or dry areas statewide. Leaves are basal, broadly arrow-shaped, and lobed at the base. Flowers are violet-purple and appear in late April.

Native Americans used the arrow-leaved violet as a witchcraft medicine.

Viola tricolor (heart's ease pansy, Johnny-jump-up) is a 4- to 12-inch escaped annual weed found in lawns and waste areas statewide. Leaves are toothed and roundish on the lower part of the plants and oblong above. Leaflike stipules are large and divided. Flowers are pansylike, in purple, white, and yellow, appearing in mid-April.

Native Americans apparently did not use Johnny-jump-up as a medicinal plant. In Europe, the plant tea is used for colds and as a gargle for sore throat. It is a sedative and febrifuge, and is mildly laxative and diuretic. It was used for asthma, as a heart medicine, and as a wash for skin eruptions.

111 *Vitaceae*

The grape family of woody vines with tendrils. The leaves are simple, pinnate or palmate, and alternate. The family is primarily tropical and subtropical, but extends into the cooler regions.

Parthenocissus quinquefolia (Virginia creeper, woodbine) is a climbing or creeping native, woody vine found in rich-soiled, moist areas statewide. Stems cling by branched tendrils, and leaves are divided into

Vitaceae

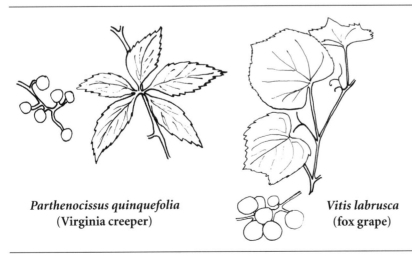

Parthenocissus quinquefolia
(Virginia creeper)

Vitis labrusca
(fox grape)

Xyridaceae

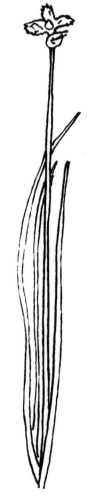

**Xyris caroliniana
(Carolina yellow-eyed-
grass)**

five toothed leaflets. Flowers are whitish, in branching clusters, and appear in late June, giving rise to bluish black fruit in late September.

Native Americans used a Virginia creeper infusion for yellow jaundice. The root decoction was taken for diarrhea. A poultice of crushed leaves and vinegar was applied to wounds and to the face for lockjaw. A vine poultice was applied to wrist swellings, and a hot decoction prepared from stems and leaves was applied to other swellings. The Iroquois regarded the plant as poisonous.

Vitis aestivalis (chicken grape, pigeon grape, summer grape) is a climbing native, woody vine found in open, moist areas statewide. Stems cling by tendrils, but there is no tendril or flower cluster opposite every third leaf. Leaves are three- to five-lobed. Flowers are greenish, in clusters, appearing in late May and giving rise to acidic, black fruit in September.

Native Americans used a summer grape leaf infusion for liver ailments and as a blood medicine. Wilted leaves were applied to breasts for soreness after childbirth, and the vine "water" was taken and used as a wash to induce lactation. A bark infusion was taken for urinary problems. It was also used for the stomach, as a refrigerant, and as a fall tonic.

Vitis labrusca (fox grape) is a climbing native, woody vine, found in rich-soiled, wet areas statewide, with the exception of the central pinelands. Stems cling by tendrils at nearly every leaf. Leaves are obscurely three-lobed, rust-woolly beneath, and toothed. Flowers are greenish, in clusters, and appear in late May, giving rise to purple fruit in early September.

Native Americans use the fox grape as they use *V. aestivalis* and applied a leaf poultice for pains, including headache.

Vitis vulpina (frost grape, winter grape) is a climbing native, woody vine found in moist areas and along riverbanks statewide, outside of the pinelands. Leaves are heart-shaped or barely three-lobed and toothed. Flowers are greenish, in clusters and appear in early June. Shiny, black fruits develop in September, becoming sweet after frost.

Native Americans used frost grape as they use *V. labrusca.* They also chewed the vine for hiccough and used a root infusion for rheumatism and diabetes. A plant decoction was taken for kidney trouble, and a twig decoction was taken to facilitate expulsion of the afterbirth. The sap was used as a hair tonic and to treat leucorrhea. The seed, juice, or ripe grape was used to remove foreign matter from the eye.

112 *Xyridaceae*

The yellow-eyed-grass family of rushlike monocotyledonous herbs, with rhizomes sometimes forming storage organs. The leaves are sheathing (enclosing), elongate or threadlike, and usually basal. The family is composed of two genera which are found in tropical and subtropical Africa, Australia, and the Western Hemisphere.

Xyris caroliniana (Carolina yellow-eyed-grass) is a 6-inch to 3-foot native perennial found in wet, sandy or peaty areas statewide. Leaves are basal, sheathing the flower stalk, grasslike, and entire. Flowers are yellow and three-petaled, appearing in mid-June.

Native Americans used a yellow-eyed-grass root infusion for diarrhea and described it as "good for children."

Uses of Medicinal Plants by Category
Name (Family)

Abortion

Achillea millefolium (029)
Acorus calamus (009)
Aletris farinosa (059)
Angelica atropurpurea (106)
Apocynum cannabinum (007)
Apocynum medium (007)
Aralia nudicaulis (010)
Aralia racemosa (010)
Aristolochia serpentaria (011)
Armoracia rusticana (033)
Asarum canadensis (011)
Asplenium trichomanes (014)
Ceanothus americanus (090)
Celastrus orbiculatus (025)
Celastrus scandens (025)
Chenopodium ambrosioides (026)
Cimicifuga racemosa (089)
Daucus carota (106)
Echinocystis lobata (034)
Erigeron philadelphicus (029)
Erigeron pulchellus (029)

Euonymus americanus (025)
Eupatorium perfoliatum (029)
Fagus grandifolia (044)
Fragaria virginiana (091)
Hedeoma pulegioides (055)
Hepatica americana (089)
Hydrangea arborescens (097)
Hypericum perforatum (052)
Juniperus virginiana (035)
Lilium canadense (059)
Lindera benzoin (056)
Mitchella repens (092)
Monarda didyma (055)
Monarda fistulosa (055)
Nepeta cataria (055)
Pedicularis canadensis (098)
Phoradendron flavescens (062)
Platanus occidentalis (082)
Polygala senega (084)
Pycnanthemum virginianum (055)
Rhus aromatica (005)

Rhus copallinum (005)
Rhus glabra (005)
Rhus radicans (005)
Rhus typhina (005)
Rhus vernix (005)
Rosa palustris (091)
Rosa rugosa (091)
Rubus pensilvanicus (091)
Rubus pubescens (091)
Sanguinaria canadensis (078)
Sanicula canadensis (106)
Sanicula marilandica (106)
Scutellaria elliptica (055)
Scutellaria lateriflora (055)
Silphium perfoliatum (029)
Solidago odora (029)
Tanacetum vulgare (029)
Taxus canadensis (101)
Tephrosia virginiana (057)
Teucrium canadense (055)
Thuja occidentalis (035)
Triosteum perfoliatum (023)
Veratrum viride (059)
Verbena hastata (109)
Viburnum lentago (023)
Xanthoxylum americum (093)

Antiemetic

Achillea millefolium (029)
Agrimonia gryposepala (091)
Ambrosia artemisiifolia (029)

Anemonella thalictroides (089)
Anthemis cotula (029)
Asarum canadensis (011)
Baptisia tinctoria (057)

Cercis canadensis (057)
Coptis trifolia (089)
Corylus americana (017)
Gnaphalium obtusifolium (029)

Hamamelis virginiana (049)
Hydrangea arborescens (097)
Lactuca biennis (029)
Lupinus perennis (057)
Mentha arvensis (055)
Mentha piperita (055)
Mentha spicata (055)
Menyanthes trifoliata (046)
Mitchella repens (092)

Nepeta cataria (055)
Oxalis corniculata (077)
Panax quinquefolium (010)
Prunella vulgaris (055)
Prunus virginiana (091)
Pteridium aquilinum (037)
Rhus copallinum (005)
Rhus glabra (005)
Rhus typhina (005)
Ribes americanum (097)

Rubus pubescens (091)
Sanguinaria canadensis (078)
Silphium perfoliatum (029)
Solidago juncea (029)
Spiraea tomentosa (091)
Ulmus americana (105)
Vaccinium oxycoccos (042)
Xanthoxylum americum (093)

Bleeding

Achillea millefolium (029)
Agrimonia gryposepala (091)
Apocynum androsaemifolium (007)
Aralia nudicaulis (010)
Artemisia ludoviciana (029)
Gentiana quinquefolia (046)
Geranium maculatum (047)
Gymnocladus dioica (057)
Hypericum perforatum (052)
Juglans cinerea (054)
Lactuca canadensis (029)
Lobelia cardinalis (021)
Lobelia siphilitica (021)

Lycopodium clavatum (063)
Mitchella repens (092)
Monarda didyma (055)
Monarda fistulosa (055)
Nuphar advena (071)
Panax quinquefolium (010)
Panax trifolium (010)
Phytolacca americana (079)
Pinus strobus (080)
Platanus occidentalis (082)
Polygala senega (084)
Prunus virginiana (091)
Pycnanthemum incanum (055)
Ranunculus abortivus (089)
Rhus aromatica (005)
Rhus glabra (005)
Rhus typhina (005)

Rumex crispus (085)
Salix discolor (094)
Salix fragilis (094)
Salix lucida (094)
Sanguinaria canadensis (078)
Sassafras albidum (056)
Silphium perfoliatum (029)
Smilacina racemosa (059)
Symplocarpus foetidus (009)
Tsuga canadensis (080)
Typha latifolia (104)
Ulmus rubra (105)
Urtica dioica (107)
Verbena hastata (109)
Xanthoxylum americum (093)

Blood Pressure

Allium vineale (059)
Alnus serrulata (017)

Hydrangea aborescens (097)
Juglans nigra (054)

Rubus strigosus (091)
Sassafras albidum (056)

Burns

Achillea millefolium (029)
Acorus calamus (009)
Althaea officinalis (066)
Anemone cylindrica (089)
Aralia nudicaulis (010)
Chenopodium album (026)
Clintonia borealis (059)
Eupatorium purpureum (029)

Geranium maculatum (047)
Goodyera pubescens (075)
Hydrangea arborescens (097)
Iris versicolor (053)
Larix laricina (080)
Ledum groenlandicum (042)
Monarda fistulosa (055)

Oxybaphus nyctagineus (070)
Physalis heterophylla (100)
Plantago aristata (081)
Plantago lanceolata (081)
Plantago major (081)
Prunella vulgaris (055)
Prunus serotina (091)
Pteridium aquilinum (037)

Rhus aromatica (005)
Rhus copallinum (005)
Rhus glabra (005)
Rhus typhina (005)
Rudbeckia laciniata (029)
Rumex crispus (085)

Sambucus canadensis (023)
Sanguinaria canadensis
(078)
Sassafras albidum (056)
Smilax glauca (059)
Smilax rotundifolia (059)

Thuja occidentalis (035)
Tilia americana (103)
Typha latifolia (104)
Ulmus rubra (105)
Xanthoxylum americum
(093)

Cancer

Agrostemma githago (024)
Aralia nudicaulis (010)
Boehmeria cylindrica (107)
Cacalia atriplicifolia (029)
Celastrus scandens (025)
Chelidonium majus (078)
Chimaphila maculata
(042)
Chimaphila umbellata
(042)

Cornus alternifolia (031)
Cynoglossum officinale
(019)
Epilobium angustifolium
(073)
Euphorbia corollata (043)
Hydrangea arborescens
(097)
Hydrastis canadensis (089)
Lonicera japonica (023)

Oxalis corniculata (077)
Pedicularis canadensis
(098)
Pyrola elliptica (042)
Stylophorum diphyllum
(078)
Tradescantia virginiana
(028)
Trifolium pratense (057)
Trillium erectum (059)

Cathartic/Laxative

Acer pensylvanicum (001)
Acorus calamus (009)
Actaea rubra (089)
Allium vineale (059)
Apocynum cannabinum
(007)
Artemisia ludoviciana
(029)
Asarum canadense (011)
Asclepias incarnata (012)
Asclepias syriaca (012)
Asclepias tuberosa (012)
Asimina triloba (006)
Baptisia tinctoria (057)
Caltha palustris (089)
Cassia hebecarpa (057)
Cassia marilandica (057)
Ceanothus americanus (090)
Celastrus orbiculatus (025)
Chelone glabra (098)
Chimaphila umbellata
(042)
Cimicifuga racemosa (089)
Convolvulus sepium (030)
Cornus rugosa (031)
Cytisus scoparius (057)
Daucus carota (106)

Dirca palustris (102)
Erechtites hieracifolia (029)
Eupatorium perfoliatum
(029)
Eupatorium purpureum
(029)
Eupatorium rugosum (029)
Euphorbia corollata (043)
Fraxinus americana (072)
Galium aparine (092)
Gentiana quinquefolia
(046)
Geranium maculatum
(047)
Gillenia trifoliata (091)
Gymnocladus dioica (057)
Hydrangea arborescens
(097)
Inula helenium (029)
Iris versicolor (053)
Juglans cinerea (054)
Juglans nigra (054)
Juniperus communis (035)
Juniperus virginiana (035)
Lobelia inflata (021)
Matricaria matricarioides
(029)

Menispermum canadense
(067)
Menyanthes trifoliata (046)
Mitchella repens (092)
Monarda fistulosa (055)
Morus alba (068)
Morus rubra (068)
Nepeta cataria (055)
Pedicularis canadensis
(098)
Physocarpus opulifolius
(091)
Phytolacca americana (079)
Pinus echinata (080)
Plantago major (081)
Platanus occidentalis (082)
Podophyllum peltatum
(016)
Polygala senega (084)
Polygonatum biflorum
(059)
Populus tremuloides (094)
Prunella vulgaris (055)
Prunus virginiana (091)
Rhamnus catharticus (090)
Rubus occidentalis (091)
Rubus odoratus (091)

Rubus strigosus (091)
Rumex crispus (085)
Sagittaria latifolia (003)
Salvia lyrata (055)
Sambucus canadensis (023)
Sanguinaria canadensis (078)
Sanicula marilandica (106)
Sisyrinchium angustifolium (053)
Smilacina racemosa (059)
Symphytum officinale (019)
Taraxacum officinale (029)
Tradescantia virginiana (028)
Triosteum perfoliatum (023)
Ulmus rubra (105)
Veratrum viride (059)
Verbascum thapsus (098)
Veronicastrum virginicum (098)
Viburnum opulus (023)

Contraception

Chelone glabra (098)
Cicuta maculata (106)
Erythronium albidum (059)
Erythronium americanum (059)
Smilacina racemosa (059)
Tanacetum vulgare (029)

Coughs/Colds/Expectorants

Acer pensylvanicum (001)
Acer saccharinum (001)
Acer saccharum (001)
Achillea millefolium (029)
Acorus calamus (009)
Actaea rubra (089)
Aletris farinosa (059)
Allium canadense (059)
Allium cernuum (059)
Allium tricoccum (059)
Allium vineale (059)
Alnus serrulata (017)
Anaphalis margaritacae (029)
Angelica atropurpurea (106)
Anthemis cotula (029)
Apocynum androsaemifolium (007)
Apocynum cannabinum (007)
Aralia nudicaulis (010)
Aralia racemosa (010)
Arctium minus (029)
Arisaema triphyllum (009)
Aristolochia serpentaria (011)
Armoracia rusticana (033)
Artemisia annua (029)
Artemisia campestris (029)
Artemisia ludoviciana (029)
Asarum canadensis (011)

Asclepias tuberosa (012)
Asplenium trichomanes (014)
Barbarea vulgaris (033)
Betula lenta (017)
Botrychium virginianum (074)
Brassica nigra (033)
Caltha palustris (089)
Castilleja coccinea (098)
Ceanothus americanus (090)
Celastrus orbiculatus (025)
Celastrus scandens (025)
Chimaphila maculata (042)
Chimaphila umbellata (042)
Cimicifuga racemosa (089)
Cornus alternifolia (031)
Cornus canadensis (031)
Cunila origanoides (055)
Cypripedium acaule (075)
Cypripedium calceolus (075)
Dentaria diphylla (033)
Duchesneu indica (091)
Erigeron philadelphicus (029)
Erigeron pulchellus (029)
Eryngium aquaticum (106)
Euonymus americanus (025)

Eupatorium maculatum (029)
Eupatorium perfoliatum (029)
Eupatorium purpureum (029)
Euphorbia ipecacuanhae (043)
Foeniculum vulgare (106)
Gaultheria procumbens (042)
Geum rivale (091)
Gillenia trifoliata (091)
Glecoma hederacea (055)
Gleditsia triacanthos (057)
Gnaphalium obtusifolium (029)
Goodyera pubescens (075)
Hamamelis virginiana (049)
Hedeoma pulegioides (055)
Helenium autumnale (029)
Heracleum lanatum (106)
Humulus lupulus (022)
Hypericum perforatum (052)
Inula helenium (029)
Ipomoea pandurata (030)
Iris versicolor (053)
Juniperus communis (035)
Juniperus virginiana (035)
Kalmia angustifolia (042)

Larix laricina (080)
Ledum groenlandicum (042)
Lilium philadelphicum (059)
Lindera benzoin (056)
Linum usitatissimum (060)
Liriodendron tulipifera (065)
Lobelia cardinalis (021)
Lobelia siphilitica (021)
Malva sylvestris (066)
Marrubium vulgare (055)
Matricaria matricarioides (029)
Melilotus officinalis (057)
Melissa officinalis (055)
Mentha aquatica (055)
Mentha arvensis (055)
Mentha piperita (055)
Mentha spicata (055)
Monarda didyma (055)
Monarda fistulosa (055)
Monarda punctata (055)
Monotropa uniflora (042)
Nepeta cataria (055)
Nymphaea odorata (071)
Pedicularis canadensis (098)
Penthorum sedoides (032)
Perilla frutescens (055)
Phytolacca americana (079)
Picea mariana (080)
Pinus strobus (080)

Plantago major (081)
Platanus occidentalis (082)
Polygala polygama (084)
Polygala senega (084)
Polygonatum biflorum (059)
Populus alba (094)
Populus candicans (094)
Populus tremuloides (094)
Prunella vulgaris (055)
Prunus americana (091)
Prunus cerasus (091)
Prunus serotina (091)
Prunus virginiana (091)
Pycnanthemum incanum (055)
Pycnanthemum virginianum (055)
Quercus alba (044)
Quercus borealis (044)
Rhus aromatica (005)
Rhus typhina (005)
Rubus allegheniensis (091)
Rubus odoratus (091)
Rubus strigosus (091)
Rudbeckia hirta (029)
Salix nigra (094)
Salvia lyrata (055)
Sanguinaria canadensis (078)
Sassafras albidum (056)
Silphium perfoliatum (029)

Smilacina racemosa (059)
Solidago odora (029)
Symplocarpus foetidus (009)
Tanacetum vulgare (029)
Taxus canadensis (101)
Thuja occidentalis (035)
Tilia americana (103)
Trifolium repens (057)
Trillium erectum (059)
Triosteum perfoliatum (023)
Tsuga canadensis (080)
Tussilago farfara (029)
Ulmus americana (105)
Ulmus rubra (105)
Urtica dioica (107)
Veratrum viride (059)
Verbascum thapsus (098)
Verbena hastata (109)
Veronica officinalis (098)
Veronicastrum virginicum (098)
Viburnum opulus (023)
Viola cucullata (110)
Viola papilionacea (110)
Viola pedata (110)
Viola pubescens (110)
Viola rafinesquii (110)
Viola rotundifolia (110)
Viola tricolor (110)
Xanthoxylum americum (093)

Cure-All

Achillea millefolium (029)
Acorus calamus (009)
Alnus glutinosa (017)
Anemone canadensis (089)
Anthemis cotula (029)
Apocynum cannabinum (007)
Arctostaphylos uva-ursi (042)
Artemisia vulgaris (029)
Asarum canadensis (011)
Chenopodium ambrosioides (026)
Collinsonia canadensis (055)

Cypripedium acaule (075)
Echinocystis lobata (034)
Epilobium angustifolium (073)
Eupatorium perfoliatum (029)
Eupatorium rugosum (029)
Geum canadense (091)
Gleditsia triacanthos (057)
Hamamelis virginiana (049)
Heuchera americana (097)
Inula helenium (029)
Ipomoea pandurata (030)
Iris versicolor (053)

Juniperus communis (035)
Kalmia angustifolia (042)
Kalmia latifolia (042)
Lindera benzoin (056)
Lobelia cardinalis (021)
Matricaria matricarioides (029)
Medeola virginiana (059)
Mentha arvensis (055)
Morus rubra (068)
Osmorhiza longistylis (106)
Panax quinquefolium (010)
Phoradendron flavescens (062)

Pinus strobus (080)
Populus alba (094)
Portulaca oleracea (087)
Prunella vulgaris (055)
Ptelea trifoliata (093)
Pycnanthemum incanum
(055)

Quercus alba (044)
Rhus typhina (005)
Rumex crispus (085)
Sabatia angularis (046)
Salix discolor (094)
Sanguinaria canadensis (078)
Saururus cernuus (096)

Tanacetum vulgare (029)
Thuja occidentalis (035)
Tilia americana (103)
Urtica dioica (107)
Veratrum viride (059)
Veronicastrum virginicum
(098)

Diarrhea

Abutilon theophrasti (066)
Acer rubrum (001)
Acer saccharinum (001)
Achillea millefolium (029)
Acorus calamus (009)
Adiantum pedatum (002)
Agrimonia gryposepala
(091)
Agrimonia parviflora (091)
Agrimonia pubescens (091)
Ailanthus altissima (099)
Aletris farinosa (059)
Ambrosia artemisiifolia
(029)
Ambrosia trifida (029)
Amelanchier arborea (091)
Amelanchier canadensis
(091)
Anaphalis margaritacae
(029)
Anemone virginiana (089)
Anemonella thalictroides
(089)
Anthemis cotula (029)
Apocynum cannabinum
(007)
Aquilegia canadensis (089)
Aralia racemosa (010)
Arisaema triphyllum (009)
Artemisia annua (029)
Artemisia ludoviciana
(029)
Asarum canadensis (011)
Asclepias tuberosa (012)
Aster novae-angliae (029)
Betula lenta (017)
Capsella bursa-pastoris
(033)
Carex brevior (036)
Carex pensylvanica (036)

Ceanothus americanus
(090)
Celastrus orbiculatus (025)
Cephalanthus occidentalis
(092)
Chenopodium album (026)
Collinsonia canadensis
(055)
Commelina communis
(028)
Conyza canadensis (029)
Cornus alternifolia (031)
Cornus florida (031)
Corylus americana (017)
Diospyros virginiana (040)
Epifagus virginiana (076)
Epigaea repens (042)
Eupatorium rugosum (029)
Fragaria virginiana (091)
Gaultheria procumbens
(042)
Geranium maculatum
(047)
Geum rivale (091)
Gillenia trifoliata (091)
Hamamelis virginiana
(049)
Hedeoma pulegioides (055)
Hepatica americana (089)
Heuchera americana (097)
Hieracium pilosella (029)
Hydrastis canadensis (089)
Hydrophyllum virginianum
(051)
Hypericum perforatum
(052)
Jeffersonia diphylla (016)
Juglans cinerea (054)
Juglans nigra (054)
Juniperus communis (035)

Kalmia latifolia (042)
Lactuca biennis (029)
Lilium canadense (059)
Linaria vulgaris (098)
Liquidamber styraciflua
(049)
Liriodendron tulipifera
(065)
Magnolia acuminata (065)
Marrubium vulgare (055)
Matricaria matricarioides
(029)
Menispermum canadense
(067)
Mentha arvensis (055)
Mitchella repens (092)
Morus alba (068)
Morus rubra (068)
Nepeta cataria (055)
Parthenocissus quinquefolia
(111)
Pedicularis canadensis
(098)
Phytolacca americana (079)
Plantago lanceolata (081)
Plantago major (081)
Platanus occidentalis (082)
Polygonatum biflorum
(059)
Polygonum aviculare (085)
Polygonum hydropiper
(085)
Polygonum pensylvanicum
(085)
Polystichum acrostichoides
(013)
Potentilla arguta (091)
Potentilla canadensis (091)
Potentilla simplex (091)
Prunella vulgaris (055)

Prunus americana (091)
Prunus serotina (091)
Prunus virginiana (091)
Pteridium aquilinum (037)
Pycnanthemum incanum
  (055)
Quercus alba (044)
Quercus borealis (044)
Ranunculus acris (089)
Rhus aromatica (005)
Rhus copallinum (005)
Rhus glabra (005)
Rhus typhina (005)
Rosa palustris (091)
Rubus allegheniensis (091)
Rubus canadensis (091)
Rubus flagellaris (091)
Rubus occidentalis (091)
Rubus odoratus (091)
Rubus strigosus (091)

Rumex acetosa (085)
Rumex crispus (085)
Salix alba (094)
Salix babylonica (094)
Salix nigra (094)
Salvia lyrata (055)
Sanguinaria canadensis
  (078)
Sassafras albidum (056)
Scutellaria elliptica (055)
Scutellaria lateriflora (055)
Sisyrinchium angustifolium
  (053)
Solidago juncea (029)
Solidago odora (029)
Spiraea tomentosa (091)
Symphytum officinale (019)
Tanacetum vulgare (029)
Tiarella cordifolia (097)
Tilia americana (103)

Tsuga canadensis (080)
Typha latifolia (104)
Ulmus americana (105)
Ulmus rubra (105)
Uvularia sessilifolia (059)
Verbascum thapsus (098)
Verbena hastata (109)
Veronicastrum virginicum
  (098)
Viola cucullata (110)
Viola papilionacea (110)
Viola pedata (110)
Viola pubescens (110)
Viola rafinesquii (110)
Viola rotundifolia (110)
Vitis aestivalis (111)
Vitis labrusca (111)
Vitis vulpina (111)
Xyris caroliniana (112)

Disinfectant

Ambrosia artemisiifolia
  (029)
Ambrosia trifida (029)
Amelanchier canadensis
  (091)
Anaphalis margaritacae
  (029)
Apocynum medium (007)
Aralia nudicaulis (010)
Aralia racemosa (010)
Aristolochia serpentaria
  (011)
Artemisia ludoviciana (029)
Asarum canadensis (011)
Carex pensylvanica (036)
Chionanthus virginicus
  (072)

Cicuta maculata (106)
Cornus alternifolia (031)
Cornus florida (031)
Equisetum hyemale (041)
Erodium cicutarium (047)
Euonymus americanus
  (025)
Eupatorium perfoliatum
  (029)
Gnapthalium obtusifolium
  (029)
Hydrangea arborescens
  (097)
Juniperus communis (035)
Juniperus virginiana (035)
Larix laricina (080)
Marrubium vulgare (055)

Matricaria matricarioides
  (029)
Mentha arvensis (055)
Picea mariana (080)
Plantago major (081)
Populus tremuloides (094)
Prunus americana (091)
Prunus serotina (091)
Prunus virginiana (091)
Pteridium aquilinum
  (037)
Quercus alba (044)
Quercus borealis (044)
Sambucus canadensis (023)
Tanacetum vulgare (029)
Veronicastrum virginicum
  (098)

Ear/Eye

Acer rubrum (001)
Acer saccharinum (001)
Acer saccharum (001)
Achillea millefolium (029)
Acorus calamus (009)
Allium canadense (059)

Allium tricoccum (059)
Allium vineale (059)
Alnus serrulata (017)
Anaphalis margaritacae
  (029)
Anemone canadensis (089)

Anemone cylindrica (089)
Anthemis cotula (029)
Apocynum cannabinum
  (007)
Aralia nudicaulis (010)
Aralia racemosa (010)

Aralia spinosa (010)
Arctostaphylos uva-ursi (042)
Arisaema triphyllum (009)
Artemisia ludoviciana (029)
Asarum canadensis (011)
Calla palustris (009)
Chimaphila umbellata (042)
Conyza canadensis (029)
Coptis trifolia (089)
Cornus alternifolia (031)
Cornus canadensis (031)
Dirca palustris (102)
Equisetum hyemale (041)
Erigeron philadelphicus (029)
Erigeron pulchellus (029)
Euonymus atropurpureus (025)
Goodyera pubescens (075)
Hamamelis virginiana (049)
Hedeoma pulegioides (055)

Humulus lupulus (022)
Hydrastis canadensis (089)
Ilex opaca (008)
Impatiens biflora (015)
Impatiens pallida (015)
Iris versicolor (053)
Juniperus communis (035)
Ledum groenlandicum (042)
Maclura pomifera (068)
Medicago sativa (057)
Monarda fistulosa (055)
Monotropa uniflora (042)
Osmorhiza claytoni (106)
Osmorhiza longistylis (106)
Panax quinquefolium (010)
Plantago aristata (081)
Plantago lanceolata (081)
Plantago major (081)
Podophyllum peltatum (016)
Portulaca oleracea (087)
Prunus virginiana (091)
Pyrola elliptica (042)
Ranunculus abortivus (089)

Rhamnus catharticus (090)
Rhus glabra (005)
Rosa blanda (091)
Rosa virginiana (091)
Rubus allegheniensis (091)
Rubus occidentalis (091)
Rubus strigosus (091)
Rudbeckia hirta (029)
Sanguinaria canadensis (078)
Sassafras albidum (056)
Smilacina racemosa (059)
Stellaria media (024)
Tanacetum vulgare (029)
Taraxacum officinale (029)
Tiarella cordifolia (097)
Trifolium repens (057)
Ulmus americana (105)
Ulmus rubra (105)
Uvularia perfoliata (059)
Verbascum thapsus (098)
Verbena hastata (109)
Veronica officinalis (098)
Viburnum opulus (023)
Vitis vulpina (111)

Emetic

Acer negundo (001)
Acer pensylvanicum (001)
Achillea millefolium (029)
Acorus calamus (009)
Adiantum pedatum (002)
Agrimonia gryposepala (091)
Allium tricoccum (059)
Alnus serrulata (017)
Ambrosia artemisiifolia (029)
Anemone virginiana (089)
Anthemis cotula (029)
Apocynum cannabinum (007)
Apocynum medium (007)
Aralia spinosa (010)
Arctostaphylos uva-ursi (042)
Asarum canadensis (011)
Asclepias incarnata (012)

Asimina triloba (006)
Baptisia tinctoria (057)
Botrychium virginianum (074)
Brassica nigra (033)
Caltha palustris (089)
Caulophyllum thalictroides (016)
Chimaphila maculata (042)
Collinsonia canadensis (055)
Convallaria majalis (059)
Coptis trifolia (089)
Cornus alternifolia (031)
Cornus rugosa (031)
Corylus americana (017)
Cytisus scoparius (057)
Epigaea repens (042)
Erechtites hieracifolia (029)
Eryngium aquaticum (106)

Eupatorium perfoliatum (029)
Euphorbia corollata (043)
Euphorbia ipecacuanhae (043)
Fraxinus americana (072)
Galium aparine (092)
Geranium maculatum (047)
Gillenia trifoliata (091)
Goodyera pubescens (075)
Hamamelis virginiana (049)
Hydrangea arborescens (097)
Hydrastis canadensis (089)
Iris versicolor (053)
Juglans nigra (054)
Juniperus communis (035)
Lactuca serriola (029)
Lindera benzoin (056)
Lobelia inflata (021)

Lobelia spicata (021)
Lysimachia quadrifolia
  (088)
Malva neglecta (066)
Mentha arvensis (055)
Mentha spicata (055)
Morus rubra (068)
Pedicularis canadensis
  (098)
Physocarpus opulifolius
  (091)
Phytolacca americana (079)
Pinus echinata (080)
Pinus strobus (080)
Platanus occidentalis (082)
Podophyllum peltatum
  (016)
Polystichum acrostichoides
  (013)
Prunella vulgaris (055)
Prunus serotina (091)

Prunus virginiana (091)
Quercus alba (044)
Quercus borealis (044)
Ranunculus abortivus (089)
Rhus glabra (005)
Rhus radicans (005)
Rhus vernix (005)
Robinia pseudoacacia (057)
Rubus occidentalis (091)
Rubus odoratus (091)
Rubus strigosus (091)
Rudbeckia laciniata (029)
Rumex crispus (085)
Salix discolor (094)
Sambucus canadensis (023)
Sanguinaria canadensis
  (078)
Sanicula marilandica (106)
Scutellaria lateriflora (055)
Silphium perfoliatum (029)
Solanum nigrum (100)

Solidago canadensis (029)
Solidago juncea (029)
Sorbus americana (091)
Tanacetum vulgare (029)
Taraxacum officinale (029)
Tilia americana (103)
Triosteum perfoliatum
  (023)
Typha latifolia (104)
Ulmus rubra (105)
Veratrum viride (059)
Verbena hastata (109)
Veronica officinalis (098)
Veronicastrum virginicum
  (098)
Viburnum lentago (023)
Viburnum opulus (023)
Xanthoxylum americum
  (093)
Zygadenus leimanthoides
  (059)

Fever

Abutilon theophrasti (066)
Achillea millefolium (029)
Acorus calamus (009)
Adiantum pedatum (002)
Agrimonia gryposepala
  (091)
Agrimonia parviflora (091)
Aletris farinosa (059)
Allium cernuum (059)
Alnus serrulata (017)
Ambrosia artemisiifolia
  (029)
Ambrosia trifida (029)
Andropogon gerardi (048)
Angelica atropurpurea
  (106)
Anthemis cotula (029)
Aquilegia canadensis (089)
Aralia spinosa (010)
Arisaema triphyllum (009)
Aristolochia serpentaria
  (011)
Artemisia ludoviciana
  (029)
Asarum canadense (011)

Aster novae-angliae (029)
Berberis vulgaris (016)
Betula lenta (017)
Brassica nigra (033)
Cassia hebecarpa (057)
Cassia marilandica (057)
Catalpa bignonioides (018)
Caulophyllum thalictroides
  (016)
Celastrus scandens (025)
Cercis canadensis (057)
Chelone glabra (098)
Chenopodium ambrosioides
  (026)
Chimaphila maculata (042)
Chimaphila umbellata
  (042)
Chrysanthemum
  leucanthemum (029)
Cornus alternifolia (031)
Cornus canadensis (031)
Cornus florida (031)
Cunila origanoides (055)
Cypripedium calceolus
  (075)

Datura stramonium (100)
Echinocystis lobata (034)
Erigeron philadelphicus
  (029)
Erodium cicutarium (047)
Erythronium americanum
  (059)
Eupatorium maculatum
  (029)
Eupatorium perfoliatum
  (029)
Eupatorium rugosum (029)
Gaultheria procumbens
  (042)
Geum rivale (091)
Gillenia trifoliata (091)
Gleditsia triacanthos (057)
Gnaphalium obtusifolium
  (029)
Hamamelis virginiana
  (049)
Hedeoma pulegioides (055)
Helenium autumnale (029)
Helianthus annuus (029)
Hepatica americana (089)

Humulus lupulus (022)
Hydrastis canadensis (089)
Hypericum perforatum (052)
Impatiens biflora (015)
Impatiens pallida (015)
Inula helenium (029)
Juglans nigra (054)
Juniperus communis (035)
Larix laricina (080)
Ledum groenlandicum (042)
Lilium philadelphicum (059)
Lindera benzoin (056)
Linum usitatissimum (060)
Liquidamber styraciflua (049)
Liriodendron tulipifera (065)
Lithospermum canescens (019)
Lobelia cardinalis (021)
Lobelia siphilitica (021)
Lycopodium clavatum (063)
Lythrum salicaria (064)
Magnolia virginiana (065)
Malva moschata (066)
Malva sylvestris (066)
Matricaria matricarioides (029)
Melissa officinalis (055)
Mentha arvensis (055)

Mentha piperita (055)
Mentha spicata (055)
Mitchella repens (092)
Monarda didyma (055)
Monarda fistulosa (055)
Monarda punctata (055)
Monotropa uniflora (042)
Myrica cerifera (069)
Nasturtium officinale (033)
Nepeta cataria (055)
Nuphar advena (071)
Oxybaphus nyctagineus (070)
Panax quinquefolium (010)
Paulownia tomentosa (098)
Phytolacca americana (079)
Plantago major (081)
Polygonum hydropiper (085)
Polystichum acrostichoides (013)
Potentilla simplex (091)
Prunella vulgaris (055)
Prunus cerasus (091)
Prunus serotina (091)
Prunus virginiana (091)
Pycnanthemum incanum (055)
Pycnanthemum virginianum (055)
Quercus alba (044)
Quercus borealis (044)
Rhus vernix (005)

Sagittaria latifolia (003)
Salix alba (094)
Salix nigra (094)
Sambucus canadensis (023)
Sanguinaria canadensis (078)
Sanicula marilandica (106)
Sarracenia purpurea (095)
Sassafras albidum (056)
Senecio aureus (029)
Solanum dulcamara (100)
Solidago canadensis (029)
Solidago juncea (029)
Solidago odora (029)
Tanacetum vulgare (029)
Tephrosia virginiana (057)
Thuja occidentalis (035)
Thymus serpyllum (055)
Trifolium pratense (057)
Triosteum perfoliatum (023)
Tsuga canadensis (080)
Urtica dioica (107)
Verbascum thapsus (098)
Veronicastrum virginicum (098)
Viburnum opulus (023)
Viburnum prunifolium (023)
Vitis aestivalis (111)
Vitis labrusca (111)
Xanthoxylum americum (093)
Zizia aurea (106)

Gynecology

Acer rubrum (001)
Acer saccharinum (001)
Achillea millefolium (029)
Actaea alba (089)
Actaea rubra (089)
Adiantum pedatum (002)
Agrimonia gryposepala (091)
Agrimonia parviflora (091)
Aletris farinosa (059)
Alisma plantago-aquatica (003)

Alnus serrulata (017)
Amelanchier canadensis (091)
Amelanchier laevis (091)
Angelica atropurpurea (106)
Antennaria plantaginifolia (029)
Anthemis cotula (029)
Apocynum androsaemifolium (007)
Aquilegia canadensis (089)
Aralia racemosa (010)

Arctium lappa (029)
Arctium minus (029)
Arisaema dracontium (009)
Arisaema triphyllum (009)
Artemisia ludoviciana (029)
Artemisia vulgaris (029)
Asarum canadensis (011)
Asclepias syriaca (012)
Asclepias tuberosa (012)
Athyrium filix-femina (013)

Baptisia tinctoria (057)
Betula lenta (017)
Caltha palustris (089)
Carex brevior (036)
Caulophyllum thalictroides
(016)
Celastrus scandens (025)
Chenopodium album (026)
Chimaphila umbellata (042)
Cimicifuga racemosa (089)
Clintonia borealis (059)
Convolvulus arvensis (030)
Cornus alternifolia (031)
Cornus florida (031)
Corylus americana (017)
Cunila origanoides (055)
Cypripedium acaule (075)
Cypripedium calceolus
(075)
Daucus carota (106)
Dioscorea villosa (038)
Dirca palustris (102)
Echium vulgare (019)
Epigaea repens (042)
Erigeron philadelphicus
(029)
Euonymus americanus
(025)
Euonymus atropurpureus
(025)
Eupatorium maculatum
(029)
Eupatorium purpureum
(029)
Eupatorium rugosum (029)
Euphorbia corollata (043)
Euphorbia ipecacuanhae
(043)
Foeniculum vulgare (106)
Fraxinus americana (072)
Geum canadense (091)
Goodyera pubescens (075)
Gymnocladus dioica (057)
Hamamelis virginiana
(049)
Hedeoma pulegioides (055)
Helenium autumnale (029)
Helianthus annuus (029)
Helonias bullata (059)
Heuchera americana (097)

Humulus lupulus (022)
Hydrangea arborescens
(097)
Impatiens biflora (015)
Impatiens pallida (015)
Inula helenium (029)
Iris versicolor (053)
Juglans cinerea (054)
Juniperus communis (035)
Lactuca biennis (029)
Lactuca serriola (029)
Leonurus cardiaca (055)
Lilium philadelphicum
(059)
Lindera benzoin (056)
Liquidamber styraciflua
(049)
Lobelia cardinalis (021)
Lycopodium clavatum
(063)
Lysimachia quadrifolia
(088)
Maianthemum canadense
(059)
Marrubium vulgare (055)
Matricaria chamomilla
(029)
Menispermum canadense
(067)
Mitchella repens (092)
Monotropa uniflora (042)
Myrica asplenifolia (069)
Osmorhiza claytoni (106)
Osmorhiza longistylis (106)
Oxybaphus nyctagineus
(070)
Panax quinquefolium (010)
Pastinaca sativa (106)
Phytolacca americana (079)
Plantago aristata (081)
Plantago lanceolata (081)
Plantago major (081)
Platanus occidentalis (082)
Polygonatum biflorum
(059)
Polygonum aviculare (085)
Polygonum pensylvanicum
(085)
Polystichum acrostichoides
(013)

Populus deltoides (094)
Populus tremuloides (094)
Prenanthes alba (029)
Prunella vulgaris (055)
Prunus cerasus (091)
Prunus serotina (091)
Prunus virginiana (091)
Pteridium aquilinum (037)
Quercus alba (044)
Rhus aromatica (005)
Rhus copallinum (005)
Rhus glabra (005)
Rhus typhina (005)
Ribes americanum (097)
Rubus allegheniensis (091)
Rubus occidentalis (091)
Rubus odoratus (091)
Rubus strigosus (091)
Rudbeckia hirta (029)
Salvia lyrata (055)
Sambucus canadensis (023)
Sanguinaria canadensis
(078)
Sanicula canadensis (106)
Sanicula marilandica (106)
Sarracenia purpurea (095)
Sassafras albidum (056)
Scrophularia lanceolata
(098)
Scrophularia marilandica
(098)
Scutellaria elliptica (055)
Scutellaria lateriflora (055)
Senecio aureus (029)
Silphium perfoliatum (029)
Smilacina racemosa (059)
Smilax glauca (059)
Smilax rotundifolia (059)
Solidago canadensis (029)
Sonchus arvensis (029)
Sorbus americana (091)
Spiraea tomentosa (091)
Stylophorum diphyllum
(078)
Symphytum officinale (019)
Symplocarpus foetidus
(009)
Tanacetum vulgare (029)
Taraxacum officinale (029)
Tephrosia virginiana (057)

Thuja occidentalis (035)
Tradescantia virginiana (028)
Trifolium pratense (057)
Trifolium repens (057)
Trillium erectum (059)
Triosteum perfoliatum (023)
Tsuga canadensis (080)

Typha latifolia (104)
Ulmus americana (105)
Ulmus rubra (105)
Urtica dioica (107)
Verbascum thapsus (098)
Vernonia glauca (029)
Vernonia noveboracensis (029)
Veronica officinalis (098)

Veronicastrum virginicum (098)
Viburnum opulus (023)
Viburnum prunifolium (023)
Vitis aestivalis (111)
Vitis labrusca (111)
Vitis vulpina (111)
Xanthoxylum americum (093)

Hallucinogens

Acorus calamus (009)
Clematis virginiana (089)

Cypripedium calceolus (075)

Magnolia virginiana (065)

Heart

Achillea millefolium (029)
Adiantum pedatum (002)
Alnus serrulata (017)
Ambrosia artemisiifolia (029)
Apocynum androsaemifolium (007)
Aquilegia canadensis (089)
Asarum canadensis (011)
Asclepias tuberosa (012)
Cassia hebecarpa (057)
Cassia marilandica (057)
Clintonia borealis (059)
Collinsonia canadensis (055)
Convallaria majalis (059)
Crataegus crus-galli (091)
Cytisus scoparius (057)
Digitalis purpurea (098)
Erigeron strigosus (029)

Filipendula rubra (091)
Filipendula ulmaria (091)
Geranium maculatum (047)
Hamamelis virginiana (049)
Hydrastis canadensis (089)
Inula helenium (029)
Lactuca biennis (029)
Matricaria matricarioides (029)
Mentha arvensis (055)
Monarda didyma (055)
Monarda fistulosa (055)
Pedicularis canadensis (098)
Polygala senega (084)
Populus tremuloides (094)
Prunella vulgaris (055)
Pycnanthemum incanum (055)

Quercus borealis (044)
Rhododendron maximum (042)
Rudbeckia hirta (029)
Sambucus canadensis (023)
Sanguinaria canadensis (078)
Sanicula canadensis (106)
Sassafras albidum (056)
Senecio aureus (029)
Symplocarpus foetidus (009)
Veratrum viride (059)
Veronicastrum virginicum (098)
Viburnum opulus (023)
Viola conspersa (110)
Viola pubescens (110)
Viola tricolor (110)
Xanthoxylum americum (093)

Hemorrhoids

Achillea millefolium (029)
Alnus serrulata (017)
Cornus alternifolia (031)
Diospyros virginiana (040)
Eupatorium perfoliatum (029)

Geranium maculatum (047)
Heuchera americana (097)
Mentha arvensis (055)
Mentha piperita (055)
Mentha spicata (055)
Mitchella repens (092)
Oenothera biennis (073)

Phytolacca americana (079)
Prunella vulgaris (055)
Prunus virginiana (091)
Quercus alba (044)
Rhus typhina (005)
Rosa blanda (091)
Rubus allegheniensis (091)

Rubus argutus (091)
Rubus flagellaris (091)
Rumex crispus (085)

Salix discolor (094)
Sanguinaria canadensis
  (078)

Ulmus americana (105)
Verbascum thapsus (098)

Herbal Steam

Achillea millefolium (029)
Anaphalis margaritacea
  (029)
Artemisia ludoviciana
  (029)
Artemisia vulgaris (029)
Conyza canadensis (029)

Iris versicolor (053)
Juniperus communis (035)
Juniperus virginiana (035)
Lindera benzoin (056)
Mentha arvensis (055)
Mitchella repens (092)
Phytolacca americana (079)

Pinus strobus (080)
Prunus virginiana (091)
Silphium perfoliatum (029)
Smilacina racemosa (059)
Taxus canadensis (101)
Tsuga canadensis (080)

Insecticides

Asimina triloba (006)
Cicuta maculata (106)
Hedeoma pulegioides
  (055)
Ipomoea pandurata (030)
Juglans nigra (054)

Oxybaphus nyctagineus
  (070)
Podophyllum peltatum (016)
Pyrola elliptica (042)
Sambucus canadensis (023)
Solanum carolinense (100)

Viola cucullata (110)
Viola papilionacea (110)
Viola pedata (110)
Viola pubescens (110)
Viola rafinesquii (110)
Viola rotundifolia (110)

Intestinal Worms

Achillea millefolium (029)
Acorus calamus (009)
Agrimonia pubescens (091)
Agrostemma githago (024)
Ailanthus altissima (099)
Allium tricoccum (059)
Amelanchier canadensis
  (091)
Anemone canadensis (089)
Angelica atropurpurea
  (106)
Apocynum
  androsaemifolium (007)
Apocynum cannabinum
  (007)
Aralia racemosa (010)
Aristolochia serpentaria
  (011)
Artemisia absinthum (029)
Artemisia vulgaris (029)
Asarum canadensis (011)
Asclepias incarnata (012)
Bidens bipinnata (029)

Capsella bursa-pastoris
  (033)
Cassia marilandica (057)
Chamaelirium luteum (059)
Chelone glabra (098)
Chenopodium ambrosioides
  (026)
Chimaphila umbellata
  (042)
Coptis trifolia (089)
Cornus alternifolia (031)
Cornus florida (031)
Cypripedium acaule (075)
Cypripedium calceolus
  (075)
Eupatorium perfoliatum
  (029)
Euphorbia corollata (043)
Fagus grandifolia (044)
Gaultheria procumbens
  (042)
Gleditsia triacanthos (057)
Helianthus annuus (029)

Juglans cinerea (054)
Juglans nigra (054)
Juniperus virginiana (035)
Lindera benzoin (056)
Liriodendron tulipifera
  (065)
Lobelia cardinalis (021)
Lobelia siphilitica (021)
Magnolia acuminata
  (065)
Mentha piperita (055)
Mentha spicata (055)
Monarda fistulosa (055)
Morus alba (068)
Morus rubra (068)
Myrica asplenifolia (069)
Nepeta cataria (055)
Panax quinquefolium
  (010)
Pinus echinata (080)
Podophyllum peltatum
  (016)
Populus tremuloides (094)

Portulaca oleracea (087)
Prunus americana (091)
Prunus serotina (091)
Rhus typhina (005)
Ribes americanum (097)
Rosa palustris (091)
Rosa virginiana (091)
Rudbeckia hirta (029)

Sanguinaria canadensis
   (078)
Sassafras albidum (056)
Sisyrinchium angustifolium
   (053)
Smilacina racemosa (059)
Solanum carolinense
   (100)

Symplocarpus foetidus
   (009)
Tanacetum vulgare (029)
Tephrosia virginiana (057)
Tilia americana (103)
Verbena hastata (109)
Xanthoxylum americum
   (093)

Kidney/Diuretics

Abutilon theophrasti (066)
Acer pensylvanicum (001)
Acer saccharinum (001)
Achillea millefolium (029)
Acorus calamus (009)
Adiantum pedatum (002)
Agrimonia pubescens (091)
Agropyron repens (048)
Agrostemma githago (024)
Alisma plantago-aquatica
   (003)
Allium canadense (059)
Allium cernuum (059)
Allium vineale (059)
Alnus serrulata (017)
Andropogon gerardi (048)
Anthemis cotula (029)
Apocynum
   androsaemifolium (007)
Apocynum cannabinum
   (007)
Aquilegia canadensis (089)
Aralia hispida (010)
Aralia racemosa (010)
Arctostaphylos uva-ursi
   (042)
Aristolochia serpentaria
   (011)
Armoracia rusticana (033)
Artemisia annua (029)
Arundinaria gigantea (048)
Asclepias incarnata (012)
Asclepias syriaca (012)
Asiminia triloba (006)
Athyrium filix-femina
   (013)
Baptisia tinctoria (057)
Brassica nigra (033)

Buddleia davidi (061)
Caltha palustris (089)
Caulophyllum thalictroides
   (016)
Celastrus orbiculatus (025)
Celastrus scandens (025)
Chimaphila umbellata (042)
Cimicifuga racemosa (089)
Clematis virginiana (089)
Collinsonia canadensis (055)
Commelina communis
   (028)
Convallaria majalis (059)
Cornus rugosa (031)
Cynoglossum officinale
   (019)
Cypripedium acaule (075)
Cypripedium calceolus
   (075)
Cytisus scoparius (057)
Daucus carota (106)
Digitalis purpurea (098)
Dirca palustris (102)
Echinocystis lobata (034)
Echium vulgare (019)
Epigaea repens (042)
Epilobium angustifolium
   (073)
Equisetum arvense (041)
Equisetum hyemale (041)
Erigeron philadelphicus
   (029)
Erigeron pulchellus (029)
Eryngium aquaticum (106)
Eupatorium maculatum
   (029)
Eupatorium perfoliatum
   (029)

Eupatorium purpureum
   (029)
Eupatorium rugosum (029)
Fragaria virginiana (091)
Galium aparine (092)
Galium triflorum (092)
Gaultheria procumbens
   (042)
Gillenia trifoliata (091)
Goodyera pubescens (075)
Gymnocladus dioica (057)
Hamamelis virginiana
   (049)
Hedeoma pulegioides (055)
Hedera helix (010)
Helianthemum canadense
   (027)
Hemerocallis fulva (059)
Hibiscus palustris (066)
Houstonia caerulea (092)
Humulus lupulus (068)
Impatiens biflora (015)
Inula helenium (029)
Ipomoea pandurata (030)
Iris versicolor (053)
Jeffersonia diphylla (016)
Juniperus communis (035)
Juniperus virginiana (035)
Lactuca canadensis (029)
Ledum groenlandicum (042)
Lonicera canadensis (023)
Lysimachia quadrifolia
   (088)
Maianthemum canadense
   (059)
Mitchella repens (092)
Monarda didyma (055)
Monarda fistulosa (055)

Myrica gale (069)
Myrica pensylvanica (069)
Nasturtium officinale (033)
Osmorhiza longistylis (106)
Panax trifolium (010)
Phytolacca americana (079)
Pinus strobus (080)
Plantago major (081)
Polemonium reptans (083)
Polygala senega (084)
Populus candicans (094)
Prenanthes alba (029)
Prunus americana (091)
Rhus aromatica (005)
Rhus glabra (005)
Ribes americanum (097)
Rosa eglanteria (091)
Rubus allegheniensis (091)
Rubus odoratus (091)
Rubus strigosus (091)
Rudbeckia hirta (029)
Rumex crispus (085)

Sambucus canadensis (023)
Sanguinaria canadensis
   (078)
Sanicula marilandica (106)
Sarracenia purpurea (095)
Scrophularia lanceolata
   (098)
Scutellaria elliptica (055)
Scutellaria lateriflora (055)
Senecio aureus (029)
Smilacina racemosa (059)
Spiranthes cernua (075)
Spiranthes lucida (075)
Tanacetum vulgare (029)
Taraxacum officinale (029)
Taxus canadensis (101)
Tephrosia virginiana (057)
Teucrium canadense (055)
Tilia americana (103)
Tradescantia virginiana
   (028)
Trifolium pratense (057)

Triosteum perfoliatum
   (023)
Tsuga canadensis (080)
Typha angustifolia (104)
Typha latifolia (104)
Ulmus rubra (105)
Utricularia (058)
Verbascum thapsus (098)
Verbena hastata (109)
Veronicastrum virginicum
   (098)
Viburnum lentago (023)
Viburnum nudum (023)
Viburnum opulus (023)
Viola canadensis (110)
Vitis aestivalis (111)
Vitis labrusca (111)
Vitis vulpina (111)
Xanthium strumarium
   (029)
Xanthoxylum americum
   (093)

Mouth

Acorus calamus (009)
Alnus serrulata (017)
Anagallis arvensis (088)
Angelica atropurpurea (106)
Apocynum
   androsaemifolium (007)
Armoracia rusticana (033)
Berberis vulgaris (016)
Bidens bipinnata (029)
Ceanothus americanus
   (090)
Cephalanthus occidentalis
   (092)
Cirsium arvense (029)
Commelina communis
   (028)
Coptis trifolia (089)
Desmodium nudiflorum
   (057)
Diospyros virginiana (040)

Gaultheria procumbens
   (042)
Geranium maculatum (047)
Gnaphalium obtusifolium
   (029)
Goodyera pubescens (075)
Heracleum lanatum (106)
Heuchera americana (097)
Hydrophyllum virginianum
   (051)
Juglans cinerea (054)
Juniperus virginiana (035)
Nymphaea odorata (071)
Oxalis corniculata (077)
Oxybaphus nyctagineus
   (070)
Panax quinquefolium (010)
Populus candicans (094)
Potentilla simplex (091)
Prunus americana (091)

Prunus cerasus (091)
Prunus serotina (091)
Prunus virginiana (091)
Pyrola elliptica (042)
Quercus alba (044)
Quercus borealis (044)
Ranunculus abortivus (089)
Ranunculus acris (089)
Rhus copallinum (005)
Rhus glabra (005)
Rhus radicans (005)
Rubus allegheniensis (091)
Rubus argutus (091)
Rubus flagellaris (091)
Rumex crispus (085)
Salix sericea (094)
Solidago odora (029)
Tiarella cordifolia (097)
Viburnum prunifolium
   (023)

Narcotics

Arctostaphylos uva-ursi (042)

Cannabis sativa (022)
Catalpa bignonioides (018)

Ledum groenlandicum (042)

Perspirants

Achillea millefolium (029)
Acorus calamus (009)
Angelica atropurpurea (106)
Anthemis cotula (029)
Aralia racemosa (010)
Aralia spinosa (010)
Arisaema triphyllum (009)
Artemisia ludoviciana (029)
Asarum canadensis (011)
Botrychium virginianum (074)
Caltha palustris (089)
Chimaphila umbellata (042)
Cornus alternifolia (031)
Cornus florida (031)
Cunila origanoides (055)
Erigeron philadelphicus (029)
Erigeron pulchellus (029)
Eupatorium perfoliatum (029)

Eupatorium purpureum (029)
Eupatorium rugosum (029)
Euphorbia ipecacuanhae (043)
Gillenia trifoliata (091)
Hedeoma pulegioides (055)
Juniperus virginiana (035)
Lindera benzoin (056)
Liquidamber styraciflua (049)
Mentha arvensis (055)
Mitchella repens (092)
Monarda didyma (055)
Monarda fistulosa (055)
Nepeta cataria (055)
Panax quinquefolium (010)
Plantago major (081)
Polygala senega (084)
Populus tremuloides (094)
Salvia lyrata (055)
Sambucus canadensis (023)

Senecio aureus (029)
Solidago odora (029)
Tanacetum vulgare (029)
Taxus canadensis (101)
Teucrium canadense (055)
Thuja occidentalis (035)
Triosteum perfoliatum (023)
Tsuga canadensis (080)
Urtica dioica (107)
Verbascum thapsus (098)
Verbena hastata (109)
Veronicastrum virginicum (098)
Viburnum prunifolium (023)
Viola papilionacea (110)
Viola pedata (110)
Viola pubescens (110)
Viola rafinesquii (110)
Viola rotundifolia (110)
Vitis vulpina (111)
Xanthoxylum americum (093)
Yucca filamentosa (059)

Poison

Actaea rubra (089)
Amianthium muscaetoxicum (059)
Anagallis arvensis (088)
Angelica atropurpurea (106)
Angelica venosa (106)
Anthemis cotula (029)
Aralia spinosa (010)
Arisaema triphyllum (009)
Castilleja coccinea (098)
Celastrus scandens (025)
Chimaphila maculata (042)
Cicuta maculata (106)

Conium maculatum (106)
Datura stramonium (100)
Epilobium angustifolium (073)
Eupatorium perfoliatum (029)
Galium aparine (092)
Helenium autumnale (029)
Juglans nigra (054)
Kalmia angustifolia (042)
Kalmia latifolia (042)
Lespedeza capitata (057)
Lycopus virginicus (055)

Parthenocissus quinquefolia (111)
Pastinaca sativa (106)
Phoradendron flavescens (062)
Morus rubra (068)
Phytolacca americana (079)
Podophyllum peltatum (016)
Polygonum aviculare (085)
Polygonum hydropiper (085)
Prunus serotina (091)
Rhus glabra (005)
Rhus radicans (005)

Rhus vernix (005)
Senecio vulgaris (029)

Solanum nigrum (100)
Veratrum viride (059)

Veronicastrum virginicum (098)

Psychological Aids

Acorus calamus (009)
Actaea rubra (089)
Ambrosia trifida (029)
Anemone cylindrica (089)
Apocynum
   androsaemifolium (007)
Arctostaphylos uva-ursi
   (042)
Artemisia ludoviciana (029)
Asarum canadensis (011)
Cannabis sativa (022)
Cichorium intybus (029)
Cynoglossum virginiana
   (019)

Eupatorium perfoliatum
   (029)
Fragaria virginiana (091)
Gnaphalium obtusifolium
   (029)
Gymnocladus dioica (057)
Juglans cinerea (054)
Juglans nigra (054)
Lobelia cardinalis (021)
Lobelia inflata (021)
Lonicera canadensis (023)
Matricaria chamomilla
   (029)
Mitchella repens (092)

Panax quinquefolium (010)
Pinus strobus (080)
Prunella vulgaris (055)
Ranunculus abortivus (089)
Smilacina racemosa (059)
Solanum nigrum (100)
Solidago canadensis (029)
Vaccinium angustifolium
   (042)
Valeriana officinalis (108)
Verbascum thapsus (098)
Vitis vulpina (111)

Pulmonary/Respiratory Aids

Achillea millefolium (029)
Acorus calamus (009)
Adiantum pedatum (002)
Aesculus hippocastanum
   (050)
Aletris farinosa (059)
Alisma plantago-aquatica
   (003)
Allium canadense (059)
Allium cernuum (059)
Allium tricoccum (059)
Allium vineale (059)
Althaea officinalis (066)
Ambrosia artemisiifolia
   (029)
Ambrosia trifida (029)
Anaphalis margaritacea
   (029)
Anemone cylindrica (089)
Anemone virginiana (089)
Anemonella thalictroides
   (089)
Angelica atropurpurea
   (106)
Anthemis cotula (029)
Apocynum cannabinum
   (007)

Aralia nudicaulis (010)
Aralia racemosa (010)
Arctium minus (029)
Arisaema triphyllum (009)
Aristolochia serpentaria
   (011)
Armoracia rusticana (033)
Artemisia ludoviciana
   (029)
Artemisia vulgaris (029)
Asarum canadensis (011)
Asclepias syriaca (012)
Asclepias tuberosa (012)
Aster novae-angliae (029)
Betula lenta (017)
Botrychium virginianum
   (074)
Brassica nigra (033)
Calla palustris (009)
Cassia hebecarpa (057)
Cassia marilandica (057)
Cassia nictitans (057)
Catalpa bignonioides (018)
Caulophyllum thalictroides
   (016)
Ceanothus americanus (090)
Cercis canadensis (057)

Circium arvense (029)
Corallorhiza maculata
   (075)
Cornus alternifolia (031)
Corylus americana (017)
Datura stramonium (100)
Dirca palustris (102)
Epigaea repens (042)
Erigeron philadelphicus
   (029)
Euonymus americanus
   (025)
Eupatorium perfoliatum
   (029)
Euphorbia ipecacuanhae
   (043)
Fagus grandifolia (044)
Gentiana quinquefolia
   (046)
Gillenia trifoliata (091)
Gleditsia triacanthos (057)
Gnaphalium obtusifolium
   (029)
Goodyera pubescens (075)
Hamamelis virginiana
   (049)
Hedeoma pulegioides (055)

Hedera helix (010)
Helenium autumnale (029)
Helianthus annuus (029)
Humulus lupulus (022)
Hydrastis canadensis (089)
Impatiens biflora (015)
Inula helenium (029)
Ipomoea pandurata (030)
Iris versicolor (053)
Juniperus communis (035)
Juniperus virginiana (035)
Ledum groenlandicum
   (042)
Lepidium virginicum (033)
Lindera benzoin (056)
Linum usitatissimum (060)
Lobelia cardinalis (021)
Lobelia inflata (021)
Lobelia siphilitica (021)
Magnolia acuminata (065)
Marrubium vulgare (055)
Mentha arvensis (055)
Mentha piperita (055)
Mentha spicata (055)
Menyanthes trifoliata (046)
Mertensia virginica (019)
Mitchella repens (092)
Monarda fistulosa (055)
Monarda punctata (055)
Nepeta cataria (055)

Panax quinquefolium (010)
Panax trifolium (010)
Phoradendron flavescens
   (062)
Pinus strobus (080)
Plantago major (081)
Platanus occidentalis (082)
Polygala senega (084)
Polygonatum biflorum
   (059)
Polystichum acrostichoides
   (013)
Potentilla simplex (091)
Prenanthes alba (029)
Prunella vulgaris (055)
Prunus americana (091)
Prunus serotina (091)
Prunus virginiana (091)
Ptelea trifoliata (093)
Quercus alba (044)
Quercus borealis (044)
Rhus glabra (005)
Rhus typhina (005)
Rhus vernix (005)
Rubus allegheniensis (091)
Rubus occidentalis (091)
Rumex crispus (085)
Salix alba (094)
Salix babylonica (094)
Salix lucida (094)

Salix nigra (094)
Salvia lyrata (055)
Sambucus canadensis (023)
Sanguinaria canadensis
   (078)
Sarracenia purpurea (095)
Silphium perfoliatum (029)
Smilacina racemosa (059)
Taraxacum officinale (029)
Taxus canadensis (101)
Tilia americana (103)
Trillium erectum (059)
Triosteum perfoliatum
   (023)
Typha latifolia (104)
Ulmus americana (105)
Ulmus rubra (105)
Veratrum viride (059)
Verbascum thapsus (098)
Veronicastrum virginicum
   (098)
Viburnum opulus (023)
Viola cucullata (110)
Viola papilionacea (110)
Viola pedata (110)
Viola pubescens (110)
Viola rafinesquii (110)
Viola rotundifolia (110)
Xanthoxylum americum
   (093)

Reproductive Aids

Amelanchier arborea (091)
Chamaelirium luteum
   (059)
Fraxinus americana (072)

Hypericum perforatum
   (052)
Panax quinquefolium (010)
Rhus aromatica (005)

Rumex crispus (085)
Spiranthes cernua (075)
Spiranthes lucida (075)
Tephrosia virginiana (057)

Sedatives

Achillea millefolium (029)
Acorus calamus (009)
Angelica atropurpurea
   (106)
Anthemis cotula (029)
Arisaema triphyllum (009)
Asarum canadensis (011)
Caulophyllum thalictroides
   (016)

Cimicifuga racemosa
   (089)
Convallaria majalis (059)
Cypripedium acaule (075)
Cypripedium calceolus
   (075)
Dentaria diphylla (033)
Eupatorium maculatum
   (029)

Gentiana quinquefolia
   (046)
Glaux maritima (088)
Gnaphalium obtusifolium
   (029)
Humulus lupulus (022)
Juniperus communis (035)
Juniperus virginiana (035)
Lactuca canadensis (029)

Leonurus cardiaca (055)
Linaria vulgaris (098)
Liriodendron tulipifera (065)
Lithospermum canescens (019)
Lonicera canadensis (023)
Matricaria chamomilla (029)
Mentha arvensis (055)
Mentha piperita (055)
Mentha spicata (055)

Mitchella repens (092)
Monarda didyma (055)
Monarda fistulosa (055)
Nepeta cataria (055)
Polygonatum biflorum (059)
Prunella vulgaris (055)
Prunus virginiana (091)
Ranunculus abortivus (089)
Ranunuculus acris (089)
Rhus vernix (005)
Salix candida (094)

Salix discolor (094)
Salvia lyrata (055)
Sambucus canadensis (023)
Smilacina racemosa (059)
Solanum nigrum (100)
Solidago canadensis (029)
Taraxacum officinale (029)
Viola tricolor (110)
Xanthoxylum americum (093)
Yucca filamentosa (059)

Skin

Abutilon theophrasti (066)
Acer pensylvanicum (001)
Acer rubrum (001)
Acer saccharinum (001)
Achillea millefolium (029)
Acorus calamus (009)
Actaea alba (089)
Actaea rubra (089)
Agastache nepetoides (055)
Agrimonia gryposepala (091)
Agrimonia parviflora (091)
Agrostemma githago (024)
Alisma subcordatum (003)
Allium canadense (059)
Allium cernuum (059)
Allium tricoccum (059)
Allium vineale (059)
Amaranthus retroflexus (004)
Ambrosia artemisiifolia (029)
Ambrosia trifida (029)
Amianthium muscaetoxicum (059)
Anaphalis margaritacae (029)
Anemone canadensis (089)
Anemone virginiana (089)
Angelica atropurpurea (106)
Anthemis cotula (029)
Apios americana (057)
Aplectrum hyemale (075)

Apocynum androsaemifolium (007)
Apocynum cannabinum (007)
Aquilegia canadensis (089)
Aralia nudicaulis (010)
Aralia racemosa (010)
Aralia spinosa (010)
Arctium lappa (029)
Arctium minus (029)
Arctostaphylos uva-ursi (042)
Arisaema triphyllum (009)
Aristolochia serpentaria (011)
Artemisia ludoviciana (029)
Artemisia vulgaris (029)
Asarum canadensis (011)
Asclepias incarnata (012)
Asclepias syriaca (012)
Asclepias tuberosa (012)
Asplenium trichomanes (014)
Aster novae-angliae (029)
Athyrium filix-femina (013)
Baptisia tinctoria (057)
Barbarea vulgaris (033)
Betula lenta (017)
Botrychium virginianum (074)
Brassica nigra (033)
Buddleia davidi (061)
Cacalia atriplicifolia (029)

Calla palustris (009)
Caltha palustris (089)
Capsella bursa-pastoris (033)
Cassia hebecarpa (057)
Cassia marilandica (057)
Caulophyllum thalictroides (016)
Ceanothus americanus (090)
Celastrus orbiculatus (025)
Celastrus scandens (025)
Chelidonium majus (078)
Chelone glabra (098)
Chenopodium album (026)
Chimaphila maculata (042)
Chimaphila umbellata (042)
Chionanthus virginicus (072)
Chrysanthemum leucanthemum (029)
Cichorium intybus (029)
Cicuta maculata (106)
Cimicifuga racemosa (089)
Clematis virginiana (089)
Clintonia borealis (059)
Collinsonia canadensis (055)
Conyza canadensis (029)
Cornus alternifolia (031)
Cornus canadensis (031)
Cornus florida (031)
Corylus americana (017)

Cunila origanoides (055)
Cuscuta gronovii (030)
Cynoglossum officinale (019)
Cynoglossum virginiana (019)
Cypripedium acaule (075)
Daucus carota (106)
Diospyros virginiana (040)
Drosera rotundifolia (039)
Duchesnea indica (091)
Epilobium angustifolium (073)
Equisetum arvense (041)
Erigeron philadelphicus (029)
Erigeron pulchellus (029)
Erythronium americanum (059)
Euonymus americanus (025)
Euonymus atropurpureus (025)
Eupatorium maculatum (029)
Eupatorium perfoliatum (029)
Eupatorium purpureum (029)
Euphorbia corollata (043)
Fagus grandifolia (044)
Fraxinus americana (072)
Galium aparine (092)
Geranium maculatum (047)
Geum rivale (091)
Gillenia trifoliata (091)
Glecoma hederacea (055)
Hamamelis virginiana (049)
Helianthus annuus (029)
Hemerocallis fulva (059)
Hepatica americana (089)
Heracleum lanatum (106)
Heuchera americana (097)
Hierochloe odorata (048)
Humulus lupulus (022)
Hydrangea arborescens (097)
Hydrastis canadensis (089)

Hypericum perforatum (052)
Impatiens biflora (015)
Impatiens pallida (015)
Inula helenium (029)
Iris versicolor (053)
Jeffersonia diphylla (016)
Juglans cinerea (054)
Juglans nigra (054)
Juniperus communis (035)
Juniperus virginiana (035)
Kalmia angustifolia (042)
Kalmia latifolia (042)
Larix laricina (080)
Ledum groenlandicum (042)
Lepidium virginicum (033)
Ligustrum vulgare (072)
Lilium philadelphicum (059)
Lindera benzoin (056)
Liquidamber styraciflua (049)
Liriodendron tulipifera (065)
Lobelia cardinalis (021)
Lobelia inflata (021)
Lobelia siphilitica (021)
Lobelia spicata (021)
Lonicera canadensis (023)
Lonicera japonica (023)
Lyonia mariana (042)
Malva neglecta (066)
Marrubium vulgare (055)
Matricaria matricarioides (029)
Melilotus officinalis (057)
Menispermum canadense (067)
Mentha arvensis (055)
Mitchella repens (092)
Monarda fistulosa (055)
Monotropa uniflora (042)
Morus rubra (068)
Myrica cerifera (069)
Nepeta cataria (055)
Nuphar advena (071)
Nymphaea odorata (071)
Oenothera biennis (073)
Opuntia compressa (020)
Osmorhiza claytoni (106)

Osmorhiza longistylis (106)
Oxalis corniculata (077)
Oxalis stricta (077)
Panax quinquefolium (010)
Panax trifolium (010)
Parthenocissus quinquefolia (111)
Pastinaca sativa (106)
Paulownia tomentosa (098)
Pedicularis canadensis (098)
Physocarpus opulifolius (091)
Phytolacca americana (079)
Pinus echinata (080)
Pinus strobus (080)
Plantago aristata (081)
Plantago lanceolata (081)
Plantago major (081)
Platanus occidentalis (082)
Podophyllum peltatum (016)
Polygala paucifolia (084)
Polygonatum biflorum (059)
Polygonum aviculare (085)
Polygonum hydropiper (085)
Polygonum persicaria (085)
Polystichum acrostichoides (013)
Populus candicans (094)
Populus tremuloides (094)
Portulaca oleracea (087)
Potentilla arguta (091)
Potentilla simplex (091)
Prenanthes alba (029)
Prunella vulgaris (055)
Prunus americana (091)
Prunus cerasus (091)
Prunus serotina (091)
Prunus virginiana (091)
Pteridium aquilinum (037)
Pycnanthemum incanum (055)
Pyrola elliptica (042)
Pyrola rotundifolia (042)
Quercus alba (044)
Quercus borealis (044)
Ranunculus abortivus (089)
Ranunculus acris (089)

Rhamnus catharticus (090)
Rhus aromatica (005)
Rhus copallinum (005)
Rhus glabra (005)
Rhus radicans (005)
Rhus typhina (005)
Rhus vernix (005)
Ribes americanum (097)
Rosa blanda (091)
Rosa virginiana (091)
Rubus allegheniensis (091)
Rubus argutus (091)
Rubus flagellaris (091)
Rubus occidentalis (091)
Rubus odoratus (091)
Rubus strigosus (091)
Rudbeckia hirta (029)
Rumex acetosella (085)
Rumex crispus (085)
Sagittaria latifolia (003)
Salix alba (094)
Salix babylonica (094)
Salix fragilis (094)
Salsola kali (026)
Salvia lyrata (055)
Sambucus canadensis (023)

Sanguinaria canadensis (078)
Sanicula marilandica (106)
Saponaria officinalis (024)
Sassafras albidum (056)
Saururus cernuus (096)
Silene stellata (024)
Smilax glauca (059)
Solanum dulcamara (100)
Solanum nigrum (100)
Stylophorum diphyllum (078)
Symplocarpus foetidus (009)
Tanacetum vulgare (029)
Taraxacum officinale (029)
Tephrosia virginiana (057)
Thuja occidentalis (035)
Tiarella cordifolia (097)
Tilia americana (103)
Tradescantia virginiana (028)
Trifolium repens (057)
Trillium erectum (059)
Triosteum perfoliatum (023)

Tsuga canadensis (080)
Tussilago farfara (029)
Typha latifolia (104)
Ulmus americana (105)
Ulmus rubra (105)
Urtica dioica (107)
Uvularia sessilifolia (059)
Veratrum viride (059)
Verbascum thapsus (098)
Verbena hastata (109)
Veronica officinalis (098)
Veronicastrum virginicum (098)
Viola cucullata (110)
Viola papilionacea (110)
Viola pedata (110)
Viola pubescens (110)
Viola rafinesquii (110)
Viola rotundifolia (110)
Viola tricolor (110)
Vitis vulpina (111)
Xanthoxylum americum (093)
Yucca filamentosa (059)
Zygadenus leimanthoides (059)

Stimulants

Achillea millefolium (029)
Acorus calamus (009)
Actaea alba (089)
Allium canadense (059)
Allium vineale (059)
Anaphalis margaritacae (029)
Andropogon gerardi (048)
Anemone cylindrica (089)
Anemone virginiana (089)
Apocynum androsaemifolium (007)
Aralia nudicaulis (010)
Aralia racemosa (010)
Arctium minus (029)
Arisaema triphyllum (009)
Aristolochia serpentaria (011)
Asarum canadensis (011)
Aster novae-angliae (029)

Betula lenta (017)
Brassica nigra (033)
Cannabis sativa (022)
Cassia fasciculata (057)
Cassia hebecarpa (057)
Cassia marilandica (057)
Cassia nictitans (057)
Chimaphila umbellata (042)
Cimicifuga racemosa (089)
Collinsonia canadensis (055)
Cornus alternifolia (031)
Cornus florida (031)
Cunila origanoides (055)
Cypripedium calceolus (075)
Eryngium aquaticum (106)
Erythronium americanum (059)

Eupatorium perfoliatum (029)
Eupatorium rugosum (029)
Gentiana quinquefolia (046)
Gnaphalium obtusifolium (029)
Gymnocladus dioica (057)
Hedeoma pulegioides (055)
Helianthus annuus (029)
Humulus lupulus (022)
Hydrangea arborescens (097)
Hydrastis canadensis (089)
Juniperus virginiana (035)
Lactuca canadensis (029)
Larix laricina (080)
Leonurus cardiaca (055)
Liriodendron tulipifera (065)

Lycopodium clavatum
(063)
Malva moschata (066)
Malva neglecta (066)
Melissa officinalis (055)
Menispermum canadense
(067)
Mentha arvensis (055)
Mentha piperita (055)
Mentha spicata (055)
Monarda punctata (055)
Morus rubra (068)
Myrica cerifera (069)
Nepeta cataria (055)
Oenothera biennis (073)
Osmorhiza longistylis (106)
Panax quinquefolium (010)
Phytolacca americana (079)
Picea mariana (080)

Pinus strobus (080)
Polygala senega (084)
Polygala verticilleta (084)
Polygonatum biflorum
(059)
Polystichum acrostichoides
(013)
Prenanthes alba (029)
Prunus serotina (091)
Pteridium aquilinum (037)
Pycnanthemum incanum
(055)
Pycnanthemum
virginianum (055)
Pyrola elliptica (042)
Rubus allegheniensis (091)
Rubus argutus (091)
Rubus canadensis (091)
Rubus flagellaris (091)

Rubus strigosus (091)
Rumex crispus (085)
Salix candida (094)
Salix discolor (094)
Salvia lyrata (055)
Sanguinaria canadensis
(078)
Sassafras albidum (056)
Smilacina racemosa (059)
Solidago odora (029)
Tephrosia virginiana (057)
Thuja occidentalis (035)
Tilia americana (103)
Tsuga canadensis (080)
Ulmus rubra (105)
Veratrum viride (059)
Verbascum thapsus (098)
Veronicastrum virginicum
(098)

Stomach

Achillea millefolium (029)
Acorus calamus (009)
Actaea rubra (089)
Adiantum pedatum (002)
Agrimonia gryposepala
(091)
Agrimonia parviflora (091)
Aletris farinosa (059)
Alisma subcordatum (003)
Allium cernuum (059)
Alnus serrulata (017)
Anaphalis margaritacae
(029)
Anethum graveolens (106)
Angelica atropurpurea (106)
Angelica venosa (106)
Antennaria plantaginifolia
(029)
Anthemis cotula (029)
Apocynum
androsaemifolium (007)
Apocynum cannabinum
(007)
Aplectrum hyemale (075)
Aquilegia canadensis (089)
Aralia nudicaulis (010)
Aralia racemosa (010)

Arctium lappa (029)
Arctium minus (029)
Aristolochia serpentaria
(011)
Armoracia rusticana (033)
Artemisia ludoviciana
(029)
Asarum canadensis (011)
Asclepias syriaca (012)
Baptisia tinctoria (057)
Betula lenta (017)
Capsella bursa-pastoris
(033)
Caulophyllum thalictroides
(016)
Ceanothus americanus
(090)
Celastrus scandens (025)
Chamaelirium luteum
(059)
Chelone glabra (098)
Chenopodium album (026)
Chimaphila umbellata
(042)
Clematis virginiana (089)
Conyza canadensis (029)
Coptis trifolia (089)

Cornus alternifolia (031)
Cornus canadensis (031)
Cornus florida (031)
Corylus americana (017)
Cypripedium acaule (075)
Cypripedium calceolus
(075)
Daucus carota (106)
Diospyros virginiana (040)
Dryopteris cristata (013)
Epigaea repens (042)
Epilobium angustifolium
(073)
Eupatorium maculatum
(029)
Eupatorium perfoliatum
(029)
Fragaria vesca (091)
Fragaria virginiana (091)
Fraxinus americana (072)
Gaultheria procumbens
(042)
Gentiana crinita (046)
Gentiana quinquefolia (046)
Gleditsia triacanthos (057)
Gnaphalium obtusifolium
(029)

Goodyera pubescens (075)
Hamamelis virginiana (049)
Hedeoma pulegioides (055)
Helenium autumnale (029)
Helianthus annuus (029)
Heuchera americana (097)
Hieracium venosum (029)
Humulus lupulus (022)
Hydrangea arborescens (097)
Hydrastis canadensis (089)
Hypericum perforatum (052)
Ilex opaca (008)
Impatiens pallida (015)
Ipomoea pandurata (030)
Juglans nigra (054)
Juniperus communis (035)
Kalmia angustifolia (042)
Ledum groenlandicum (042)
Leonurus cardiaca (055)
Ligustrum vulgare (072)
Lilium canadense (059)
Liriodendron tulipifera (065)
Lobelia cardinalis (021)
Lobelia inflata (021)
Lobelia siphilitica (021)
Lycopus americanus (055)
Lysimachia quadrifolia (088)
Magnolia acuminata (065)
Malva neglecta (066)
Marrubium vulgare (055)
Matricaria chamomilla (029)
Matricaria matricarioides (029)
Melissa officinalis (055)
Menispermum canadense (067)
Mentha aquatica (055)
Mentha arvensis (055)
Mentha piperita (055)
Mentha spicata (055)
Menyanthes trifoliata (046)
Mitchella repens (092)
Monarda didyma (055)

Monarda fistulosa (055)
Monarda punctata (055)
Morus rubra (068)
Myrica cerifera (069)
Nepeta cataria (055)
Oenothera biennis (073)
Osmorhiza claytoni (106)
Osmorhiza longistylis (106)
Panax quinquefolium (010)
Panax trifolium (010)
Pedicularis canadensis (098)
Pinus strobus (080)
Plantago aristata (081)
Plantago lanceolata (081)
Plantago major (081)
Platanus occidentalis (082)
Polygala senega (084)
Polygonatum biflorum (059)
Polygonum aviculare (085)
Polygonum hydropiper (085)
Polygonum persicaria (085)
Polypodium vulgare (086)
Polystichum acrostichoides (013)
Populus candicans (094)
Populus tremuloides (094)
Portulaca oleracea (087)
Prunella vulgaris (055)
Prunus cerasus (091)
Prunus serotina (091)
Prunus virginiana (091)
Pycnanthemum incanum (055)
Pyrola elliptica (042)
Quercus alba (044)
Quercus borealis (044)
Ranunculus abortivus (089)
Rhus aromatica (005)
Rhus typhina (005)
Rosa blanda (091)
Rosa rugosa (091)
Rubus allegheniensis (091)
Rubus occidentalis (091)
Rubus odoratus (091)
Rubus pubescens (091)
Rubus strigosus (091)
Rudbeckia laciniata (029)
Rumex acetosella (085)

Rumex crispus (085)
Sagittaria latifolia (003)
Salix candida (094)
Salix discolor (094)
Salix nigra (094)
Sambucus canadensis (023)
Sanguinaria canadensis (078)
Sassafras albidum (056)
Saururus cernuus (096)
Silphium perfoliatum (029)
Sisyrinchium angustifolium (053)
Smilacina racemosa (059)
Smilax glauca (059)
Smilax rotundifolia (059)
Solanum dulcamara (100)
Solanum nigrum (100)
Solidago canadensis (029)
Solidago juncea (029)
Sorbus americana (091)
Symphytum officinale (019)
Symplocarpus foetidus (009)
Tanacetum vulgare (029)
Taraxacum officinale (029)
Tiarella cordifolia (097)
Tilia americana (103)
Tradescantia virginiana (028)
Trillium erectum (059)
Triosteum perfoliatum (023)
Tsuga canadensis (080)
Typha latifolia (104)
Ulmus americana (105)
Ulmus rubra (105)
Urtica dioica (107)
Veratrum viride (059)
Verbena hastata (109)
Veronicastrum virginicum (098)
Viburnum opulus (023)
Viola eriocarpa (110)
Vitis aestivalis (111)
Vitis labrusca (111)
Vitis vulpina (111)
Xanthoxylum americum (093)

Glossary

abortifacient An agent that causes abortion.

achene A dry, one-seeded fruit such as in sunflower.

allelopathy Biochemical interactions between plants.

alluvial A soil type found in floodplains.

alterative An agent that causes change or improvement in health.

amenorrhea Absence or suppression of the menstrual discharge by any cause other than pregnancy or the menopause.

analgesic An agent that relieves pain; also called an anodyne.

anemia A condition of deficiency of red blood cells or hemoglobin.

ancyclostomaisis An intestinal infestation of blood-sucking worms of or related to the genus *Ancyclostoma.*

anthelmintic (anthelminthic) A substance that expels or destroys intestinal worms.

annuals A plant that lives for one season and is germinated from seed annually.

anodyne An agent that relieves pain; also called an analgesic.

anorexia Loss of appetite not accompanied by a loathing of food.

anticaries Effective in preventing tooth cavities.

apetalous Flowers that lack distinct petals.

aquatic Freshwater plants.

arillate Having an aril, an external covering of certain seeds such as the scarlet coating of the seeds of bittersweet (*Celastrus scandens*).

astringent A substance that drives fluid from and shrinks tissues.

auricle An ear-shaped appendage.

axil The angle between leaf and stem.

bark The external covering of a woody stem or root.

basal Located at or forming the base of the stem.

berry Any pulpy fruit of small size.

calculus Solid matter such as gravel or stones formed in the body.

calyx The sepals (the outer series of floral leaves) collectively; it is usually green.

canker A gangrenous ulcer in or around the mouth.

carcinogenic Causing cancer.

carminative Causing the expulsion of gas.

caryopsis A small, dry fruit such as found in grasses.

catamenia The menses.

catarrh Inflamation of a mucous membrane.

cathartic A mild purgative medicine.

catkin A cattail-like inflorescence.

chancre The venereal lesion of syphilis.

clasping A leaf attachment in which the leaf attaches directly to the stem without a stalk.

cold infusion Extraction of plant nutrients with cold water.

colic Abdominal pain usually due to gas.

convulsant Causing convulsions.

cordate A heart-shaped leaf with a notched base.

corm A short bulblike stem.

costiveness Constipation.

croup Any affectation of the larynx or trachea accompanied by difficult breathing and a hoarse, ringing cough.

cynanche Any disease of the tonsils, throat, or windpipe attended with inflammation and difficult breathing and swallowing.

decoction An extract prepared by boiling plants or plant organs in water.

demulcent A soothing substance for mucous membranes.

diaphoretic A substance that increases perspiration; also called a sudorific.

dicotyledonous A group of plants characterized by two seed leaves, for example, beans.

dioecious Having male and female flowers on separate plants.

diuretic A substance that increases urine flow.

downy Covered with soft hairs.

dropsy An abnormal accumulation of fluid in the body.

drupe A fruit consisting of a stone surrounded by usually fleshy tissue, for example, a peach.

dyspepsia Indigestion.

dysuria Reduced urine production.

emetic a substance that causes vomiting.

emmenagogue A substance that promotes menstruation (abortifacient).

emollient A soothing and softening agent.

enteritis Inflammation of the intestine.

erysipelas A disease associated with reddish inflammation of the skin of the face.

escape A plant that has become wild from cultivation or has developed from self-sown seed of a cultivated plant.

expectorant A substance that facilitates discharge of phlegm.

febrifuge A substance that reduces fever.

felon A painful inflammation of the finger.

female obstruction Menstrual failure (pregnancy).

flatulence Gases generated in the stomach or intestines.

follicle A dry fruit with a single suture such as found in a milkweed.

frond The leaf of a fern.

glabrous Smooth, without hairs.

glaucous Bluish green in color.

gleet A persistent, transparent mucous discharge.

glutinous Moist, sticky.

gout A metabolic disease of the joints.

hemicrania Headache affecting one side of the head.

hepatotoxic A liver toxin.

hydrophobia Rabies.

hypertensive Increases blood pressure.

hypotensive Decreases blood pressure.

imbricated Overlapping in regular order.

indolent ulcer A painless ulcer.

inflorescence The flowering portion of a plant; may be one or more flowers.

infusion An extract prepared by steeping plants or plant organs in hot water.

inner bark The moist, inner layer of root or stem bark.

intermittent fever Malaria.

inulin A tasteless, white polysaccharide resembling starch.

involucre A whorl or rosette of bracts subtending a flower cluster or fruit.

jaundice A disease condition characterized by yellow skin, eyes, and urine.

lactation The production of milk.

laryngitis Inflammation of the larynx.

leucorrhea A vaginal discharge of white, yellowish, or greenish white, viscid mucous.

lumbrici Parasitic roundworms of the intestine.

malodorous Ill smelling.

marasmus Progressive emaciation.

mitogenic Stimulating mitosis (cell division).

monocotyledonous A group of plants characterized by having one seed leaf, for example, corn.

monoecious Having separate male and female flowers on the same plant.

moxa Any plant material burned on the skin for therapeutic purposes.

moxibustion The use of a moxa in medicine.

native A plant growing in its original area.

naturalized A plant completely established in one area but native to another area.

neuralgia A pain tracing the path of a nerve.

palliative Serving to relieve.

palmate A leaf having lobes radiating from a common point.

panacea A cure-all.

peltate A leaf attachment in which the stalk joins the leaf at or near the center of the leaf, as, for example, the leaf of the water lily.

perennial A plant that continues to live from year to year.

perfect A flower having both male and female parts (both staminate and pistillate flowers).

perigynium The bracts subtending the pistillate flower in *Carex* becoming the flask-shaped envelope of the fruit.

pertussis Whooping cough.

petiole The leaf stalk.

pharmacognosy The study of drugs.

phthisis Pulmonary tuberculosis.

pinnate A leaf divided into leaflets.

pistillate Having female flowers.

pith The spongy center of the stem in dicotyledonous plants.

pityriasis Any skin disease characterized by the shedding of flaky scales.

poultice A soft pad to be applied externally.

pubescent Hairy.

prostrate Low growing.

psora An itching disease of the skin.

psoriasis A chronic skin disease characterized by scaly red plaques.

ptomaine Poisoning caused by spoiled food.

purgative A strong cathartic or laxative.

quinate A compound leaf with five leaflets.

quinsies Severe inflammation of the throat.

raceme An elongated type of inflorescence.

rhizome An underground stem.

rubefacient A substance that causes the skin to become red.

sagittate Shaped like an arrowhead.

salubrious Promoting health.

samara A dry, winged fruit.

scrofula A tuberculous disease.

sedative Having a calming, soothing, or tranquilizing effect.

sepal Floral leaves forming the calyx.

serrate A saw-toothed leaf edge.

simple An untoothed leaf edge.

smudge To burn so as to produce smoke and little or no flame.

soporific Sleep inducing.

spadix A clublike flower spike.

spasmodic A substance that produces spasms.

stalk Leaf- or flower-bearing structure.

staminate Producing male flowers.

stipule One of the usually small, paired, leaflike appendages at the base of a leaf or leaf stalk.

stomachic A remedy for mild stomach ailments.

strangury Slow, painful urination associated with spasms of the urethra and bladder.

stricture A narrowing of the urethra such as that caused by an enlarged prostate gland.

strobilus A conelike fruiting structure.

subtend To be located underneath.

sudorific A substance that causes perspiration; also called a diaphoretic.

suppurate To form or discharge pus.

thrush An oral infection caused by the yeast *Candida albicans.*

tic douloureux Trigeminal neuralgia; a painful spasmodic muscular contraction usually of the face or extremities.

tincture A dilute alcoholic extract.

tonic A substance that restores or increases bodily tone.

tuber A swollen, usually underground stem, for example, a potato.

umbel A flower cluster in which the flower stalks arise from or near the same point.

vermifuge An agent that destroys or causes the expulsion of intestinal worms.

vulnerary A substance used in treating or healing wounds.

whorl Leaves or flowers arising circumferentially from the same area on the stem.

Sources

Ahluwalia, R., and B. Mechin. 1980. *Traditional Medicine in Zaire*. International Development Research Centre, Ottawa, Canada.

American Medical Association. 1925. *Useful Drugs*. American Medical Association, Chicago.

Asprey, G. F., and P. Thornton. 1953. "Medicinal Plants of Jamaica." *West Indies Medical Journal* 2:253.

Ayensu, E. S. 1978. *Medicinal Plants of West Africa*. Reference Publications, Algonac, Michigan.

Bailey, L. H. 1935. *The Standard Cyclopedia of Horticulture*. Macmillan, New York.

Barton, B. S. 1798 and 1804. "Collections for an Essay towards a Materia Medica of the United States." Bulletin of the Lloyd Library, no. 1, 1900. Lloyd Library, Cincinnati, Ohio.

Bell, E. A. and B. V. Charlwood. 1980. *Secondary Plant Products*. Springer-Verlag, Berlin.

Bigelow, J. 1822. *Materia Medica*. Charles Ewer, Boston.

Boulos, L. 1983. *Medicinal Plants of North Africa*. Reference Publications, Algonac, Michigan.

Boyd, H. P. 1991. *A Field Guide to the Pine Barrens of New Jersey*. Plexus, Medford, New Jersey.

Brock, T. D., ed. 1961. *Milestones in Microbiology*. Science Tech, Madison, Wisconsin.

Bruneton, J. 1995. *Pharmacognosy, Phytochemistry, Medicinal Plants*. Trans. C. K. Hatton. Lavoisier, Paris.

Buchman, D. D. 1980. *Herbal Medicine*. Gramercy, New York.

Chesnut, V. K. 1898a. *Plants Poisonous to Stock*. U.S. Department of Agriculture, Washington, D.C.

Chesnut, V. K. 1898b. *Principal Poisonous Plants of the United States*. U.S. Department of Agriculture, Washington, D.C.

Chiej, R. 1984. *Medicinal Plants*. Macdonald, London.

Chopra, R. N., I. C. Chopra, and B. S. Varma. 1969. *Supplement to Glossary of Indian Medicinal Plants*. Publications and Information Directorate, New Delhi.

Chopra, R. N., S. L. Nayar, and I. C. Chopra. 1956. *Glossary of Indian Medicinal Plants*. Publications and Information Directorate, New Delhi.

Coffey, T. 1993. *Wildflowers*. Houghton Mifflin, New York.

Culpeper, N. 1826. *Culpeper's Complete Herbal*, facsimile ed. Pitman Press, England.

Dastur, J. F. 1962. *Medicinal Plants of India and Pakistan*. Taraporevala, Bombay, India.

Densmore, F. 1928. *How Indians Use Plants for Food, Medicine and Crafts*. Reprint 1974. Dover, New York.

de Padua, L. S., G. C. Lugod, and J. V. Pancho. *Handbook on Philippine Medicinal Plants*, vol. 2. University of the Philippines, Los Banos.

Dols, M. W. and Gamal, A. S. 1984. *Medieval Islamic Medicine*. University of California Press, Berkeley.

Duke, J. A. 1985. *Handbook of Medicinal Herbs*. CRC Press, Boca Raton, Florida.

Ewan, J., ed. 1969. *Botany in the United States*. Hafner, New York and London.

Fiske, J. G. 1932. *Some Poisonous Plants of New Jersey*. New Jersey Agricultural Experiment Station, New Brunswick.

Foster, S., and J. A. Duke. 1990. *Medicinal Plants*. Houghton Mifflin, Boston.

Gerard, J. 1633. *The Herbal*. Revised and enlarged by T. Johnson. Dover, New York.

Gress, E. M. 1935. *Poisonous Plants of Pennsylvania*, vol. 18, no. 5. Pennsylvania Department of Agriculture, Harrisburg.

Grieve, M. 1931. *A Modern Herbal*, vols. 1 and 2. Reprint 1971. Dover, New York.

Harris, B. C. 1985. *The Compleat Herbal*. Bell, New York.

Harshberger, J. W. 1916. *The Vegetation of the New Jersey Pine-Barrens*. Reprint 1970. Dover, Mineola, New York.

Hough, M. Y. 1983. *New Jersey Wild Plants*. Harmony Press, Harmony, New Jersey.

Hungry Wolf, B. 1980. *The Ways of My Grandmothers*. Quill, New York.

Hutchens, A. R. 1973. *Indian Herbology of North America*. Merco, Windsor, Ontario, Canada.

Josselyn, J. 1672. "New-England Rarities Discovered and Two Voyages to New-England." Bulletin of the Lloyd Library, no. 26. Reproduction Series no. 8, 1927. Lloyd Library, Cincinnati, Ohio.

Kohlstedt, S. G., ed. 1991. *The Origins of Natural Science in America*. Smithsonian Institution Press, Washington, D.C.

Kokwaro, J. O. 1976. *Medicinal Plants of East Africa*. East African Literature Bureau, Nairobi, Kenya.

Lewis, W. H., and M.P.F. Elvin-Lewis. 1977. *Medical Botany*. Wiley, New York.

Lucas, R. 1977. *Secrets of the Chinese Herbalists*. Cornerstone Library, New York.

Luckner, M. 1984. *Secondary Metabolism in Microorganisms, Plants, and Animals*. Springer-Verlag, Berlin.

Mann, J., R. S. Davidson, J. B. Hobbs, D. V. Banthorpe, and J. B. Harborne. 1994. *Natural Products*. Longman Scientific and Technical, England, and Wiley, New York.

Marderosian, A. D., and L. Leberti. 1988. *Natural Product Medicine*. Stickley, Philadelphia.

Millspaugh, C. F. 1892. *American Medicinal Plants*. Reprint 1974. Dover, New York.

Mitsuoka, T. 1992. Intestinal Flora and Aging. *Nutrition Reviews*. 50:438–446.

Moerman, D. E. 1986. *Medicinal Plants of Native America*, vols. 1 and 2. University of Michigan Museum of Anthropology, Ann Arbor.

Montgomery, J. D., and D. E. Fairbrothers. 1992. *New Jersey Ferns and Fern Allies*. Rutgers University Press, New Brunswick, New Jersey.

Morton, J. F. 1981. *Atlas of Medicinal Plants of Middle America*. Thomas, Springfield, Illinois.

Mugera, G. M. 1977. *Useful Drugs and Cancer Causing Chemicals in Kenya Medicinal and Toxic Plants*. University of Nairobi, Kenya.

Newcomb, L. 1977. *Wildflower Guide*. Little, Brown, Boston.

"New Jersey Medicine in the Revolutionary Era." 1976. Exhibition of the New Jersey Historical Society, Newark.

Newton, P., and N. Wolfe. 1992. "Can Animals Teach Us Medicine?" *British Medical Journal* 350:1517–1518.

Oliver-Bever, B. 1986. *Medicinal Plants in Tropical West Africa*. Cambridge University Press, Cambridge.

Ortiz de Montellano, B. 1990. *Aztec Medicine, Health, and Nutrition*. Rutgers University Press, New Brunswick, New Jersey.

Pavy, A. 1987. *Treatment and Cures with Local Herbs*. Paria, Trinidad, West Indies.

Putnam, A. R., and C-S. Tang, eds. 1986. *The Science of Allelopathy*. Wiley, New York.

Reed, H. S. 1942. *A Short History of the Plant Sciences*. Chronica Botanica, Waltham, Massachusetts.

Rice, E. L. 1984. *Allelopathy*. Academic Press, Orlando, Florida.

Robichaud, B. and M. F. Buell. 1983. *Vegetation of New Jersey*. Rutgers University Press, New Brunswick, New Jersey.

Robinson, S. 1830. *A Course of Fifteen Lectures on Medical Botany, Denominated Thomson's New Theory of Medical Practice*. J. Howe, Printer, Boston.

Rodriguez, E., and R. Wrangham. 1993. "Zoopharmacognosy: The Use of Medicinal Plants by Animals." In *Phytochemical Potential of Tropical Plants*, ed. K. R. Downum, J. Romeo, and H. A. Stafford, pp. 89–106. Plenum Press, New York.

Seigler, D. S., ed. 1977. *Crop Resources*. Academic Press, New York.

Sidel, V. W. 1985. *A Barefoot Doctor's Manual*. Gramercy, New York.

Sigerist, H. E. 1951. *A History of Medicine*. Oxford University Press, New York.

Singha, S. C. 1965. *Medicinal Plants of Nigeria*. Nigerian National Press, Lagos.

Squibb, E. R. 1866. "An Appeal for the Materia Medica." Extracted from the *Transactions of the Medical Society of the State of New York*, Albany.

Steiner, R. P., ed. 1986. *Folk Medicine*. American Chemical Society, Washington, D.C.

Stewart, F. H. 1932. *Indians of Southern New Jersey*. Gloucester County Historical Society, Woodbury, New Jersey.

Still, J. 1877. *Early Recollections and Life of Dr. James Still*. Lippincott, Philadelphia.

Stone, W. 1973. *The Plants of Southern New Jersey*. (Originally published 1911.) Quarterman Publications, Boston.

Swain, T., ed. 1972. *Plants in the Development of Modern Medicine*. Harvard University Press, Cambridge, Massachusetts.

Takemi, T., M. Hasagawa, A. Kumagai, and Y. Otsuka, eds. 1985. *Herbal Medicine: Kampo, Past and Present*. Tsumura Juntendo, Tokyo.

Tantaquidgeon, G. 1971. *Folk Medicine of the Delaware and Related Algonkian Indians*. Pennsylvania Historical and Museum Commission, Harrisburg.

Thomson, S. 1835. *Botanic Family Physician*. J. Q. Adams, Printer, Boston.

Torssell, K.B.G. 1983. *Natural Product Chemistry*. Wiley, London.

Tyler, V. E. 1987. *The New Honest Herbal*. Stickley, Philadelphia.

Weiner, M. A. 1980. *Earth Medicine—Earth Food*. Collier Macmillan, New York and London.

Wherry, E. T. 1937. *Guide to Eastern Ferns*. Science Press, Lancaster, Pennsylvania.

Wherry, E. T. 1948. *Wild Flower Guide*. Doubleday, New York.

Wichtl, Max, ed. 1994. *Herbal Drugs*. Trans. N. G. Bisset. Medpharm, Stuttgart, and CRC Press, Boca Raton, Florida.

Wood, G. B. 1837. *Introductory Lecture to the Course of Materia Medica*. J. G. Auner, Philadelphia.

Wood, G. B. 1848. *Introductory Lecture to the Course of Materia Medica and Pharmacy*. T. K. and P. G. Collins, Printers, Philadelphia.

Wyeth Laboratories. 1966. *The Sinister Garden*. Wyeth Laboratories, New York.

Young, J. H. 1961. *The Toadstool Millionaires*. Princeton University Press, Princeton, New Jersey.

Index

About the Author

Cecil C. Still is a professor in the plant science department of Cook College, Rutgers University, New Brunswick, and received his doctorate in biology from Temple University. He teaches courses in the area of medicinal plants and alternative therapies. He has published several scientific articles in professional journals and continues his research on the isolation and identification of novel, biologically active chemicals from plants. Dr. Still is a New Jersey native with roots in the pinelands of the southern half of the state. He is an amateur photographer with plants and natural scenes as his subjects. He also cultivates native medicinal plants as a hobby.